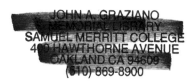

NURSING EDUCATION CHALLENGES IN THE 21ST CENTURY

NURSING EDUCATION CHALLENGES IN THE 21ST CENTURY

LEANA R. CALLARA
EDITOR

Nova Science Publishers, Inc.
New York

LIBRARY OF CONGRESS CATALOGING-IN-PUBLICATION DATA
Available Upon Request

ISBN 1-60021-661-7

Published by Nova Science Publishers, Inc. ✤ New York

CONTENTS

PREFACE

Nursing education is facing a massive set of obstacles as the fields of medicine continues to progress at warp speed at the same time hospitals do not have enough doctors and depend more on nurses than anytime before. The result is overworked nurses running to keep it with the fields in which they must work. This new book presents some analyses of nursing education at a critical juncture in the field.

Expert Commentary A - Transforming clinical education for psychiatric nursing students is a must given the changing patterns of health care delivery. Hospitals are not longer the only hub where nursing care is provided; therefore contemporary nursing clinical education must evolve to include not only acute care but home care, community health, and primary care experiences. Healthy People 2010 has identified determinants of illnesses that are influenced by multiple dimensions. Therefore, nursing students will need to assess clients' mental health needs from varied perspectives: biophysical, psychological, social, as well as environmental. As the authors move forward in this commentary several concepts need to be examined: Why should we care about including high quality psychiatric mental health component in clinical nursing education? How can we promote effective and innovative strategies for clinical experiences and learning?

Expert Commentary B – People with mental illness are a vulnerable group and more needs to be done to promote high quality research to ensure access to the best treatment options. For example, psychosocial interventions, such as cognitive behavioural therapy or motivational interviewing, are becoming increasingly common treatments for people with mental health problems and substance misuse, but the efficacy of these interventions requires continuous assessment and review. That said, mental health is not an easy area to evaluate and can present many challenges to seasoned researchers, let alone those embarking on research. No area is more challenging than the randomised controlled trial (RCT). This commentary aims to provide some guidance to assist those contemplating research in this important area in order to ensure the quality and success of their trial.

Expert Commentary C – When speaking of quality, it is easy to revert back to such managerial concepts as quality control, quality mechanisms, quality management, etc. These concepts, however, are not neutral. They convey a technocratic and top-down approach that will only backfire in academic settings. Therefore, the term "culture" was chosen to convey a connotation of quality as a shared value and a collective responsibility for all members of an profession, including students and nurses staff. To talk more precisely about quality culture, the authors need to operationally define the term. Heritage® Dictionary of the English

Language says quality "a degree or grade of excellence or worth." The Random House Unabridged Dictionary says: culture "the attitudes and behavior that are characteristic of a particular social group or organization." Here's a definition of culture: It's the shared beliefs, values, attitudes, institutions, and behavior patterns that characterize the members of a community or organization. Professional culture emerges from that which is shared between colleagues in an profession, including shared attitudes and norms of behaviour. Quality culture means that the profession as a whole has accepted the quality elements of the functions the authors would like to enhance. A quality culture was a shared value and a collective responsibility for all members of a social group and/or an institution. A quality culture is characterized by specific attitudes, abilities, and behavior of each member of. a particular social group or organization. The concept of quality culture has been used to describe the extent to which quality is important and valued in an organization – i.e. how much organizational culture supports and values quality. Quality culture is perceived as a composition of elements of profession culture, which determine the quality of teaching and career most strongly (facilitate or act as an obstacle in the process of achieving high teaching quality). A culture that is supportive of quality maybe particularly important in service nursing, where simultaneous production and consumption of the service makes close control impossible. Functioning as nurses, autonomously and interdependently, requires the development and acquisition of an appropriate set of personal, professional, profession and organizational values.

Chapter 1 – Assessment is an integral component of nurse education. The authors are of the opinion that assessment is in fact more important than the learning and teaching in nurse education today. This chapter attempts to move away from the conventional and restrictive forms of assessment, which still dominates many Higher Educational Institutes, to a more innovative and creative form of assessment which has its roots strongly embedded in clinical nursing practice. The assessment model offered is multifaceted in use and can be used as an academic assessment model across both the range and levels of post registration nursing but is equally useful as an assessment model for awarding formative and summative assessments at pre registration. It can also be used successfully for awarding the acquisition of knowledge, skills and attitudes which do not necessarily need to be related to the achievement of academic credit ratings. The raison d'etre of the model is its capacity to assess a performance of understanding in which it can be demonstrated that students have acquired a thorough integration of knowledge, reflexivity and intuitive action required for exceptional nursing practice at all levels.

Chapter 2 – Gardner identified eight intelligences that the brain can use in learning. Student engagement with learning and their retention of new information can be improved by engaging these multiple intelligences. A five-phase model – the Multiple Intelligence Teaching Approach [MITA] –can be employed in the classroom and in clinical settings to reinforce learning and enhance the students' professional development and clinical practice. This chapter explores the concept of multiple intelligences [MI] and the use of MITA to enhance nurse education.

Part one of this chapter explores early developmental theories and the relationship between development and intelligence and how MI impacts on teaching and learning. Many gaps remain the evidence base pertaining to conceptual and educational aspects of learning. The part two of the chapter examines how MITA is a means of initiating change within an integrated studies context. It exemplifies multiple ways of knowing and is a new departure from the traditional teaching approaches to present day post technocratic advances in education.

Chapter 3 – Central government has placed an emphasis on providing education within the National Health Service (NHS) close to the employees' workplace, which is clinical practice. Subsequently, there has been an emergence of new roles defined as 'educators in practice' in particular the roles of lecturer practitioner and practice educator have been promoted as being the most noteworthy. Despite this there is evidence of an earlier role advocated as providing education within practice that of the clinical nurse specialist. With the drive to meet central government policy it is possible the newer roles of the lecturer practitioner and practice educator have led to the demise of the clinical nurse specialist as a 'recognised' educator in clinical practice. The purpose of this research therefore was to measure, describe and compare the activity and experiences of clinical nurse specialists, lecturer practitioners and practice educators in providing education within an acute NHS trust hospital.

A non-experimental design using mixed methods was adopted. A questionnaire generated both the quantitative and the qualitative data. The mixed methods approach was used in order to capture the 'complete' view of both educational activity and personal experiences of the participants. Voluntary participants were obtained by postage of the questionnaire to the study population. A response rate of 70.5% provided 60 research participants. Because a small number of practice educators and large group called 'trainers' contributed to the study these were combined to form a group of 'educators in practice'. This group was used in the comparative analysis.

The results of this research found similarities between all the roles identified including their biographical profile and teaching activity. However, a small number of differences were found, these focused mainly on activity relating to a local university. Lecturer practitioners were found to be more involved with constructing and marking educational assessments and clinical nurse specialists in particular identified they would like to have been given the opportunity to contribute to university curriculum. Within clinical practice the clinical nurse specialists were found to be more involved in providing education for patients and carers.

It has been shown that the clinical nurse specialists within this research were motivated educationalists within clinical practice alongside the roles of lecturer practitioners and other educators in practice. Therefore one of the recommendations of this study has been that the educative aspect of the clinical nurse specialist role is formally recognised and subsequently valued.

Chapter 4 – With direct reference to how student nurses acquire, apply and evaluate theory for practical purposes this chapter highlights a number of key lessons for nursing education. The first of which is that educators must acknowledge the personal knowledge and personal experience of each student. Preconceptions must be highly valued and incorporated into the programme of study. This means that as far as is practicable the student must be involved in the design of an individualised programme which must maximise personal experiences and preconceptions. A second implication is that educators must acknowledge that there are three forms of theory to which a student nurse will be exposed and educators must explain those forms of theory to the student. In addition it must be emphasised that all of these forms of theory may be considered as equally valid and that any apparent variance between them should be regarded as an energising force that aids rather than inhibits learning. Third, students should be prepared to expect dissonance and to manage the associated psychological discomfort. As the process of learning to apply theory in practical contexts is an experience that involved emotions, educators must clearly appreciate the importance of emotions in learning and provide opportunities for intra-practicum and post practicum debriefing. Emotional responses should not be viewed as a barrier to learning, but rather as a catalyst to the enhancement of learning. The final lesson for nursing education is that formal, practical and private theories have different roots and any understanding of those different forms of theory cannot be evaluated by the same criteria. Therefore, when educators determine the method that will be used to assess students during a practicum they must involve the student as an active partner. The student should be able to select a means of assessment that most closely corresponds with criteria that relate to related to each of the different forms of theory.

Chapter 5 – This chapter focuses on the idea that the development of mental health nursing as a profession in the United Kingdom depends on the strength of our ability to train our students interpersonally to a high level. The chapter gives the historical context of the development of a therapeutically active role for mental health nurses since the 1940s and the end of the asylum system. It goes on to argue that the development of interpersonal skills and the values and attitudes that are required for their effective use is essential if mental health nursing is to meet the challenges of this new role. Further background is given covering the social and political forces that have led to the development of mental health service user movement since the 1970s hospital scandals. The authors go on to discuss why these factors have impacted on the unique nature and development of mental health nursing as a profession, and user involvement as a political and social force.

The chapter puts forward a definition of interpersonal skills as the point of delivery for nursing care, reviews the literature on service user involvement in interpersonal skills training and assessment across medical and nursing professions and provide a commentary on and direction for nursing research and curriculum development in this area as developed by the authors.

"The words we choose matter, and will serve either to perpetuate the problem or resolve it".

Chapter 6 – This chapter draws upon on a study carried out with B.S.N. students during psychiatric clinical experience in which the concentration on interpersonal relationships and therapeutic conversation encouraged students to look beyond the diagnostic label.

Coudriet describes how the nurse enters an instant with his or her own life spinning and full of stresses and doubts, "constelling themselves with the suffering of her patients.". It is this "constelling" by nursing students that this study sought to tap into. For each week of a seven or eight week clinical rotation in psychiatric settings, students were asked to reflect upon their experiences and to write these experiences in the form of a poem. Coudriet suggests that when the nurse and patient meet they bear witness to each other regarding not only the story of their lives, but also to the moment of meeting itself. "It is this very act, this fundamental act of witness, of compassion, that becomes emotion, becomes memory, becomes sound, becomes voice, and becomes a poem.".

The content of the 179 poems generated in this study was subjected to thematic analysis. A number of themes were identified from the poems including initial uncertainty and fear of the students ; ways in which the students come to terms with caring for the clients; feelings of confusion and helplessness experienced by the students during the clinical rotation; and issues relating to moving beyond that particular clinical experience

At the conclusion of the clinical rotation the students were asked to provide an anonymous evaluation on the use of poetry. Most students reported that the experience made them "think deeper" and get in touch with their own feelings, even although they might never have written poetry before. They did not report any disadvantages in using poetry as a reflective tool compared to other methods they had been exposed to, and most preferred it as a means of assessment. They reported enjoying the creative aspects of the poetry and enjoyed "a new way of thinking" that enabled them to view the "clinical experience as a whole."

Chapter 7 – Background: Working in a team has become a significant component of modern healthcare practice and pre-qualification education must prepare students for this role. Interprofessional learning is increasingly regarded as key to achieving this although there remains considerable debate about the value of it. In particular there is concern that students need to develop their own professional identity before they can learn to work with others.

Aim: To use social identity theory as a vehicle to examine and compare nursing, dental, medical and pharmacy students' perceptions of the professional identity of their discipline and to consider the implications for developments in interprofessional education.

Method: Focus groups were carried out with pre-qualification students from four healthcare professions in the first semester of the first year of their course in order to gain an insight into the shared understandings, attitudes and values of becoming a healthcare professional. Focus group data were analysed using an ethnographic approach where interaction is analysed as being negotiated through sequenced talk.

Results: Some common themes emerged with all groups indicating that their knowledge of the identity of their discipline, and their motivation to join the profession, came from contact with professionals in healthcare settings or having a member of their family involved in healthcare. Analogies were made between the process of becoming a professional and the developmental process of moving from childhood to adulthood. Differences emerged between the professions with regard to students' perceptions of their future professional role, of other healthcare professionals and others' perceptions of them. In-group and out-group identities were apparent with nursing students located in the out-group of the other professions and also placing themselves in this group. The focus group process itself reinforced the group identity.

Conclusion: A greater understanding of students' perceptions of their professional identity and the processes involved in becoming a professional can help to inform developments in pre-qualification healthcare education. Pre-qualification interprofessional learning should be developed to encourage students to have an inclusive rather than an exclusive professional identity if effective team workers are to emerge.

Chapter 8 – This chapter reports on an Action Research study, conducted at a university based school of nursing in Brisbane, Australia, with the aim of improving interaction in tutorials and subsequently encouraging intellectual growth and social and personal development in learners. The study was directed by the following two questions: 1) from a student perspective, what constitutes a useful learning experience in a tutorial context and what factors contribute to that usefulness? and 2) what strategies can be incorporated into tutorials to encourage student attendance and active participation? Composite pictures of what makes a useful learning experience and what factors contribute to that usefulness were developed from information gathered from students. The information – the students' voice - was then used to direct quality improvement and curriculum development within the tutorials of a large undergraduate mental health nursing unit. Strategies developed and used to enhance teaching and learning within the tutorials of this unit are described along with the pragmatic, pedagogical and professional reasons that supported the innovations. Outcomes for both teachers and learners are detailed and some recommendations made for future thinking and planning for encouraging the intellectual growth and social and personal development in learners.

Chapter 9 – This article addresses subjects that are also vitally important to understanding what moves the hearth of nursing: What are values? What kinds of values? What are personal values? What are professional values? What is profession values? What are the main values that govern nurses and nursing? What are the kind of values that guide nursing as a profession. How can the values we hold and promote also ensure that nurses are and become persons of integrity, and nursing a profession of integrity? The kind of values nurses hold in practice, and what happens to the nurses? Are the values we hold and promote the relevant ones? Are there certain values that are more valuable, more right, more desirable than others? What should this be so? Are nurses change their behaviours and attitudes as a result of changing values? Why should we challenge the values we hold? To what should they be changed? Can education change our values? Should we expect nurse education to change values?

In this issue the authors scrutinize the values in and of education, practice, and the very existence of nursing: those we come with, those we acquire and those we promote. Nursing educators have a professional obligation to teach and reinforce professional nursing values that are consistent with the professional nursing role. Especially today, there is a definite need for values education in nursing education programs.

Chapter 10 – Background: Traditionally, health services and academia have viewed themselves as discrete sectors, with different agendas and priorities. Health services have focused on patient care, while academia has concerned itself with the advancement of knowledge through research and teaching. Although health services often incorporate research and teaching into their activities, it is generally not their primary focus.

Objectives: Using the example of a modern mental health service, this chapter sets out some opportunities for collaboration between health services and academia. These include a multidisciplinary approach, mentoring and peer support, practical steps to start bridge building, opportunities for publication, grant applications, and student supervision. The authors also briefly highlight some possible risks associated with attempting to bring the clinical and academic sectors closer together, and ways these might be addressed.

Discussion: A range of activities can help to bridge the divide between the academic and clinical sectors. These activities include: forums that promote constructive feedback and scholarly dialogue, negotiating relationships with universities to provide role orientation, positive teaching experiences and gaining insight into the realities of academia and the clinical setting. All these activities can be readily provided by a range of disciplines based on realistic and fair workloads. Building research capacity is not only beneficial for clinical staff, but enhances opportunity for clinically relevant academic research programs. This approach is not without risks, such as confusion among staff about roles and the time required to negotiate bureaucratic requirements; but, on balance, the advantages to staff and patients outweigh these potential disadvantages.

Conclusion: With careful planning, risks associated with forging partnerships between the clinical and academic sectors can be overcome to promote clinical and research excellence, and contribute to innovative career pathways.

Chapter 11 – Reflective practice is generally accepted as a means of developing an individual's professional and scientific knowledge based upon how the individual observes and processes his experience, most especially his experience in his practice profession. In the nursing profession reflective practice has been incorporated into nursing curriculae and is regarded as being an integral element of the practice of nursing in the clinical setting both by students and by experienced nurses. In order to facilitate the acceptance of reflective practice it has been presented to nurses in the guise of various different frameworks. These frameworks attempt to formalize the reflective process so that it is accessible to those who are encountering it for the first time. 'In Search of Lost Time' is the magnum opus of the French writer Marcel Proust. In this book Proust tried to recapture time through the deployment of memory, in effect Proust's work constitutes a lengthy reflective essay. This paper seeks to show ways by which the process of reflection can be illuminated by examining in detail the reflective mechanisms that Proust utilised in writing his novel. The paper then explores how these mechanisms may be used by nurses who are experienced in the reflective process in order to further develop their practice.

Chapter 12   The overall aim of the present research was to describe the phenomenon of learning in nursing, and advanced nursing, education. More precisely, the aim was to better understand the integration of theoretical caring science with caring in practice in the context of nursing, and advanced nursing, education. This entailed studying how students learn caring science theory, based on experiences of and reflection on nursing care situations.

The theoretical perspective of the research was caring science and its educational approach, while phenomenology and a lifeworld perspective have formed the epistemological foundation of the method and the empirical realisation. The research data consisted of narratives and interviews.

The results of the analysis show that the student's process of learning is a solitary one. They are left with a knowledge gap and no equipment with which to bridge it. The students' need for reflection and their desire to understand caring science knowledge in both theory and practice is insufficiently met in the education. Unreflective model learning dominates the learning process, which means that a reflective dialogue together with teachers and carers in practice does not take place. The findings also show that when an intertwined, scientifically grounded approach to caring is lacking, the students are left with their unreflected "natural attitude" to caring, based in their own unreflected lived experiences.

Chapter 13 – Dramatic changes in personnel, positions, roles, and responsibilities are rampant within the Canadian health care system. The first-line nurse manager's (F-LNM's) role has altered significantly, despite the dependence upon this role in realizing quality of patient care, quality of work life for staff nurses, as well as organizational effectiveness and efficiency. The literature suggests that little support is afforded F-LNMs in terms of both orientation to this changing, demanding role and educational opportunities. Further, there has been little research documenting the challenges and learning needs of this important health care professional.

The question guiding the research reported here is, "What is the impact of health care system restructuring upon the roles, leadership models, knowledge, skills, and competencies of first-line nurse managers?" The research program exploring the selection, training, development, and support systems of these F-LNMs entails Personal Interviews and a Delphi Study. In-depth, personal interviews, conducted with 26 F-LNMs, provide the basis for this paper, which focuses upon their experiences regarding formal and informal learning opportunities and needs.

In:: Nursing Challenges in the 21st Century
Editor: Leana E. Callara, pp. 1-5
ISBN 1-60021-661-7
© 2008 Nova Science Publishers, Inc.

Expert Commentary A

INNOVATIVE CLINICAL TEACHING ENCOUNTERS: PSYCHIATRIC MENTAL HEALTH NURSING

Roberta Waite

College of Nursing and Health Professions
Drexel University, Philadelphia, PA 19102
Rlw26@drexel.edu

Transforming clinical education for psychiatric nursing students is a must given the changing patterns of health care delivery. Hospitals are not longer the only hub where nursing care is provided; therefore contemporary nursing clinical education must evolve to include not only acute care but home care, community health, and primary care experiences (Kline & Hodges, 2006). Healthy People 2010 (United States Department of Health, 2000) has identified determinants of illnesses that are influenced by multiple dimensions. Therefore, nursing students will need to assess clients' mental health needs from varied perspectives: biophysical, psychological, social, as well as environmental. As we move forward in this commentary several concepts need to be examined: Why should we care about including high quality psychiatric mental health component in clinical nursing education? How can we promote effective and innovative strategies for clinical experiences and learning?

THE NEED FOR HIGH QUALITY PSYCHIATRIC CLINICAL NURSING EDUCATION

From the start it is essential to emphasize the relevance of formal psychiatric mental health clinical training. We live in increasingly uncertain times surrounded by evidence of failing mental health for many people. Psychiatric illness represents a significant public health concern in almost every country in the world (Grigg, 2003), and while highly prevalent, it goes largely unrecognized and untreated. Psychiatric disorders currently account for 12% of the total global burden of diseases, an impact anticipated to grow in the next 10 years, and grow most in developing countries (World Health Organization (WHO), 2001;

2003). Over half of the top ten most disabling disorders in the world are psychiatric disorders, with unipolar depression expected to become the world's most disabling disease, across all cultures and countries, surpassing cardiac, and infectious, and accidental trauma states by the year 2020 (WHO, 2003). Given these statistics the clinical experience of learning, practicing, and developing psychiatric nursing skills is a requisite for all students during their undergraduate nursing education experience. Too often the 'non-technical' aspects of patient care are relegated last, integrated with a smattering of content here and there with no formal clinical component, and/or dismissed to include psychosocial principles taught by another discipline (i.e., social work or psychology). To do this minimizes the centrality of contemporary psychiatric nursing which examines the needs of a client from a holistic standpoint to support health promotion, prevention of mental health problems, and the management of illness. Student nurses not only learn therapeutic communication, coping, and adaptation to normative occurrences, but they also address non-normative health states. Nursing students are taught the pathophysiology of chest pain, they learn to implement nursing actions matched to bio-scientific knowledge and nursing care that helps the client from suffering further adverse cardiac events. During this process students learn how a person's changing cardiac rhythm affects their functioning, what their blood pressure tells them about the heart, and what interventions would improve those findings. These elements are taught in the clinical context of being present with the client during the unfolding of their health needs. Nursing students must also take their awareness of the normative process of mood and the pathophysiological changes that produce aberrant mood states, and apply that knowledge to nursing actions intentionally and somatically derived to address assessed patient need. This is significant given that mood and emotional states often result in physiological co-morbidities, i.e., the identified link between stress and cardiovascular health (Salyers, Hunter, & McGuire, 2006; Walling, 2005). Engagement of students in psychiatric mental health clinical links what they learn in the didactic portion of their course with assessment strategies in the clinical area. For students to realistically contribute to a clients care related to psychiatric mental health nursing there must be adequate, efficient and effective time for quality learning related to clinical education intended for individuals, families and communities. Nursing encompasses the largest number of health care professionals in the world, with psychiatric nurses being the most common providers of mental health services (WHO, 2004). Nurses are major contributors, in their respective countries, to the assessment of general health, the promotion of mental health, the prevention of psychiatric disease, and the treatment of mental illness (McCabe, 2005). Thus, it is imperative that student nurses develop the requisite skills to take upon the challenge of providing appropriate and effective psychiatric care.

PROMOTING INNOVATIVE STRATEGIES: PSYCHIATRIC NURSING CLINICAL LEARNING EXPERIENCES

The learning that student nurses incur is principled on contextual encounters with clients, families, communities, registered nurses as well as other health care providers. These potent encounters help students to read, interpret and understand client experiences and it is during clinical practice that nursing students develop the competencies and skills required for professional nursing. Because of the changing health care environment, diverse cultural backgrounds of clientele and co-morbid health care problems experienced by many individuals, students need experience with clients having mental health concerns across the life span, as well as those with highly prevalent health problems, those who are learning to manage chronic conditions, and those making significant changes in health behavior. These diverse care needs requires students to enrich their skills related to analysis, synthesis, application, and evaluation of complex real-world concerns related to psychiatric mental health illness. These areas can be addressed using varied forums (acute, community and primary care settings). However two proposed strategies will be discussed in this commentary that can supplement traditional methods of learning: use of standardized patients and service-learning experiences.

THE STANDARDIZED PATIENTS

The use of standardized patients (SP), an individual who has been carefully trained to present an illness or scenario in a systematic, unvarying manner, is more of a recent phenomenon within nursing. However, its usefulness has been documented related to teaching and evaluating clinical skills such as interpersonal communication, history taking and interviewing, physical and psychological assessment, as well as patient education (Hunt, 2006). The SP process allows faculty to shape students experiences particularly for use in training or assessment by not relying on the random patient experiences students receive in hospital or outpatient settings, developing a core set of patient-centered problems based on curricular objectives, and controlling the domain as well as the complexity of the clinical problem, while providing students with equivalent patient experiences. Clearly, the intent is not to replace the actual patient encounter with an SP encounter but to augment it in an integrative and standardized way. The SP process provides an opportunity for students to see themselves 'in action' and reinforces the concept of self-evaluation/ critique, and allows faculty/clinicians an opportunity to address and clearly identify a student's specific difficulties that may arise in areas of therapeutic interaction skills, interpersonal communication, mental status assessment, history taking, as well as in the identification of linkages between psychopathology and psychiatric symptoms. Moreover SP allows students to learn and practice formative skills in a less threatening and controlled environment, focuses students' attention on the acquisition of clinical skills, allows nursing students to develop comfort in managing sensitive patient issues, promotes a context for immediate feedback on students' performance enabling opportunities for improvement, and it makes visible the students' clinical reasoning process.

SERVICE LEARNING EXPERIENCES

Service learning, a participatory learning event, is another process that provides psychiatric nursing students with the opportunity to use critical thinking skills, communication techniques, and assessment skills in a community environment. This method provides services to a community while also providing nursing students with real-world experiences. This can take place 'in-person' at health clinics, churches, etc., or through use of telehealth promotion with telephones and/or computers. Service learning not only emphasizes, a learning-centered approach which focuses on the achievement of course and programmatic objectives and the acquisition of transferable skills related to the students' professional development but it also supports development in citizenship, social responsibility, and personal growth. This process attends to the need for awareness of diverse cultures and lifestyles, as well as the communication skills required to function in a culturally competent manner. This forum enables student nurses to understand and become familiar with community-based values, traditions, and customs when developing interventions and programs.

For example, mental health students may conduct wellness screening projects with faculty that examines depression, obsessive compulsive disorders, and anxiety. From this students can work with clients to develop educational components that will benefit the community. This can focus on preventive measures such as controlling stress and tension to more specific interventions tailored to meet the needs of community clientele. For nursing students to build cultural competence, they must move beyond the bricks and mortar of the university campus and engage with the true populations representing communities within society. To be involved in such a process reduces stereotyping and facilitates ethnic and cultural understandings associated with mental illness and health-related concerns.

Skills developed from these innovative clinical approaches to teaching assist in promoting competent nursing professionals within the healthcare arena. These approaches support and shape the knowledge of basic skill acquisition which is essential given that only 3% of the registered nurse workforce cares for this vulnerable segment of society (Hanrahan & Gerolamo, 2004).

Transforming the clinical education process for psychiatric nursing students necessitates innovative strategies that complement and enhance traditional forms of clinical teaching. Faculty assist in guiding the learning process while students engage in meaningful experiences in acute care setting, locations in the community as well as primary care. The evolving sociodemographic and epidemiological transitions necessitate a corresponding change in the student nurses' educational experiences related to psychiatric nursing. Let that change be firmly rooted in the practices that strengthen student's clinical skills as they move into an increasingly pluralistic society.

REFERENCES

Grigg, M. (2003). Working at the world health organization: An international perspective on mental health nursing. *International Journal of Mental Health Nursing, 12*, 235-236.

Hanrahan, N., & Gerolamo, A. (2004). Profiling the hospital-based psychiatric registered nurse workforce, *Journal of the American Psychiatric Nurses Association, 10*, 282–289.

Hunt, R. (2006). Developing emotional competence through service learning. *Annual Review of Nursing Education, 4,* 251-271.

Kline, K. S., & Hodges, J. (2006). A rational approach to solving the problem of competition for undergraduate clinical sites. *Nursing Education Perspectives, 27*(2), 80-83.

McCabe, S. (2005). Uniting the family of psychiatric nurses: Commonalities and divergences in the nursing lives we lead. *Perspectives in Psychiatric Care, 41*(1), 35-41.

Saylers, V., Hunter, A., & McGuire, S. (2006). Cross-cultural reliability of the health perception index and the health control and competence index. *Journal of Nursing Scholarship, 38*(4), 387-492.

United States Department of Health and Human Services (November 2000). *Healthy People 2010.* 2nd ed. With Understanding and Improving Health and Objectives for Improving Health. 2 vols. Washington, DC: U.S. Government Printing Office.

Walling, A. D. (2005). Anxiety and depression in cardiovascular disease. *American Family Physician, 71*(3), 600-602

World Health Organization (WHO). (2001). *Atlas: Mental health resources in the world 2001.* World Health Organization.

World Health Organization. (2003). *Investing in mental health.* Geneva: World Health Organization.

World Health Organization. (2004). *Mental health resources in the world: Current results of project Atlas.* Geneva: World Health Organization.

In:: Nursing Challenges in the 21st Century
Editor: Leana E. Callara, pp. 7-10

ISBN 1-60021-661-7
© 2008 Nova Science Publishers, Inc.

Expert Commentary B

RANDOMISED CONTROLLED TRIALS OF PSYCHOSOCIAL INTERVENTIONS IN A MENTAL HEALTH SETTING: HOW CAN THE GOLD STANDARD BE ACHIEVED?

Michelle Cleary[1],*, Garry Walter[2],†,
Sandy Matheson[3] and Nandi Siegfried[4]

[1] Faculty of Nursing and Midwifery, University of Sydney, and Research Unit, Sydney South West Area Mental Health Service
[2] University of Sydney, and Child and Adolescent Mental Health Services, Northern Sydney Central Coast Health.
[3] Research Unit, Sydney South West Area Mental Health Service (Eastern Zone)
[4] Dept of Clinical Medicine, University of Oxford, and UK Cochrane Centre

People with mental illness are a vulnerable group and more needs to be done to promote high quality research to ensure access to the best treatment options. For example, psychosocial interventions, such as cognitive behavioural therapy or motivational interviewing, are becoming increasingly common treatments for people with mental health problems and substance misuse, but the efficacy of these interventions requires continuous assessment and review (Ley & Jeffrey, 2003). That said, mental health is not an easy area to evaluate and can present many challenges to seasoned researchers, let alone those embarking on research. No area is more challenging than the randomised controlled trial (RCT). This commentary aims to provide some guidance to assist those contemplating research in this important area in order to ensure the quality and success of their trial.

High quality RCTs are the gold standard researchers seek to emulate when assessing treatment effectiveness (Schulz & Grimes, 2002a). Achieving such a standard when assessing

---

* Correspondence: Dr Michelle Cleary, Mailing Address: Research Unit, Sydney South West Area Mental Health Service, PO Box 1, Rozelle, New South Wales, 2039, Australia Tel: (02) 9556 9100; Fax: (02) 9818 5712, Email: michelle.cleary@email.cs.nsw.gov.au

† Mailing Address: Coral Tree Family Service, PO Box 142, North Ryde, NSW, 1670, Australia, Phone: +61 2 9887 5830; Fax: +61 2 9887 2941, Email: gwalter@mail.usyd.edu.au

psychosocial interventions is far from straightforward, but can be realized if researchers are aware of the pitfalls to avoid and the best ways to design a RCT. Adequate randomisation, allocation concealment and masking, and low attrition rates all contribute to ensuring the internal validity of a RCT, while sample representativeness ensures its external validity. These techniques must be used rigorously in modern scientific trials to reduce bias and it is imperative to adhere to them in order to enable reliable interpretation of the trial results (Schulz et al., 1995).

Many researchers believe that alternate or sequential allocation, assignment by date of birth or by case record number is adequate. However, these techniques are not random, so bias can result (Schulz & Grimes, 2002a). For example, socioeconomic factors, such as access to medical specialists, may influence the day of the week that a child is born; in turn, socioeconomic factors may influence the level of education a child goes on to receive and, conceivably through that, responsiveness to certain psychological therapies. Thus, a study investigating responses to cognitive therapy in schizophrenia may be immediately biased if subject allocation is by day of the week that a child is born. Even coin-tossing, dice-throwing or shuffling cards can be manipulated intentionally or unintentionally by investigators (Schulz & Grimes, 2002a).

Schulz and Grimes (2002a) suggest that using a computer-generated table of numbers is one "correct" randomisation technique. For example, in a trial with a predicted sample size of 100, a table of randomly ordered numbers from 1 to 100 can be generated usually using a computer. Starting with any arbitrary point on the table and working through it to allocate the first 50 numbers generated to one group and the next 50 to the other group helps ensure equal sample sizes. Each number represents a participant's position in the trial's enrolment line as they sign up for the study which then becomes their ID number. As the two group sequences involve 50 random numbers each, there is no way to know during enrolment which group a participant's ID number belongs to, unless of course they are privy to the group sequences.

Those involved in allocating ID numbers to participants as they enrol and the participants themselves must remain unaware of these pre-determined sequences (Schulz & Grimmes, 2002b). This means that those involved cannot, and are not tempted to, exclude or delay the enrolment of certain patients, perhaps based on their prognosis (Schulz et al., 1995). It is worth noting that the non-random techniques outlined above can lead to inadequate allocation concealment as they are transparent; investigators can always find out the day of the week a person was born, simply by asking them.

Masking or blinding is also integral to a bias-free RCT (Schulz & Grimmes, 2002c). Blinding ensures that trial participants, investigators and/or assessors will not be influenced by their knowledge of which treatment condition a participant is receiving or has received. During drug trials, participants can be influenced by the expectation of the effects of the trial drug and investigators may inadvertently hint that one drug is expected to do better than another. Outcome assessors may also unintentionally influence results due to their own expectations of what the results should be (Jadad et al., 1996). Blinding thus manages expectations. While this can usually be achieved in drug trials, it is much harder to achieve for psychosocial interventions such as cognitive therapies where participants and investigators cannot be blinded to the treatment condition. However, blinding assessors is possible and should be considered an important component of a RCT using psychosocial interventions.

A further consideration to ensuring internal validity is to attempt to keep attrition or drop out rates low and attempt to keep participants engaged throughout all treatment sessions. This is particularly difficult in psychosocial interventions as often the intervention is spread over several weeks, months or even years and anything may happen in that time to affect participation. An excessive attrition rate can make the results questionable as those remaining in the study may have different characteristics to those dropping out. For example, those remaining in a study looking at treatment effectiveness of substance misuse may have been less addicted to substances than those dropping out and so may respond better to treatment, exaggerating the results. This is particularly problematic if there is differential attrition between the intervention groups. One way to address this is to conduct an intention-to-treat analysis. This involves analysing data from all participants randomised to treatment, regardless of their level of treatment received; this is thought to result in an unbiased and consistent interpretation of treatment effects, unlike those done on subsamples (Nich & Carroll, 2002).

Other participants may remain in the study but fail to attend all treatment sessions (adherence is particularly problematic with mental health patients), so their treatment 'dose' may fall somewhere between the treatment and control groups, again affecting the results. It is also important to ensure that everyone involved in the treatment group receives exactly the same treatment by using experienced and well-trained staff, adhering to strict guidelines for performing the interventions.

RCT's for psychosocial interventions often have planned follow-up assessments at set times after completion of the treatment sessions, for example at 6 months and 12 months, to determine whether a particular treatment has long-lasting effects. Again, participants lost to follow-up assessments can cause problems for researchers as the results from the reduced sample may not be generalizable. It is important to encourage participation by committing adequate resources to implement procedures that minimize attrition. Schulz and Grimmes (2002d) suggest several ways to ensure participants remain available. These include: hiring a person to manage the participants and encourage follow-up; monitoring contact details; organising a suitable location for assessment; excluding, prior to randomisation, those unlikely to be available for the duration of the study; providing monetary subsidies; and, keeping the assessment instruments short.

Ensuring the sample is representative of the wider community of people it is supposed to represent is also crucial to the quality of a RCT. Eligibility criteria need to be carefully planned and carried out prior to randomisation (Schulz & Grimes, 2002d). For example, in a RCT comparing cognitive behavioural therapies to assertive community treatment (ACT) for mentally ill patients with substance abuse problems, it would be important to ensure that not only both male and female patients with acute psychosis are included in the study, but also those with other disorders across a wide age range.

Finally, once the trial is over and the writing begins, accurate and complete reporting of the design, conduct, analysis and generalizability of the trial must be included so that the processes are transparent and are able to be replicated. RCTs must report in detail inclusion/exclusion criteria, study population characteristics, how randomisation, allocation concealment and masking was achieved, participant 'flow' or engagement in treatment, and descriptive and inferential statistics to allow alternative analyses to be conducted by readers (Begg et al., 1996; Turpin, 2005).

In conclusion, while there are many hurdles to ensuring a "gold" standard RCT of psychosocial interventions, awareness of these potential problems in advance of commencement of the trial will help to minimize their occurrence. To this end, this commentary hopes to encourage discussion to promote ways of conducting high quality RCTs in mental health settings.

ACKNOWLEDGEMENTS

This commentary was supported by the McGeorge Bequest, The University of Sydney.

REFERENCES

Begg, C., Cho, M., Eastwood, S., Horton, R., Moher, D., Olkin, I., Pitkin, R., Rennie, D., Schulz, K.F., Simel, D. & Stroup, D.F. (1996). Improving the Quality of Reporting of Randomized Controlled Trials. The CONSORT Statement. *JAMA*, 276(8), 637-639.

Jadad, A.R., Moore, A., Carroll, D., Jenkinson, C., Reynolds, D.J.M., Gavaghan, D.J. & McQuay, H.J. (1996). Assessing the Quality of Reports of Randomized Clinical Trials: Is Blinding Necessary? *Controlled Clinical Trials*, 17, 1-12.

Ley, A. & Jeffrey, D. (2003). Cochrane review of treatment outcome studies and its implications for future developments. In *Substance Misuse in Psychosis: Approaches to Treatment and Service Delivery*. Eds Graham, H.L., Copello, A., Birchwood, M.J., Mueser, K.T. John Wiley & Sons, Ltd. Chapter 20, pp, 349-365.

Nich, C. & Carroll, K.M. (2002). 'Intention-to-treat' meets 'missing data': implications of alternate strategies for analyzing clinical trials data. *Drug and Alcohol Dependence,* 68, 121-130.

Schulz, K.F., Chalmers, I., Hayes, R.J. & Altman, D.G. (1995). Empirical Evidence of Bias. *JAMA*, 273(5), 408-412.

Schulz, K.F. & Grimes, D.A. (2002a). Generation of allocation sequences in randomised trials: chance, not choice. *The Lancet*, 359, 515-519.

Schulz, K.F. & Grimes, D.A. (2002b). Allocation concealment in randomised trials: defending against deciphering. *The Lancet,* 359, 614-619.

Schulz, K.F. & Grimes, D.A. (2002c). Blinding in randomized trials: hiding who got what. *The Lancet,* 359, 696-700.

Schulz, K.F. & Grimes, D.A. (2002d). Sample size slippage in randomized trials: exclusions and the lost and wayward. *The Lancet,* 359, 781-785.

Turpin, D.L. (2005). CONSORT and QUOROM guidelines for reporting randomized clinical trials and systematic reviews. *Am J Orthod Dentofacial Orthop*, 128, 681-686.

In: Nursing Education Challenges in the 21st Century
Editor: Leana E. Callara, pp. 11-13

ISBN 1-60021-661-7
© 2008 Nova Science Publishers, Inc.

Expert Commentary C

BUILDING A QUALITY CULTURE IN NURSING

Insaf Altun

Kocaeli Univ., Nursing High School, The Dept. of Fundamentals Nursing,
Kocaeli, Turkey, insafaltun@mynet.com ialtun@kou.edu.tr

When speaking of quality, it is easy to revert back to such managerial concepts as quality control, quality mechanisms, quality management, etc. These concepts, however, are not neutral. They convey a technocratic and top-down approach that will only backfire in academic settings. Therefore, the term "culture" was chosen to convey a connotation of quality as a shared value and a collective responsibility for all members of an profession, including students and nurses staff. To talk more precisely about quality culture, we need to operationally define the term. *Heritage® Dictionary of the English Language* says quality "a degree or grade of excellence or worth." T*he Random House Unabridged Dictionary* says: culture "the attitudes and behavior that are characteristic of a particular social group or organization." Here's a definition of culture: It's the shared beliefs, values, attitudes, institutions, and behavior patterns that characterize the members of a community or organization. Professional culture emerges from that which is shared between colleagues in an profession, including shared attitudes and norms of behaviour. Quality culture means that the profession as a whole has accepted the quality elements of the functions we would like to enhance. A quality culture was a shared value and a collective responsibility for all members of a social group and/or an institution. A quality culture is characterized by specific attitudes, abilities, and behavior of each member of. a particular social group or organization. The concept of quality culture has been used to describe the extent to which quality is important and valued in an organization – i.e. how much organizational culture supports and values quality. Quality culture is perceived as a composition of elements of profession culture, which determine the quality of teaching and career most strongly (facilitate or act as an obstacle in the process of achieving high teaching quality). A culture that is supportive of quality maybe particularly important in service nursing, where simultaneous production and consumption of the service makes close control impossible. Functioning as nurses, autonomously and interdependently, requires the development and acquisition of an appropriate set of personal, professional, profession and organizational values.

Building a quality culture in nursing career is required a system of shared values defining what is important, and norms, defining appropriate attitudes and behaviors, that guide members' attitudes and behaviors. This system is consisting of both cognitive values and behavioral norms. Values change with time, as does the professional culture. Redefinition of roles and functions in the healthcare systems of the future requires embracing to the value of continuing education. Thus, professional culture is reflected by a common way of making sense of the profession that allows people to see situations and events in similar and distinctive ways. Therefore we can say quality in nursing is defined as the degree to which nursing services for individuals and populations increase the likelihood of desired objectives or outcomes and are consistent with current nursing knowledge.

İnternational Council of Nurses (ICN) is the body that speaks for nurses globally. According to *ICN* (2006) Nurses have four fundamental responsibilities: to promote health, to prevent illness, to care holistically, to alleviate suffering. According *ICN* (2006) Nurses have six key roles: advocacy, promotion of a safe environment, research, participation in shaping health policy, in patient and health systems management, education. This fundamental responsibilites and roles are values of the nursing profession. These values are reflected in the practice of professional nursing. The values of the profession give nurses direction, guide nursing behaviors and are pivotal in decision making. As the visible manifestation of a profession's culture and values, nursing professionalism is under increased pressure to play its part in quality improvement. Nurses' professional responsibility is building a quality culture. Building a quality culture is not an easy task. How principals can build a culture of quality that supports standards of excellence.

Nurses can advance the development of quality culture by: points defining the scope of nursing practice, continuing to promote the nursing and nurses values, Developing and disseminating a position statement on the importance of quality culture, supporting research, collecting data for quality culture A strong, professional quality culture is important because it encourages consistency of behaviour based on shared perceptions. In particular, it provides a context in which new professional are acculturated. The education of nursing rests on a curricular foundation that reflects the nursing theory and knowledge bases, practice patterns, and unique skills. In addition, nursing education must respond to and reflect changes in technology, societal definitions of health and wellness, and broad social issues such as access to care, health care funding, and changing patient demographics. These issues are interwoven with efforts to also provide high-quality education with positive learning outcomes. Professional education at the graduate level is aimed at preparing nurses for professional roles by contributing to the development of their unique bodies of professional knowledge and skills and internalizing values needed today in professional roles. The overall goals of staff are to expand their knowledge and intellectual skills, to strengthen their practical skills and to improve their attitudes and communication skills. Well-developed group consciousness are foundation for the advancement of quality culture, points to knowledge and specialization based on scientific principles, responsibility, accountability, autonomy, inquiry, collegiality, collaboration, and innovation.

REFERENCES

The American Heritage® Dictionary of the English Language, Fourth Edition, Copyright © 2000 by Houghton Mifflin Company. *http://dictionary.reference.com/browse/quality* (Accessed: March 03, 2007).

The Random House Unabridged Dictionary, © Random House, Inc. 2006. *http://dictionary.reference.com/browse/culture*. (Accessed: March 03, 2007).

International Council of Nurses. Code of ethics for nurses. Geneva: ICN, 2006)(*Available from: URL: http://www.icn.ch/ethics.htm* [Accessed March 03, 2007].

In: Nursing Education Challenges in the 21st Century   ISBN 1-60021-661-7
Editor: Leana E. Callara, pp. 15-22   © 2008 Nova Science Publishers, Inc.

Chapter 1

TOWARDS A PERFORMANCE OF UNDERSTANDING: THE UNIFICATION OF THEORY AND PRACTICE IN NURSE EDUCATION

Jen Hawkins [1] *and Tom Foster* [2]

Faculty of Health, Wellbeing & Science. Suffolk College, Ipswich

ABSTRACT

Assessment is an integral component of nurse education. We are of the opinion that assessment is in fact more important than the learning and teaching in nurse education today. This chapter attempts to move away from the conventional and restrictive forms of assessment, which still dominates many Higher Educational Institutes, to a more innovative and creative form of assessment which has its roots strongly embedded in clinical nursing practice. The assessment model offered is multifaceted in use and can be used as an academic assessment model across both the range and levels of post registration nursing but is equally useful as an assessment model for awarding formative and summative assessments at pre registration. It can also be used successfully for awarding the acquisition of knowledge, skills and attitudes which do not necessarily need to be related to the achievement of academic credit ratings. The raison d'etre of the model is its capacity to assess a performance of understanding in which it can be demonstrated that students have acquired a thorough integration of knowledge, reflexivity and intuitive action required for exceptional nursing practice at all levels.

---

[1] Correspondence to : 65 Westerfield Road Ipswich Suffolk IP4 2XP 01473 251068 jen@jenhawkins.co.uk

[2] Correspondence to: 8 Paddock Close Belton Great Yarmouth Norfolk NR31 9NT 01493 780829 tom@tom123.demon.co.uk.

INTRODUCTION

There comes a time when all nurse educationalists need to determine whether their ambitions of encouraging, teaching, instructing, coaching and motivating their students has been realised through the assessment process. For this to be a reality a sound knowledge and understanding of the art and science of assessment and evaluation is necessary as is a creative, innovative and realistic approach to its implementation.

Higher education institutes that incorporate departments responsible for the education and training of nurses have tended to adopt a traditional standard assessment strategy of predominantly written assignments, such as essays, reports and case studies in an attempt to determine the student's acquisition, understanding and application of nursing knowledge, attitudes and skills. These forms of assessment can be prone to criticism as they are open to varied, subjective interpretations and although they may purport to give a measurement of the knowledge retained by the student, they demonstrate little evidence of the student's understanding related to that knowledge.

Part of the curriculum design process of any educational pursuit is to ensure that the chosen method of assessment not only best suits the content, delivery method and learning outcomes of the course or programme to be presented but also contributes to the personal and professional development of those being assessed. This is particularly the case in vocational courses. The notion that nursing is a vocation as well as an art and science remains a contentious debate and it is not the purpose of this chapter to pursue this, rather our interest lies in the choice of assessment procedures used to assess vocational education and training. It is our belief that the model we present in this chapter is a more accurate and appropriate form of assessment in which to assess all student's knowledge attitudes, skills and performance of understanding. Furthermore, it captures the control knowledge advocated by Eraut (1994) who suggests that 'self-knowledge about one's strengths and weaknesses, the gap between what one says and what one does, and what one knows and doesn't know'. We feel that this provides a skeletal outline for our 'Performance of Understanding'.model.

In the case of nurse education, a move away from the traditional academic forms of assessment to a more creative and innovative assessment procedure for both individuals and groups is clearly needed, specifically to allow the student to demonstrate a strong knowledge base which informs and determines skill competence within the clinical setting. Kenny (2004) claims that education provision has failed to provide newly qualified nurses with the skills to function effectively in a complex and constantly changing National Health Service organisation. This is a clear indication that the move away from the 3,000 word assignment which merely describes skilled practice towards the observation of skilled practice in the clinical setting is essential. A move away from the skill of recalling what has been taught to one of facilitating the innate humanistic skills required when nursing the vulnerable patient is not merely a fanciful notion but rather a compelling reality.

Within nurse education, the question of appropriate assessment procedures is paramount. Here, along with knowledge retained, the emphasis must be on the understanding of the implications of that knowledge in the delivery of clinical practice. How appropriate or safe is it to grade a practical clinical skill with an academic assessment tool? An assessment procedure based on a 'Performance of Understanding' offers a unique way of determining, not only the level of knowledge developed by the student over a specific period of study, but also the application of that knowledge as it relates to professional development and practice. This enables the student to be assessed more accurately through both real and simulated clinical exercises during actual nursing practice and not just in the confines of a skills laboratory. Our assessment strategy grew out of a strong recognition that one could not give a percentage grade to a nurse taking a patient's blood pressure. This activity requires an assessment related to an understanding of what is taking place rather than the emphasis being on the psychomotor skill being observed.

The 'Performance of Understanding' assessment model is multifaceted in its use, unlike the traditional methods of assessment which are strongly linked to academic credit ratings. This model works equally as well for those wishing to undertake a course of study but not wishing to collect academic credits. There may be a number of reasons for nurses not wanting to collect academic credits. For example, there are those who already hold a higher degree, those unable to cope with the anxieties which can beset some students at assessment time, also the many nurses who want to keep updating their knowledge and nursing skills outside the formal courses such as degrees and diplomas of nursing. The use of the 'Performance of Understanding' assessment model enables them to receive an authentic acknowledgment of their professional informed clinical practice. On completion of the period of study the model requires the student to be observed in clinical practice performing a specific nursing task related to the area of study. The task may be observed by the academic tutor responsible for the delivery of the area of study and it may also be prudent to involve, in the assessment process, the student's clinical manager (or another significant and approved clinician.) Both should be required to assess the student's performance of the clinical skill against a set of criteria based on knowledge, reflection and skill competence within the clinical setting. The model identifies five stages of understanding and enables an assessment appropriate to clinical expertise at all five levels.

The first level of the model evidences that the student's performance is dependant upon instruction. The student 'knows something but it is insufficient and not fully understood'. This lack of knowledge and understanding will impede autonomous practice.

The second level evidences that the student is constrained by limited knowledge and understanding. Here, the student 'knows a little about something which is right but has limited understanding', again restricting autonomous practice through limited knowledge and understanding.

At the third level the student's performance is underpinned by limited but increasing knowledge and understanding. Here the student 'knows a little about a lot of things' Understanding is increasing leading to the start of informed autonomous practice through increased knowledge and understanding.

The fourth level evidences a performance of understanding informed by both sound knowledge, understanding and reflective practice. Here the student 'knows a lot about a lot of things'. This leads to a sound knowledge and understanding of reflective autonomous practice.

At the fifth level the student gives 'a performance of understanding guided by tacit knowledge and reflexivity' demonstrating a thorough integration of knowledge, understanding, reflexivity and intuitive action required for exceptional clinical practice.

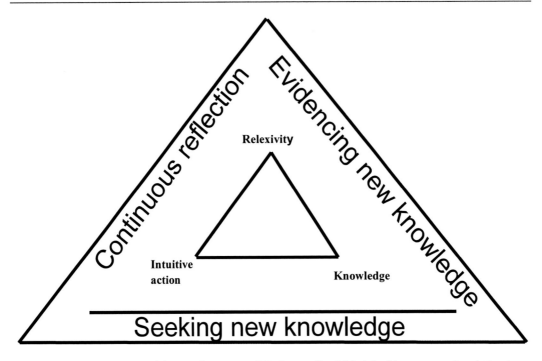

Figure 1. Shows an aspect of the 'Performance of Understanding' Model of Assessment in relation to the increasing knowledge, understanding, reflexivity and intuitive action of the skilled practitioner.

In order to fully understand this model we offer the following examples of its varied and multifaceted use. Let us take a senior nurse in pain control management who is already in possession of a higher degree but as part of continuing professional development and updating knowledge may choose to undertake a post registration module on aspects of pain relief. The academic credits attached to this module would be of little benefit to this student, as would a certificate of attendance. However, a certificate of a 'Performance of Understanding' assessed using the 'Performance of Understanding' model awarded on completion of the assessment procedure would enable the student to clearly demonstrate not only an increased knowledge base, but also how this new knowledge informs clinical practice and the student's reflections on that practice. Certification would reflect the level of assessed performance but would clearly state that no academic credit rating had been included

Equally a pre-registration nursing student during training may be awarded a number of certificates evidencing a range of performances of understanding which would then form a major part of their required professional portfolio. Clinical managers, mentors and academic staff would observe the student involved in a series of nursing activities, preferably with patients in clinical settings, where they are able to perform nursing activities, reflect on the process and report on the nursing theories and principles informing each of the skilled activities. Examples such as taking and reporting a patient's blood pressure, completing required patient documentation, feeding or bathing a patient, all require the student to work at a level of competence demonstrating increasing knowledge, understanding and reflective practice, which can be assessed using a 'Performance of Understanding' assessment model.

A Performance Of Understanding Assessment Model			
Degree Classification			
Refer	Experiential knowledge small and decisions tentative. Practice not informed by knowledge. *Performance depends upon instruction*	Knowing something but it's insufficient and not understood	✗
3rd	Experiential knowledge increases. An indicator towards performance. Knowledge informs practice. *Limited understanding of their performance and of the knowledge informing that performance*	Knowing something and it's right	✔
2:2	Performance of understanding increasing and knowledge informs practice. *Increasing understanding of their performance and actions are informed by knowledge*	Knowing a little about a lot of things	✔ ✔
2:1	*Increased performance of understanding. Practice informed by knowledge and reflective practice*	Knowing a lot about a lot of things	✔ ✔ ✔
1st	*A performance of understanding guided by tacit knowledge and reflexivity*		

.Figure 2. Demonstrates the 'Performance of Understanding' assessment model in its totality from degree classification through to a system of symbols in the form of ticks and crosses which can be used in place of traditional academic tools.

The ease with which academic subjects can be assessed does not readily lend itself to the assessment of a clinical situation where the emphasis needs to be less on the assessment of knowledge alone but more on its implementation and consequences for clinical practice leading to a greater understanding of that practice. For example, rather than a written assignment on the subject of suicide, a nursing module based on 'the management of suicide' could have, as its summative assessment, a simulated interaction with a suicidal patient. This would encourage students to make obvious the extent of their learning gained through attending lectures, private study, and the seeking of evidenced based research which informs day-to-day practice. As well as knowledge gained, the assessors will also be seeking evidence of apposite, considered and responsive interventions which are sensitive, empathetic and patient centred applicable to the vulnerable patient. On completion, the student would be required to demonstrate reflection on the practice, highlighting those elements of the interaction which were considered good practice and those needing further consideration. This is self-development in its broadest sense, including knowing how to learn and control one's own learning and the ability to reflect and self evaluate, that is to provide oneself with feedback (Eraut 1994). The 'Performance of Understanding' assessment model. would accurately reflect the importance and value of the transference of theories, knowledge and understanding of suicide into the student's clinical practice. We believe that the module leader and a clinical practitioner, with expertise in nursing suicidal patients, need to be present jointly for the student's assessment. The student will be expected to have talked through the patient's history, presenting problem and possible interventions using appropriate research and referencing while demonstrating an empathetic attitude. This assessment procedure has some links with the oral and practical assessment methods used in languages and the sciences where some subjective judgement is needed but criteria for performance are clearly stated (Childs 1993). It differs in one major aspect, where students in general report finding face-to-face assessments intimidating. Nursing students are expected to work face-to-face with their patients in the performance of their duties on a daily basis and as such should be empowered and enabled, by this method of assessment, to give a performance of understanding, which demonstrates both their knowledge and the application of that knowledge in simulated or real clinical practice situations.

More and more nurses update their clinical practice through attendance at study days and workshops. On completion of this form of study many are left with little or no formal recognition of their increased knowledge, improved skills and greater understanding. Often the people delivering this form of study are expert clinicians demonstrating and sharing both their knowledge, and clinical excellence thus empowering and enabling participants to strive for excellence in their clinical practice. More often than not a certificate of attendance is all that is on offer on completion of the study. This is frustrating not only for the participants but also for those delivering the teaching. The whole of the educational and learning experience is reduced to a mere 'certificate of attendance' which does not give any indication of the increased understanding that has taken place. The Performance of Understanding model would facilitate both those attending and delivering the workshops. Participants who wished to be assessed in relation to the new information and how it relates to their clinical duties could request the workshop facilitator to undertake a performance of understanding assessment at a convenient time during their clinical practice.

Clear guidelines allow the assessor to determine the level of understanding which can be demonstrated in a number of creative and innovative ways dependant on the topic being studied. As can be seen in the 'Performance of Understanding' model of assessment, we have made every effort to move away from the traditional assessment grades A, B, C or 50%. These are felt to be restrictive and can add to student's distress at assessment time. Assessment tends to dominate the students experience of learning and can be more influential than the learning process itself. Instead, the model uses statements of competence and/or symbols related to the individual student's performance. This will clearly identify how the decision was made thus allowing the student, through feedback, to see were improvements need to be made. Here, the feedback focuses on the students learning rather than on the marks or grades awarded.

Collaboration between academic and clinical staff in the assessment of students work is not unusual. However, in most cases the assessment is undertaken individually in the classroom and in the clinical practice area. The 'Performance of Understanding' model of assessment requires a partnership, the tutor and clinician working jointly alongside the student in the pursuit of excellence in practice at all levels of nursing, and this has the potential to greatly reduce the theory / practice gap.

It is accepted by many educationalists, specifically those involved in a vocational curriculum, that all learning is best done through active involvement. The old Chinese proverb

> I hear and I forget
> I see and I remember
> I do and I understand

is particularly relevant here as most nurses are strongly motivated to acquire the knowledge, skills and attitudes that can influence their work in an immediate and practical way. Therefore, the nearer we can make the learning fit the real world of nursing the more acceptable and compelling the need to assess the performance of understanding within the clinical setting. After all, students have a right to expect that any form of nurse education assessment reflects a true picture of the reality of modern day nursing and that the knowledge, skills and competences that they have acquired are immediately applicable and realistic in relation to their clinical practice.

Changing the assessment procedures may be a long drawn out task and getting academic and clinical staff to work collaboratively on the assessment procedure may prove difficult and expensive. However, change is long over due and necessary to address the deficits which are being highlighted daily by educationalists, nurses, their managers, patients and government papers.

CONCLUSION

In conclusion we have identified four key characteristics which highlight the need for improved assessment in nurse education today.

Many nurses enrolling on courses of study, workshops and modules do so not for academic accreditation but rather for professional development.

All nurses are strongly motivated, wishing to acquire knowledge and skills that they can use in immediate and practical ways the performance of understanding assessment model facilitates and promotes this method of learning.

An assessment procedure based on a performance of understanding offers a unique way of determining, not only the level of knowledge developed by the student over a period of study, but also the application of that knowledge as it relates to professional development and practice.

Within nurse education the question of appropriate assessment is paramount.

The performance of understanding assessment model requires a true collaboration between the academic tutor and the clinician from practice working alongside the student in pursuit of excellence in practice at all levels of nursing, working to reduce the theory / practice gap.

The excellence which we seek from our students comes not in the knowing of the principles and theories which underpin the practice of nursing but rather in the complexity of the contexts in which the principles and theories are applied.

The excellence in practice which we seek from our students comes not in the knowing of the principles and theories which underpin the practice of nursing but rather in the complexity of the contexts in which the principles and theories are applied. It is our belief that the use of the 'Performance of Understanding' assessment model will capture the very essence and sophistication of nursing practice. Equally this assessment model has potential as an instrument of assessment in any educational and training establishment that offers study days, modules, workshops, courses and other forms of educational activities that require students to demonstrate not only academic attainment but also vocational expertise demonstrated through a performance of understanding. Such a performance of understanding would evidence the knowledge which informs that performance, the skills used in the performance and the reflexivity which is integral to that performance.

REFERENCES

Child, D. 1993 *Psychology and the Teacher.* Cassell London

Eraut, M. 1994 *Developing Professional Knowledge and Competence.* The Falmer Press, London

Kenny, G. 2004 The tensions between education and models of nurse education. *British Journal of Nursing 13 (2)*

In: Nursing Education Challenges in the 21st Century
Editor: Leana E. Callara, pp. 23-48
ISBN 1-60021-661-7
© 2008 Nova Science Publishers, Inc.

Chapter 2

THE LEARNING EXPERIENCE: A NEW APPROACH TO OPTIMIZE STUDENT LEARNING

*Margaret Denny[1], Olga Redmond Stokes[1], John Wells[1,2],
Ellen F. Weber[2,3] R. McMaster[2,4]
Maxwell Taylor[3,5] and Kathleen O'Sullivan[4,6]*

[1] Department of Nursing,Waterford Institute of Technology
[2] MITA Center for Brain Based Education Renewal, PO Box 347 Pittsford, NY
[3] Applied Psychology,University College Cork.Ireland
[4] Department of Statistics,University College,Cork.Ireland

ABSTRACT

Gardner [1983] identified eight intelligences that the brain can use in learning. Student engagement with learning and their retention of new information can be improved by engaging these multiple intelligences. A five-phase model – the Multiple Intelligence Teaching Approach [MITA] – developed by Weber [1995; 1999], can be employed in the classroom and in clinical settings to reinforce learning and enhance the students' professional development and clinical practice. This chapter explores the concept of multiple intelligences [MI] and the use of MITA to enhance nurse education. Part one of this chapter explores early developmental theories and the relationship between development and intelligence and how MI impacts on teaching and learning.

[1] Correspondence to : Department of Nursing,Waterford Institute of Technology Landline: 00-353-51-845537 Email: olgaredmondstokes@wit.ie

[2] Correspondence to : Head of the Department of Nursing,Waterford Institute of Technology Landline:00-353-51-845542,, Email: jswells@wit.ie

[3] Correspondence to : Director of MITA Center for Brain Based Educaton Renewal PO Box 347 Pittsford, NY 14534 Email: eweber1@frontiernet.net Web: www.mitaleadership.com [585] 421-3656

[4] Correspondence to : Assistant Director of MITA Center for Brain Based Education Renewal PO Box 347 Pittsford, NY 14534 Web: www.mitaleadershp.com

[5] Correspondence : Department of Applied Psychology,Univerrsity College Cork Ireland

[6] Consultant Statistician Department of Statistics,University College,Cork.Ireland

Many gaps remain the evidence base pertaining to conceptual and educational aspects of learning. The part two of the chapter examines how MITA is a means of initiating change within an integrated studies context. It exemplifies multiple ways of knowing and is a new departure from the traditional teaching approaches to present day post technocratic advances in education.

SECTION 1- HISTORICAL OVERVIEW OF DEVELOPMENTAL PSYCHOLOGY

Introduction

The purpose of higher education according to Duff, Hegarty and Hussey [2000, p.13] is to achieve effective learning or advanced knowledge acquisition by students through a variety of learning activities. Therefore, the interaction that takes place between student and the lecturer is pivotal to the overall success of this goal, "since teaching without learning would be pointless, working to improve teaching is the key." Therefore, educators need to use a variety of educational approaches to support life long learning [Rushford and Ireland, 1997].

It is crucial that lecturers promote positive learning environments through the enhancement of teaching and learning strategies, which will improve the performance of all socio-economic groups accessing third level education. In addressing the antithesis to a positive learning environment Jensen, [1998 p.16] posits that a typical classroom tapers thinking strategies and answer options. "Educators who insist on singular approaches and the 'right answer' are ignoring what's kept our species around for centuries."

Learners may be exposed to traditional modes of instruction and so teaching can be aimed at meeting the needs of two types of intelligence, that is, logical mathematical and verbal linguistic. It is very important for educators to be aware of multiple intelligence [MI] teaching strategies because understanding such brain-based learning approaches can enhance teaching and learning in third level education and, in so doing, enable positive educational outcomes for all students [Schofield 1972].

Gardner [1993] proposes that if existing teaching approaches are modified in order to accommodate MI, educators can address the learning needs of all students. MI facilitates instructional environments where students' and teachers' dominant intelligence can be represented, thereby, allowing both parties to become actively engaged in the learning process.

Indeed, a significant amount of theoretical work has been undertaken on MI approaches to teaching and learning. However, an interesting application of this work is based on the success of Howard Gardner's [1983] appreciative work on intelligence and his ongoing quest to help people to develop all their intelligences. At present, teaching approaches mainly focus on knowledge acquisition and consequently more emphasis is placed by students and indeed educators on memorisation, repetition and, to some degree, rote learning. MI theory highlights the fact that individuals are born with multiple intelligences, linguistic and logical mathematical being dominant while other types of intelligence remain recessive [Gardner 1993].

Therefore, androgogical styles of learning and teaching must adapt and change in response to contemporary educational developments. MI facilitates student motivation and learning in the classroom and beyond. Implementing MI teaching approaches using a multiple intelligence teaching approach [MITA] in conjunction with problem based learning [PBL] and enquiry based learning [EBL] is a juxtaposition of many contemporary learning and teaching approaches. The MITA model by itself enables students to extract their past knowledge and experiences, combining it with curriculum content to solve problems and think critically [Weber 1999].

Teaching for MI using MITA is a contemporary way to progress from neo-traditional approaches to teaching and learning and yields a greater understanding of brain-based approaches to learning/teaching. The outcomes for students and educators are new approaches to teaching and learning, which are lifelines for learners and are crucial to ongoing growth and development within faculties of education.

Lifespan and Development of Intelligence

In order to understand intelligence and consequently how learning takes place an introduction to developmental psychology [DP] is required. DP is concerned with the study of individual development [ontogenesis] of a person throughout the lifespan [Baltes Rees & Lipsitt 1980; Baltes, 1997; Baltes & Lindenberger, 1997; Baltes, 1999; Staudinger & Lindenberger, 1999]. Slater and Bremner [2006,p.4] define DP as an attempt to describe and explain the changes that occur over time in thought, behaviour, reasoning and functioning of a person due to biological, individual and environmental influences.

Developmental psychologists are concerned with age-related changes in behaviour and development but aging alone does not produce change as there are many other factors that impact on development of the person and, consequently, intelligence [Slater and Bremner, 2003]. Research and theory on lifespan development and the phylogenetic aspect of DP has generated knowledge pertaining to three aspects of individual development:

- Interindividual commonalities [regularities] in development
- Interindividual differences in development
- Interindividual plasticity [malleability] in development

[Baltes et al 1999,p. 472].

Baltes et al [1999] suggests that combined attention to these components and their age-related interaction are the conceptual and methodological fundamentals of developmental activity [Baltes et al 1999]. Lifespan ontogenesis is constructed as person-centered [holistic] and function-centered [Baltes et al 1999]. Magnusson [1996] and Smith and Baltes [1997] offer a more holistic approach suggesting that the person is a system from which one can ascertain a knowledge base about lifespan development, by describing stages of development or age- related activities. Erickson's [1959] theory of lifespan development emphasises the importance of culture and history, and rests on the epigenetic principle, which is the view that physiological development and personality unfolds to an internal plan. Therefore, growth is viewed as a set of sequential changes continuing throughout the life span. The person centered thesis has been criticised because it is overly broad and difficult to explore experimentally [Baltes,1999]. Whereas, the function-centered approach addresses changes in behaviour and processes associated with, for example, perception, information processing action control, attachment, identity, personality traits and so on. Incorporation of these approaches is one conceptual framework for understanding the ontogenetic nature of development [Baltes et al, 1999].

Contemporary Developmental Theories

Developmental theories today are classified under two world-views or paradigms, organismic and mechanistic. The organismic theory views the person as a biological organism that is 'inherently active and continually interacting with the environment, and therefore helping to shape its own development" [Slater and Bremner, 2003, p.7; Lerner, 1986]. The central tenet of organismic theory is the connection between maturation and experience, which is the means by which the process and variables involved in development occur. Piaget's [1960] general theoretical framework, which he called genetic epistemology of development, exemplifies this analysis. Piaget, made detailed observation studies of children, and subsequently developed a stage theory of cognitive development. He posited that all children pass through a series of distinct developmental cognitive stages and intellectual growth occurs as a result of primarily two processes, which he called assimilation and accommodation. He subsequently explained intelligence as the result of the interaction between the person and the environment [Piaget 1970]. Piaget's stage theory connects with observed cycles of brain growth or maturation in infancy.

In contrast, the mechanistic theory views the person as a machine that is inert until stimulated by the environment [Slater and Bremner, 2003]. So development is viewed as a more continuous process with the person as a passive recipient rather than an active beneficiary in shaping lifespan development. Behaviourists such as Skinner [1953] would represent this paradigm. Behaviour psychology rests on the principle that extrinsic motivators such as incentives, rewards and punishment shape behaviour. A contemporary view of mechanistic theory is put forward by Baltes [1980] who theorises that three factors influenced development

- Normative age-graded life events
- Normative history-graded life events
- Non-normative life-events

Normative age-graded life events are influenced by chronological age; normative history-graded influences are events such as wars or earthquake disaster that happened at a particular juncture in time; nonnormative life events are events that influence a person at a particular stage, for example bereavement, separation, or accidents. These events are dependent on the interplay or interaction of biological and environmental factors [Malim & Birch, 1998].

Therefore, development of the person occurs through a complex interplay between biological factors such as genetic programming and the quality of the social environment [Horowitz, 1987]. Bronfenbrenner [1979] suggests that the influence of the ecology of the environment on a person is much more complex then originally thought, and impacts on development through the interchange of four nested systems.

Table 1. The Ecology of Development in Context [Bronfenbrenner, 1979]

Microsystem	Mesosystem	Exosystem	Macrosystem
Interactions that occur when a child is in nursery	Interactions thatoccur when a child is at home or at school	Interactions that occur when a child is with parents or other social systems	Interactions that occur later in life, for example, third level education

Bronfenbrenner's [1979] model highlights the importance of ontogenetic and phylogenetic processes of lifespan development. These influences are a means of understanding the complexities of contemporary lifespan development, which unquestionably influence intelligence.

In terms of the development of intelligence genetic theories serves to explain some aspects of human ability, which are confirmed by brain imaging and neuropsychology examinations. However, the relationship between genetics, brain structure and intelligence remains contentious. Explaining the workings of the brain in order to understand intelligence is almost bewildering, considering the many influences that impact on this almost elusive ability. Most arguments centre on how intelligence is affected by nature [genetics] and nurture [environment] and these theories continue to pervade the literature and capture many of the salient debates on this truly intriguing topic [Weinberg, 1989]. Sternberg [1994, p. 3] appropriately referred to these theories as "a motley collection of models and metaphors'[that] serve to explain some of the unanswered questions, but intelligence remains to some degree indefinable in the structure of the brain"

It is generally accepted that environmental determinants play a key role in the early development of childhood intelligence. These factors have been identified as, socio-economic status, maternal ethnicity, smoking during pregnancy, breast feeding, childhood height, body mass index, sub-optimal nutrition, and parental education [Lawlor et al 2006; Turkheimer, 1991;Turkheimer, et al 2003;]. Altogether, they posit that these early life predictors explained just 13% of the variation in intelligence at age 5 and just 8% at age 14 but they question whether the approximations may have been greater had they been able to allow for within-subject variation. They propose that results demonstrate the importance of indicators of socio-economic position as predictors of intelligence and 'may reflect the broad effects of early life social disadvantage on intellectual ability' [p149]. Similar research on intelligence can be evidenced in the literature of such disciplines as phrenology, sociology, education, neuroscience and politics [Toga & Thompson 2005].

Alfred Binet and the Birth of a Scientific Term for Intelligence

Early concepts of intelligence viewed it as a unitary concept supporting nativistic theories, which viewed intelligence as a qualitatively unique faculty with a relatively fixed quantity [Schlinger, 2003, p.15]. Nevertheless, the study of intelligence began with the instruments employed to measure it [Kassin, 2004]. In 1905 Alfred Binet [1857-1911] a French psychologist and Theodore Simon [1873-1961], his co-researcher, developed the first intelligence test, the Simon Binet test. Binet was asked by the French Government to devise a test that would enable the identification of children who required special education [Malim & Birch 1998]. This test required students to undertake tasks in different ascending orders. When children failed at a particular level this was deemed to be their intelligence quotient [IQ].

In 1916, the Simon-Binet test was revised by Lewis Terman of Stanford University and became known as the Stanford–Binet test. The Stanford-Binet test compared individual intelligences using age correlation methods. Charles Spearman [1927] scientifically developed a new category of intelligence test that was based on factor analysis, which he included in his historic book *The Abilities of Man*. Factor analysis is a statistical method which enables one to find several independent primary mental abilities. Within the psychometric custom, versions of factor analysis have provided the major techniques for determining components of intelligence [Perkins & Tishman 1998] by reducing the number of variables under investigation while capitalising on the amount of information in the analysis [Gorsuch, 1983]. This became know as 'general factor' or 'g', which is a numerical outcome or algebraic factor and specific factors or 's', which are the specific skills and knowledge needed to answer questions on a particular test. These analyses resulted from an intricate series of statistical manipulations or factor analyses [Schlinger, 2003].

Spearman [1927] postulated that these two factors measured the intercorrelation observations between tests of mental functioning by employing a method of tetrad differences. This pioneering work generated a new body of knowledge pertaining to the existence of a general intelligence or general cognitive ability. Psychometric 'g' and 's' factors were perceived as the two most important factors in predicting educational and work-related achievement[Brand, 1996]. Spearman regarded 'g' as the "common and essential element in intelligence" [1904, p.126]. Some in the psychometric tradition have posited that multiple factors are involved in determining 'g' [Guilford, 1967, Guilford & Hoepfner, 1971;Jensen, 1980] while others put forward important sub factors [Carroll, 1993; Horn & Cattell, 1966; Horn, 1989]. Fancher [1985] and Gould [1981] were critical of Spearman's research approach, design and analyses and the supposition that 'g' is a statistical construct. He suggested that he committed the logical error of reification by taking abstract mathematical correlations and reifying them as 'g' intelligence. Schlinger [2003,p. 16] maintained that once this error occurs it is easy to commit another logical error, circular reasoning, which is trying to prove an assertion by simply repeating it in different words. Schinger [2003] suggests that the only evidence from Spearman's analyses for 'g' were positive correlations, which may correlate for any number of reasons, and if none existed then he could not have theorised about 'g'. Wechsler [1939] developed another set of intelligence tests, the Wechsler Adult and Children Intelligence Scale (WAIS; WISC). Wechsler's test relied on verbal subtests and performance subsets. He felt that Binet overly relied on verbal skills. Modern day IQ continue to use modified IQ tests [Kosslyn & Rosenberg, 2006].

The advent of neuroimaging has allowed researchers to correlate unitary or 'g' intelligence with physiological factors in the brain, such as, nerve conduction velocity, reaction time and glucose metabolism during problem solving [Toga, &Thompson, 2005].

These findings provide support for the nature debate on intelligence and are referred to as biological theories of intelligence.

Brody [1992], having performed a critical review of the literature on intelligence theory and its measurement, concluded that modern psychometric analyses 'provides clear support for a theory that assigns fluid ability, or 'g' to a singular position at the apex of a hierarchy of abilities' [p.349]. Brand [2001] suggests that Spearman's 'g' factor remains the all-pervading test of intelligence in current day psychological test. However, psychometric analysis has been supported by some and equally has been criticised by other researchers, who suggest that a 'g' factor is not sensitive enough to individual differences and should not predict ability or educational attainment [Gould 1996; Kamin, 1997].The reliability of measurement of intelligence only using a 'g' factor is dependent on many issues, such as culture and contextual issues.

Horn and Cattell [1966] developed a theory of intelligence that specified fluid and crystallized abilities, which they regarded as two broad factors that determine intelligence. Fluid intelligence they represents the ability to explain and solve problems in new or unknown situations. While in contrast, crystallised intelligence is the extent to which an individual has attained the knowledge of a culture. According to Horn [1989], fluid and crystallised 'theory can also be thought of as a theory of multiple intelligences because of the relative independence of fluid and crystallized abilities [characterized by distinctly separate patterns of covariation]. Horn [1989] states that these abilities "... are outcroppings of distinct influences operating through development, brain function, genetic determination, and the adjustments, adaptations, and achievements of school and work" [Horn, 1989, p. 76].

Guilford [1956] hypothesised that several autonomous units of intelligence coexist and suggested that intelligence is better viewed as a set of independent factors. This has been supported by findings in research from neuropsychology to developmental psychology to artificial intelligence, as theorised by Gardner [1983] and MI theory.

Sternberg [1985], in his triarchic theory of intelligence, posits that intelligence is made up of three general type of processes. These three sub-theories or interacting aspects of intelligence are context-specific or pertaining to practical intelligence, and are related to

- experience or creative intelligence and
- cognitive components of information processing and metacognition

This theory according to Sternberg [1985] asserts that there are different types of intelligence such as metacomponents that control and monitor processing; performance components that process and execute plans; and knowledge acquisition components that encode and assemble new knowledge. Altogether, triarchic theory maintains different aspects or kinds of intelligence such as academic, practical ability. [Yekovich, 1994].

According to Frith [1997] the brain consists of many modules that process information relatively independently of each other and he suggests that, 'it seems likely that it will be easier to discover how one of those modules works than to explain the functioning of the brain as a whole' [p. 5]. Das [2002] suggests that Frith's thesis queries the validity of the concept that there is 'g' or general factor intelligence. He further suggests that many of the organs of the body are unambiguous and varied in terms of functioning. Therefore, the brain, even though it works as a whole, cannot be conceived to have one general intelligence function [Das, 2002, p. 28]. He states that in people who have brain damage, specific cognitive functions are often spared, while other functions remain impaired:

> In addition, individuals who have significantly damaged frontal lobe functions may have normal IQs, despite the fact that the frontal lobes are essential for higher cognitive processes. Similarly, some dyslexic children have high IQs despite their significant difficulties in reading.

Das maintains that these cases challenge the notion of 'g' factor intelligence and suggests that intelligence should be viewed as multidimensional. He cites the work of Gardner [1983] and MI theory, Sternberg's [1985] triarchic theory and the planning, attention, simultaneous, and successive [PASS] theory that he and his colleagues [Das, Kirby, & Jarman, 1975] proposed, which refers to a model [Figure 2] that conceptualises four kinds of intellectual human competence.

Table 2. PASS Theory of Intellectual Human Competence

Planning Processes	Attention or Arousal Processes	Simultaneous Processing	Successive Processing
Decisions about how to solve problems, anticipating and monitoring feedback	This allows a person to selectively attend to some stimuli while ignoring others, resist distractions, and maintain vigilance	Integrates stimuli into groups. As a result, stimuli are seen as whole, each piece being related to the others.	Includes integrating stimuli in a specific serial order

Since its inception the authors have elaborated on two of the areas originally identified namely, planning component and attention-arousal component [Das, Kar, & Parrila, 1996; Das, Naglieri, & Kirby, 1994]. Das [2002, p.29] states that the 'PASS theory was developed with the intention of predicting and explaining normal as well as atypical cognitive functions'. They have also developed practical applications of the model, including the 'Cognitive Assessment System' CAS [Naglieri & Das, 1997] and the 'PASS Reading Enhancement Program' [PREP], and a remediation programme for persons who present with reading difficulties and arithmetic problems [Das, 1999]. Das [2002] states that in PASS a link between the four areas of competence processes with particular areas of the brain. This expands on the work of Luria [1966a]. Luria [1966b] emphasised the closeness of the anterior frontal cortex to those parts of the cortex that are electrically excitable in terms of motor functions [Goldberg, 1990]. Lassen el al [1978] claim that the bulk of Luria's work was a study of the characteristic way in which various functional systems were disturbed by damage to a particular brain area. Luria himself stated that when 'a particular factor is incapacitated by a brain lesion, all the complex behavior processes that involve the factor are disturbed and all others remain normal' [p. 72].

The publication entitled *The Bell Curve* in 1994 [Herrnstein & Murray, 1994; Kamin,1995] which was a critical review of the history of research on intelligence [Hunsley and Lee, 2006] is reminiscent of earlier debates on intelligence and will undoubtedly continue to dominate this important research area, which is complex and multifaceted. Nonetheless, the contention that intelligence is in part a biological entity or a potential, which exists in the brain and can be measured, is at the forefront of many contemporary intelligence theories. Accordingly, whether one subscribes to a 'g' intelligence or to Gardner's [1983, p.8] MI interpretation as interaction between biological proclivities and opportunities for learning in a particular cultural context, or to Thorndike's [1927] aphorism that whatever exists at all exists in some amount and can be measured is acceptable. However, the solitary notion of 'g' intelligence, which Perkins and Tishman [1998, p.9] state that foregrounds ability, may hamper research in brain based learning approaches such as MI.

According to Lohman [1993, p. 14], many educators and psychologists continue to think that intelligence tests measure the innate capacity or the potential of the learner. Lowman suggests that this a personal theory that is staunchly held by professionals and, like other personal theories, is not easily altered by disconfirming evidence. Similarly, multiple intelligence variation in student performance is considered a virtue, not a vice by educators [Eisner, 2004]. According to Schlinger [2003, p.17]:

> Intelligence, then, as an essence or quality, is a myth. Intelligence is first and foremost a word that psychologists and others use to refer to various behaviors in varying contexts. It may be useful for social reasons to distinguish between behaviors that are more relevant to academic, practical, or emotional contexts, or to subdivide and categorize behaviors according to other socially relevant criteria. However, we should remember that these are not scientific distinctions, at least not yet.

These deliberations about intelligence will continue to be debated; however, a paradigm shift is required in education if learners are to benefit from a more holistic viewpoint as advocated by Gardner in his epic research on MI theory. The final word here is left to Gardner [2000] who states that there is nothing magical about intelligence and if we define it narrowly we place cognitive and academic endeavours on a pedestal instead of accepting and valuing all intelligences.

SECTION 11- THEORETICAL GROUNDWORK OF GARDNER'S THEORY

Introduction

As outlined in section one the concept of 'g' the influence of environment, culture, and the persistent debate on nature versus nurture and the very existence of intelligence remains a controversial subject [Weinberg, 1989; Howe 1990]. Gardner's [1983] original definition of intelligence was "a biopsychological potential to process information that can be activated in a cultural setting to solve problems or create products that are of value in a culture" [p. 33-34]. He then refined this definition and stated that, "intelligence is the biological potential to process information in certain ways that can be activated in a cultural setting to solve problems or make products that are value in a culture"[Gardner, 1999, p. 34].

Gardner [1983], however, was influenced by what happened to people who had sustained brain injuries or strokes. He described how these people, who were brain damaged, would lose some intellectual abilities while other abilities would remain intact. This led him to theorise that people have multiple intelligences. Gardner [1983] about brain development and synthesised many scientific findings about brain development when formulating his theory on MI and suggests certain criteria and requirements that each intelligence must meet in order to be classed as intelligence, not just a talent or a skill. The eight criteria he considered were

1. Potential isolation by brain damage or neurological evidence
2. The existence of idiots-savants, prodigies, and other exceptional individuals
3. An identifiable core operation of set of operations
4. A distinctive development history and a definable set of expert en-state performances
5. An evolutionary history and evolutionary plausibility
6. Support from experiential psychological tasks
7. Support from psychometric findings
8. Susceptibility to encoding in a symbol system

[Gardner 1983]

Gardner [1983] described seven equal and autonomous intelligences and more recently expanded the list to include naturalistic and existential and perhaps spiritual intelligence [Gardner, 2000]. His theory suggests that individuals have multiple intelligences rather than a single intelligence and the potential to harness and develop all intelligences is possible. The MI's that he proposed are linguistic, spatial, logical mathematical, musical, naturalistic, bodily kinaesthetic, intrapersonal, interpersonal and existential. What Gardner [1983] proposes is that we all learn in different ways and by different approaches and educators need to implement specific learning and teaching methods during the learning process. He describes these nine intelligences as:

Further developments in intelligence have focused on emotional intelligence [Goleman, 1995, p. xii] which is defined as the capacity to reason with emotions and consists of abilities such as self control, zeal and persistence and the ability to self motivate [Mayer & Geher, 1996;Mayer & Salovey 1993; Mayer, Caruso & Salovey,2000]

Education, Teaching, and Learning

Jerome Bruner, a psychologist, was one of the well known influential thinkers on the cognitive revolution in Psychology. His book the *Process of Education* [1960] is still highly acclaimed to this day. Bruner [1966] suggested that to teach someone is not a matter of knowledge-getting but is a participatory process that makes possible the establishment of knowledge. He said …'knowing is a process not a product' [p. 72].

He also considers a theory of cognitive growth that focuses on development in terms of the impact of experience and environment on the learner. Bruner [1996] became disillusioned by the cognitive focus and later wrote about the influences of culture on the education and schooling of children in his book the *Culture of Education* [1996,p. ix-x] where he wrote "how one conceives of education we have finally come to recognize, is a function of how one conceives of the culture and its aims, professed and otherwise."

Table 3. Gardner's Multiple Intelligences

Intelligence	Operational Definition
Linguistic	Gardner [1999 ,p. 41] states that linguistic intelligence relates to sensitivity to spoken and written language, the ability to learn languages, and the capacity to use language to accomplish certain goals.
Logical-mathematical	Logical mathematical intelligence involves the capacity to analyze problems logically carry out mathematical operations and investigate issues scientifically [Gardner 1999, p.42].
Musical	Musical intelligence is the capacity to think in music, to be able to hear patterns, recognize them, remember them, and perhaps manipulate them [Gardner 1999, p.42].
Spatial	Gardner [1999 p. 42] posits that visual spatial intelligence features the potential to recognize and manipulate the patterns of wide space as well as the patterns of more confined areas.
Bodily-kinestheic	Gardner [1999,p.42] suggests that bodily-kinaesthetic intelligence entails the potential of using one's whole body or parts of the body [like the hand or the mouth] to solve problems or fashion products.
Interpersonal	Gardner [1999,p.43] states that interpersonal intelligence, denotes a person's capacity to understand intentions, motivations, and desires of other people and, consequently, to work effectively with others.
Intrapersonal	Gardner [1999p.43] states that intrapersonal intelligence involves the capacity to understand oneself, to have an effective working model of oneself-including one's own desires, fears, and capacities-and to use such information effectively in regulating one's own life.
Naturalist	Naturalist intelligence designates the human ability to discriminate among living things [plants, animals] as well as sensitivity to other features of the natural world [clouds, rock configurations] [Gardner & Checkley,1997, p. 12].
Existential	More recently Gardner [1999,p.60] identified a ninth intelligence that he called existential intelligence, which is the capacity to locate oneself with respect to the furthest reaches of the cosmos-the infinite and the infinitesimal-and the related capacity to locate oneself with respect to such existential features of the human condition as the significance of life, the meaning of death, the ultimate fate of the physical and the psychological worlds, and such profound experiences as love of another person or total immersion in a work of art.

Gardner [2001] states that Bruner in his books "put forth his evolving ideas about the ways in which instruction actually affects the mental models of the world that students construct, elaborate on and transform"[Gardner 2001,p.93]. Gardner [2001,p.94] acclaims Bruner as "not merely one of the foremost educational thinkers of the era; he is also an inspired learner and teacher…To those who know him, Bruner remains the complete educator in the flesh…"

Contemporary definitions of education such as Jarvis [1983] suggests that education may result from both teaching and independent study. Moore, [1995] defines education as a deliberate, planned, organised activity that is undertaken with the conscious intention of changing knowledge, skills and attitudes.

To be eclectic in teaching means not relying on any single teaching or learning approach but using multiple or varied methods, thereby connecting with those learners who are more comfortable or perform better when educators use pedagogic, androgogic, didactic, or experiential methods of learning to engage students. Educators, therefore, need to create safe, secure environments for all learners so that learning can be achieved. Caine and Caine [1994,p.69] support this contention when they state that:

> The brain appears to be much like a camera lens: the brain's 'lens' opens to receive information when challenged, when interested, or when in an innocent, childlike mode and closes when it perceives threat that triggers a sense of helplessness.

The experiential method was critically acclaimed by Ausubel [1968,p.3] when he said of educational psychology:

> If I had to reduce all educational psychology to just one principle, it would be this: The most important single factor influencing learning is what the learner already knows. Ascertain this and teach him accordingly.

Kosslynn and Rosenberg [2006] describe learning as a relatively enduring change in behaviour, which occurs as the result of past experience, and which is not simply ascribable to the processes of growth. Stones [1968, p.3] asserts that "unless the child gives some evidence of a change in behaviour, we cannot tell whether or not he has learned". The simplest form of learning is habituation, which is a tendency to become familiar with a stimulus merely as a result of repeated exposure [Kassin 2004 p.169]

Gagne [1977,p. 4] theorised about the conditions of learning and argued that the best indication that learning has occurred is a change in performance or behaviour. He proposed an eclectic approach to learning and drew on major theories of learning such as a behaviourist perspective, perception, attention, information processing, concept formation, language skills and models of memory.

Gagne [1985,p.3] defined learning as, "a change in human disposition or capability which persists over a period of time, and which is not simply ascribable to a process of growth." In his theory Gagne refers to learned capabilities as verbal information and attitudes, motor skills and cognitive skills. He suggests that internal factors and external factors are necessary to acquire each learned capability. Gagne [1977] also alluded to the theory of how instruction should be operationalised. He spoke about using a variety of strategies to gain students attention [Table 4].

Table 4. Gagne's Instructional Strategies

Gaining attention	Using strategies that including loudness of the voice, gesturing, asking questions, or practically demonstrating a skill
Informing students of the objective	Informing students about the objectives of the lesson in order to motivate them to learn
Stimulating recall of prior learning	Asking students to recall previously learned material, which is relevant to the lesson.
Presenting the stimulus	This may involve using PowerPoint, printed journal articles, books, PBL scenario, or demonstration of a motor skill
Providing learning guidance	Relating new information to existing knowledge and giving concrete examples of abstract concepts
Eliciting performance	In order to assess if learning has occurred asking students to demonstrate the application of learning to a new problem
Providing feedback	Giving verbal, nonverbal or written feedback
Assessing performance	Using case scenarios or one minute papers, where student is asked to work on new examples
Enhancing retention and transfer	This can be done by simulating the work environment or assessing learning while students are in practice

Models of Learning

Knowles [1989] identified three main models of learning, pedagogy, androgogy and synergogy. Knowles [1989] suggests that androgogy is the art and science of helping adults to learn, whereas, pedagogy, is the art and science of helping children to learn. The androgogical paradigm acknowledges that the learner develops their self-concept on a continuum from dependence to independence and this is relative to the person's readiness to learn, experience of life and orientation to learning; whereas in the synergy model learning materials are managed by a learning administrator rather than having a teacher who might be seen as an authority figure. Students have responsibility for their own learning through active involvement with other students. The synergy model rests on the premise that learning that arises from team-work is greater than that done by the individual alone, which is the principle of synergy. The planned interaction with colleagues acts as a motivator for learning [Tennant 1997].

Jarvis [1983] notes that learning is the attainment of new knowledge that may not necessarily result in behaviour change, suggesting that behaviour change is not the only measure of learning. Learning is concerned with the development of new skills or the enhancement or reactivation of old skills and the attainment of new knowledge and attitudes [Figure 1].

MITA Research Significance and Application within Third Level Settings

MI using MITA extends the theory of multiple intelligences, informing learning environments with theoretical principles that allow possibilities for individual student initiative, utilising all their intelligences. MITA broadens the application of PBL in education and enables students to transfer critical thinking skills to practice. PBL alone has not always contained the solid structures within which solutions can be evidenced in the classroom [Weber, 1999]. Implementation of MITA, into existing higher education courses is not without challenges and is a mission for all educators who aspire to scholarly excellence in the classroom and beyond. MITA's phases are rooted in significant facts about the human brain, as explored by Gardner [1983;1995]. Central to implementing MITA problem solving and knowledge learning approaches are key questions that engage educators, students and the wider community with new approaches for redesigned third level education. At the core of MITA-PBL innovations, are measurable outcomes that draw from both course content and problem solving acumen.

Table 5. Knowles's Models of Learning

Model	Meaning	Assumption
Pedagogy	Pedagogy is the art and science of teaching children. It refers also to an approach to teaching that adopts a teacher-child approach, irrespective of whether it is children or adults being taught.	Pedagogy model assigns to the teacher the full responsibility for making all decisions about what will be learned; how it will be learned; when it will be learned and if it will be learned.
Androgogy	Androgogy refers to an approach to the art and science of the teaching of adults, literal meaning men, and not just adult teaching. The term was coined by a German teacher Alexander Kapp in 1833 and was revived by a German social scientist Rosenstock in 1921.	Androgogy model presupposes the learner's need to know; the learner's self-concept; learner's experience; readiness to learn; orientation to learning. It is life-centred; task-centred; problem-centred; and motivation may be external and internal.
Synergy	Synergy a systematic approach to learning in which members of small teams learn from one another through structured interactions [Mouton and Blake 1984].	Synergy model;direction; non inhibition;team work; synergy [Mouton and Blake 1984].

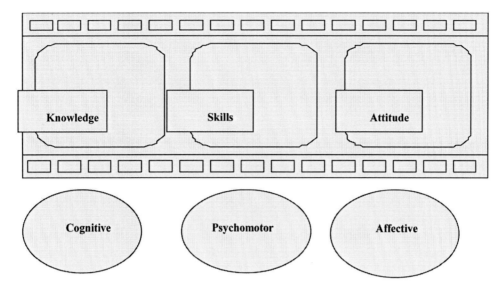

Figure 1: Conceptualising learning and the learning domains.

New Innovations in Teaching and Learning

Traditional colleges and universities tend to neglect active student involvement, and so fail to tap the rich wells of diversity in class [Weber 2005]. A 'Multiple Intelligence Teaching Approach [MITA] incorporates Gardner's [1983] vision of a wider family of intelligences and problem based learning [PBL] that enables students to learn actively using all their intelligences. MITA's introduction in third level facilities of education is designed to facilitate faculty and students in diverse populations to solve complex problems in authentic situations. In nursing this includes nursing/medical emergencies, and the ability to evaluate effectiveness of these applications. MITA/PBL enables students to extract their past knowledge and experiences together with curriculum content in order to solve problems and think critically [Weber, 1999]. MITA asks: *How are you smart,* a very different question think from the traditional, *How smart are you?* [Weber, 1999].

MITA Model

MITA's five phases provide structure which begins on day one of class, and demonstrates problem solving evidence on the final or examination day, in a Knowledge Celebration. In phase one, MITA inquiry adds dialogue for problem-solving roundtable discussions [Lieberman, 1992], using a two-footed question approach to link critical inquiry to content and experiences. Phase two identifies targets that guide students past the problem to consider possible solutions. In phase three, rubrics [scoring matrix] are created, to guide students through learning tasks and these same criteria become the checklist for faculty assessment of students' work. MITA's fourth phase offers learning and assessment tasks to convert students' multiple intelligences in order to demonstrate authentic solutions. MITA tasks fuse students' interests and abilities to content requirements and to nursing/medical problems for solutions [Jacobs Hayes, 1989]. Finally, in phase five, students and faculty reflect on knowledge gained and on the learning process itself. In this phase students explore ways to draw upon hidden or unused mental resources; to explore course topics for deeper understanding, and to integrate several fields of science as an approach to solve complex problems or handle emergencies [Brandt, 1993]. It should be noted that in the final or reflective phase, students and faculty engage a wider community in celebrating knowledge as a structured way to convert facts and investigations into evidence of nursing/medical solutions within the wider community [Weber 1999].

Research on MI and MITA will enable educators to replicate and acquire additional knowledge and competency in this important development in approaches to learning and teaching in third level education [Denny, 2006]. Bruer [1993,p.7] highlights the importance of research based practice when he said:

> Teaching methods based on research in cognitive science are the educational equivalents of the polio vaccine and penicillin. Yet, few outside the educational research community are aware of these breakthroughs or understand the research that makes them possible.

It is evident from the literature and research undertaken in the area of MI that there is a gap in the literature pertaining to teaching and learning using brain-based approaches. Questions that require further debate are whether nursing still at the neophyte stage in terms of teaching and learning, and whether education has moved beyond knowledge to measuring learning outcomes in all intelligences. In a climate where new graduates are working with unregulated health care workers there is a requirement to equip the graduate with knowledge and leadership skills, using their multiple intelligences. Nursing education and, hence, nursing knowledge is not a vale to be filled but a fire for learning to be kindled using multiple intelligences.

Mita as a Model to Enhance Student Learning

Research evidence shows that students understand deeply when they investigate authentic problems, rather than simply recite back isolated facts on standardised tests [Boyer 1987]. When students enjoy a climate where they can think critically and creatively and are empowered to generalise learning to a wider community, they prepare for meaningful contributions to humanity, especially in the caring professions [Weber, 1997; 1999]. The MITA model [Table 1] consists of a five-phase strategy to facilitate students' learning through engaging their strengths, both individually and in collaboration with others [Weber, 2005]

- Questions for Curiosity and wonder: MITA phase one
- Learning objectives for focus and vision: MITA phase two
- Rubrics for accuracy and fairness: MITA phase three
- Multiple assessments for one benchmark: MITA phase four
- Reflection and ongoing renewal: MITA phase five

At the core of the MITA model is the human brain's optimum potential for success when brain-based practices are used for teaching/learning and assessment [Pool, 1997]. This is in keeping with MITA's pattern to extend theory into practice, and to inform practice with theoretical principles. MITA's five phases provide structure that begins on day one of the learning experience. The model's first phase responds to the fact that a search for meaning is innate in the human brain [Weber,2005]. Phase two relies on the fact that learning is enhanced by challenge and inhibited by threat. Phase three addresses the fact that learning is developmental. Phase four recognises the fact that each human brain is uniquely wired and is different from other brains [Caine & Caine, 1994]. Phase five rests on the premise that the brain/mind is a complex dynamic system [Weber, 2005].

In each case this five phase model relies on MI theory as developed by Howard Gardner [1983] and constructivist teaching and learning approaches put forward by von Glasserfeld [1995]. "Constructivism is a theory of learning that claims that students construct knowledge rather than merely receive and store knowledge transmitted by the teacher" [Ben-Ari, 1998, p.257]. Weber's [1999] practical model MITA addresses diversity through engaging students actively in structured PBL tasks. MITA, is like a hologram with three distinctive images or functions,for instance, through MI ideas, students engage talents and interests; through constructivist ideas, students mine their past knowledge and experiences; through MITA ideas, students dare to risk extended possibilities for problem-solving [Weber, 1999].

In one way, the model reaches forward to include new facts about the brain's optimum capacity to learn. It enables lecturers to create innovative curriculum tasks that challenge and activate students in higher education classes [Chickering, 1995]. In another way, this model reaches back to adapt to a problem-based approach to learning, grounded in constructivist and multiple intelligence theory. These resulting brain-based approaches to learning enhance PBL and EBL because of the strong connection to students' strengths and interests [Fogarty, 1991].

Thus, it is essential that all phases are covered during the learning experience otherwise the exclusion of any one phase will give rise to confusion, sloppiness, waste or stagnation [Table 6].

Table 6. MITA Phases

---

1. Question + Target + Expect + Move + Reflect = Growth

2. Question + _____ + Expect + Move + Reflect = Confusion

3. Question + Target + _____ + Move + Reflect = Sloppiness

4. Question + Target + Expect + _____ + Reflect = Waste

5. Question + Target + Expect + Move + _____ = Stagnation

© Ellen Weber, 2000.

MITA inquiry adds dialogue for problem solving roundtables [Lieberman, 1992], using a two-footed question approach to link critical inquiry to content and experiences. In roundtable discussions, the best questions become two footed so that one foot relates to students' experiences and one relates to the lesson topic [Weber1999].MITA is rooted in Vygotsky's [1978] notion that all learning is a socially derived development. Therefore, it is essential to match learning tasks within students' zone of proximal development [ZPD], which is defined as the space between getting help to solve problems and independent performances that follow capable guidance from adults or capable peers. He challenges teachers to step back from talking in order to engage all students actively[Weber,2005,p.3].

A MITA lesson, which is taken from practice, will serve to explain how this model operates in a classroom. Phase one commences with a two-footed questions [Table7].

Table 7. Phases I -Two Footed Question

- What is mental health and how have you observed it expressed normally and abnormally?
- In this lesson, we ask: What are mental health presentations and how can interventions help?

In phase two [Table 8] targets are set that guide students past the problem to consider possible solutions.

Table 8. Phase II Target Discuss the concepts of abnormal and normal behaviour patterns and describe how mental health problems may manifest in persons with varying degrees of intellectual disability

- Describe the signs and symptoms of how mental health problems
- Discuss the concept of dual disability
- Evaluate interventions used in the treatment of mental health problems
- Implement a plan of care for a person who has and intellectual disability and a mental health problem

In phase three, [Table 9] scoring criteria or rubrics are created in order to guide students through learning tasks. These same criteria become the checklist for lecturer assessment of students' work. The scoring criteria show what is expected in this lesson on dual disability.

Table 9. Phase III –Expect

- Research on latest information on intellectual disability and dual disability
- Every team member contributes an assessment tool used to diagnose dual disability
- Each team member shares specific findings on incidence and prevalence of dual disability in people with intellectual disabilities
- Evidence showing understanding of interventions used in dual disability
- A spatial diagram representing the 'Promotion of Mental Health' in people with intellectual disabilities

MITA's fourth phase [Table 10] offers learning and assessment tasks using students' multiple intelligences as tools to present authentic solutions. MITA's tasks connect students' interests and abilities to curriculum requirements in order to resolve practice issues [Jacobs Hayes, 1989]. MITA's fourth phase [Table 10] offers learning and assessment tasks using students' multiple intelligences as tools to present authentic solutions. MITA's tasks connect students' interests and abilities to curriculum requirements in order to resolve practice issues [Jacobs Hayes, 1989].

Finally, in phase five [Table 11] students and lecturers reflect on knowledge gained and on the learning process itself . In this phase, students explore ways to draw upon hidden or unused mental resources in order to explore course topics. It should be noted that in the final or reflective phase, students and lecturer engage a wider community in celebrating knowledge through a presentation of their work. Weber [2005] stresses the importance of using the five phase approach and asks rhetorically how MITA will guarantee that growth and challenge will continue to occur in higher nurse education?

Table 10. Phase IV Move: Using Students' Multiple Intelligence

Group	Two-footed Questions	Measurable Targets	Assessment Task Ideas
Math	How often and how are people with abnormal behaviours helped to lead normal lives and how can you tell?	▪ Graph clients' rate of independence following intervention	Graphs, statistics, timelines, ratios, numeric, cause and effect, problem solving.
Music	How do you observe music's impact on a person's mental process for normal and abnormal behaviour?	▪ Compose song to motivate tasks ▪ Present music to move ▪ Depict abnormal behaviour through music	Compositions, background music, rhythms, integrate music and learning, music video, solo, duet, interpret health through music, demonstrate music as it moves the brain waves
Intra-personal	What are the lived experiences of people who are mentally challenged and how can you as person help these people?	▪ Publish one personal intervention story ▪ Express lived experience of a client ▪ Journal as an ID client might	Journal, personal reflections, personal quotes, legacy, ethical choices, personal role model, assume roles of another, personal stories, personal target-setting, personal change agents
Inter-personal	How have you engaged people who present abnormal behaviour patterns and what has been the outcome?	▪ Interview people re: contentment ▪ Teach peers through case or vignette ▪ Collaborate to share success outcomes	Shared stories, collaboration, interviews, surveys, team teaching, character descriptions, proofread, mentoring and being mentored, compete in teams.
Kinae-sthetic	How can you express mental health patterns through movement?	▪ Lie in unsafe mental health posture ▪ Create a dance /play/ that captures mental wellbeing	Choreographed dance, tableau, buildings, and travel to centre, design outdoor living sites, produce a play, use body language, and create sports for normal and abnormal behaviour.

Table 10. Phase IV Move: Using Students' Multiple Intelligence (Continued)

Group	Two-footed Questions	Measurable Targets	Assessment Task Ideas
Natural	What does nature offer to improve your mental health and behaviour patterns for all persons'?	▪ Accompany a person with intellectual disability on natural outing ▪ Recreate relaxed natural setting ▪ State nature's message to mental health	Compare and contrast natural settings, research and demonstrate nature's effect on mental health, experiment with nature, contrast nature in past and today, illustrate natural phenomena.
Spatial	How can mental health be illustrated pictorially and with what effects on a person's mental development?	▪ Create book without words ▪ Etch a disturbed development ▪ Build mobile of person's mental development	Design a poster on mental health, paint, show adjustments to a setting, draw, create patterns for three-D projects, create posters to show multiple perspectives, display bulletin boards, design webpage
Linguist	How would you use words to describe abnormal & normal behaviours and add recommendations?	▪ Read poem that expresses intervention ▪ Create a case or vignette ▪Write a disturbed letter to a friend	Write stories, poems, interview an expert, debate two sides of the issue, lecture peers, read chorally, design a book of comparisons, write a letter to the editor of local news paper with recommendations for positive mental health approaches.

Table 11. Phase 5- Reflect

Reflect	How will information on dual diagnosis help you as an intellectual disability nurse to care for with people who present with mental health problems?

Addressing the Future Teaching and Learning Portfolio

Students benefit from a range of teaching /learning approaches such as the use of the 'arts', care/case studies and patient/client simulations with actors, clinical and interpersonal skills, presentations [creative projects, thematic maps, posters, graphics, videos, diaries], clinical simulation laboratories [CSL],objective structured clinical examination/assessment [OSCE/A], WebCT as adjunct to assessment using [Multiple Choice Questions] MCQ's and team teaching as a medium of teaching/learning. Post graduate nurse education programmes can work towards collaborative endeavours built on principles of EBL that embrace empirical, ethical, personal, aesthetic and socio-political ways of knowing [White, 1995]. The general principles that this approach espouses are a focus on real cases, learning through doing, emphasis on the development and use of enquiry skills, working at an individual and group level and integrating knowledge and theory from a range of sources [Newman, 2003]. Curry and Wergin [1993] suggest that faculty need to reflect on how their teaching, research and service activities take place and should endeavour to model professional expertise, which is nowadays increasingly demanded by society.

Finally, assessment of teaching and learning using a MITA-PBL approach is essential in order to monitor development and improve teaching and learning for faculty. Educators today need to be visionaries as this drives motivation and actions. Louis and Miles [1990,p.237] remind the reader that "Visions are not a simple, unified view of what this school can be, but a complex braid of evolving themes of the change program. Visioning is a dynamic process, no more a one-time event that has a beginning and an end than is planning. Visions are developed and reinforced from action, although they may have a seed that is based simply on hope."

This also means that the educator has to redeploy or reinvent teaching and learning approaches and Senge [1990,p.237] speaks of this personal mastery as "a process of continually focusing and refocusing on what one truly wants, on one's visions" [p. 49] It does certainly involve a challenge and is an unremitting journey every educator should undertake. As Senge [1990,p.159] posits that " it's a relentless willingness to root out the ways we limit or deceive ourselves from seeing what is, and to continually challenge our theories of why things are the way they are. It means continually broadening our awareness, just as the great athlete with extraordinary peripheral vision keeps trying to see more of the playing field."

Senge [1990] suggests that people with a high level of personal mastery have several characteristics in common, such as a sense of purpose that lies behind their vision and goals and they "see current reality as an ally, not an enemy" [p.142] ... "although they may have a seed that is based simply on hope" [p.237]. In summary this requires intrapersonal intelligence, emotional intelligence and cognitive ability and as Palmer [1998,p.2] says in *The Courage to Teach*:

> When I do not know myself, I cannot know who my students are. I will see them through a glass darkly in the shadows of my own unexamined life. And when I do not see them clearly, I cannot teach them well.

CONCLUSION

Learners bring a veritable goldmine of life experiences and maturity when they enter third level education, which should be positively connected to learning. However, in tandem with this exposure is the socialisation process to this new setting, which can impact on many students' self confidence and their approach to learning. The result is often displayed through apathy and disinterest in learning. The challenge for educators is to help students to adapt to such changes. Certainly, innovative ways of learning in the classroom, such as MITA-PBL and EBL have the potential to enable students to negotiate through this maze of new experiences. Teaching and learning has become a more important and popular agenda for educators, as populations of diverse student groups enter this setting. A method of assuring that education and consequently learning is facilitated, delivered, evaluated and appropriately embraced is surely a desirable outcome. This can only be achieved if educators are willing to accept an axiom such as– it is not about teaching it's about learning.

REFERENCES

Ausubel, D. P. (1968). *Educational psychology: A cognitive view*. New York: Holt, Rinehart & Winston.

Baltes, P.B., Reese, H. W. & Lipsitt, L.P. (1980). Life-span developmental psychology.*Annual Review of Psychology*, 31,65-110.

Baltes, P.B. (1997).On the incomplete architecture of human ontogeny. Selection, optimization, and compensation as foundation of developmental theory. *The American Psychologist*, 52(4):366-80.

Baltes, P. B., & Lindenberger, U. (1997). Emergence of a powerful connection between sensory and cognitive functions across the adult life span: A new window at the study of cognitive aging? *Psychology and Aging, 12,* 12–21.

Baltes, P.B. (1999). Age and aging as incomplete architecture of human ontogenesis. *Zeitschrift Gerontoligie Geriatrie*, 3,2,6, 433-448.

Baltes, P.B., Staudinger, U.M., & Lindenberger. U. (1999). Lifespan psychology:Theory and application to intellectual functioning. *Annual Review Psychology*,50, 471-507.

Boyer, E. (1987). *College:The undergraduate experience in America*. New York: Harper and Row.

Brand , C. (2001). The G factor. Available: http://www.douance.org/qi/brandtgf.htm

Brandt, R. (1993). On Teaching for Understanding: A Conversation with Howard Gardner. *Educational Leadership*. 50,(7) ,4-7.

Brody, N. (1992) *Intelligence*. (2nd ed.). New York: Academic Press.

Bronfenbrenner, U. (1979). *The ecology of human development: Experiments by nature and design*. Harvard University Press: Cambridge, MA.

Bruer T. (1993). The mind's journey from novice to expert. *American Educator*, p. 7.

Bruner, J (1960). *The Process of Education*. Cambridge, Mass: Harvard University Bruner, J. S. (1966). *Toward a Theory of Instruction*. Cambridge, Mass: University Press.

Bruner, J.S. (1996). *The Culture of Education*. Cambridge, Mass.: Harvard University Press

Caine, R.N., & Caine, G. (1994). *Making connections: Teaching and the human brain*. New York: Addison-Wesley, Innovative Learning Publications.

Carroll, J. B. (1993). *Human cognitive abilities: A survey of factor-analytic studies*. New York: Cambridge University Press.

Chickering, A. (1995). Considering the public interest. *Liberal Education*, 81.2, p. 18.

Curry , L. & Wergin, J. (1993). *Educating professionals:Responding to new expectations for competence and accountability*. San Francisco: Jossey Bass.

Das, J.P., Kirby, J.R., & Jarman, R.F. (1975). Simultaneous and successive syntheses: An alternative model for cognitive abilities. *Psychological Bulletin*,82, 87–103.

Das, J.P., Naglieri, J.A., & Kirby, J.R. (1994). *Assessment of cognitive processes: The PASS theory of intelligence.*Boston: Allyn and Bacon.

Das, J.P., Kar, B.C., & Parrila, R.K. (1996). *Cognitive planning*. Thousand Oaks, CA: Sage.

Das J.P. (2002) *A Better Look at Intelligenc*. Current Directions in Psychological Science. American Psychological Society.

Denny, M. (2006). *Exploring intelligence theory in the context of teaching and learning in undergraduate nurse education in Ireland*. First internationl nurse education conference. Canada: Vancouver

Duff, T., Hegarty, J. & Hussey, M. (2000). *Academic quality assurance in Irish higher education.* Dublin: Blackhall Publishing.

Eisner, E. E. (2004). Multiple intelligences: Its tensions and possibilities. *Teachers College Record,* 106, (1), 31–39.

Fancher, R. E. (1985). *The intelligence men: Makers of the IQ controversy.* New York: Norton.

Fogarty, R. (1991). *The mindful school: how to integrate the curricula.* IL,Palatine: Skylight Publishing.

Frith, C.D. (1997). Linking brain and behavior. In R.S.J. Frackowiak, K.J. Friston, R.J. Dolan, & J.C. Mazziotta (Ed.), *Human brain function* (pp. 3–23). San Diego: Academic Press.

Gagne, R.M. (1977). *Conditions of Learning* (3rd ed.). New York: Holt, Rinehart and Winston.

Gagne, R.M. (1985). *The conditions of learning* (4th ed.). New York: Holt, Rinehart & Winston .

Gardner H. (1983). *Frames Of Mind.* New York: Basic Books.

Gardner, H. (1993). *Multiple Intelligences: The Theory in Practice.* New York: Basic Books.

Gardner, H. (1995). Reflections on multiple intelligences: Myths and messages. *Phi Delta Kappan,* 72, 2.

Gardner, H. & Checkley, K. (1997). The first seven...and the eighth: A conversation with Howard Gardner. *Educational Leadership,* 55,(1), 8-13.

Gardner, H. (1999). *Intelligence reframed: Multiple intelligences for the 21st century.* New York: Basic Books.

Gardner, H. (2001). Jerome S. Bruner. In J. A. Palmer (Ed.), *Fifty modern thinkers on education: From Piaget to the present.* London: Routledge.

Gardner , H. (2000) *Intelligence reframed: Multiple intelligence for the 21st Century.*New york: Basic Books.

Goldberg, E. (1990). *Contemporary neuropsychology and the legacy of Luria.* Hillsdale, NJ: Lawrence Erlbaum Associates.

Goleman, D. (1995). *Emotional intelligence.* New York: Bantam Books.

Gorsuch, R.L. (1983). *Factor analysis.* Hillsdale, New Jersey: Lawrence

Gould, S. J. (1981). *The mismeasure of man.* New York: Norton.

Gould , S.J. (1996). *The Mismeasure of man .* New York : Norton.

Guilford, J. P. (1956). The structure of intellect. *Psychological Bulletin,53,267-293.*

Guilford, J. P. (1967). *The nature of human intelligence.* New York: McGraw-Hill.

Guilford, J. P., & Hoepfner, R. (1971). *The analysis of intelligence.* New York: McGraw-Hill.

Herrnstein, R. J., & Murray, C. (1994). *The bell curve: Intelligence and class structure in American life.* New York: The Free Press.

Horn, J. (1989). Models of intelligence. In R. Linn (Ed.), *Intelligence: Measurement, theory, and public policy* (pp. 29-73). Chicago: University of Illinois Press.

Horn, J. L., & Cattell, R. B. (1966). Refinement and test of the theory of fluid and crystallized intelligence. *Journal of Educational Psychology*, 57, 253-270.

Horowitz, F.D.(1987).*Exploring developmental theories: towards a structural/behavioural model of development.* New York; Erlbaum.

Howe, M. J. A. (1990). Does intelligence exist? *The Psychologist,* 490-493.

Hunsley, J. and Lee, C.M. (2006). *Introduction to clinical psychology.*Canada:Wiley

Jacobs Hayes, H. (1989). *Interdisciplinary curriculum: design and implementation*. Virginia: Association1 for supervision and curriculum development.

Jarvis,P. (1983) *Professional Education.* London: Croom Helm.

Jensen , A. R.(1980). *Bias in mental testing* . New York : Free Press

Jensen , A.R.(1998).*The G factor: The science of mental ability*. Westport CT: Praeger.

Kassin,S. (2004). *Essentials of Psychology*. New Jersey: Pearson.

Kamin, L. J. (1995).Behind the curve. *Scientific American*, 272, 99-103.

Kamin L.J. (1997). Twin studies, heritability, and intelligence. *Science*, 278, 1385.

Knowles, M. S. (1989) *The Making of an Adult Educator: An autobiographical journey*, San Francisco: Jossey-Bass.

Kosslynn, S.M. & Rosenberg, R.S. [2006] *Psychology in context*. (3rd ed.). London: Pearson

Kornhaber, M., Krechevsky, M., and Gardner, H. (1995) Expanding Intelligence. *Educational Psychologist*, 25, 177 – 199.

Lassen, N. A., Ingvar, D.H. & Skinhoj, E. (1978). Brain function and blood flow. *Scientific American*, 239 (4), 62 - 71.

Lawlor, D.A., Najman,J.M., Batty, D.G., O'Callaghan, M.J., & Bor, W. (2006) Early life predictors of childhood intelligence: Findings from the Mater-University study of pregnancy and its outcomes.*Paediatric and perinatal epidemiology,*20,148–162

Lerner, R. (1986). *Concepts and theories of human development.* (2nd ed.) New York : Random House.

Lieberman, A. (1992).The meaning of scholarly activity and the building of community. *Educational Researcher*, 5 - 12.

Lohman, D.F. (1993). Teaching and testing to develop fluid abilities. *Educational Researcher,* 22,7, 12 – 23.

Louis, K. S., & Miles, M. B. (1990). *Improving the urban high school: What works and why.* New York: Teachers College Press.

Luria, A. R. (1966a). *Higher cortical functions in man*. New York: Basic Books.

Luria, A. R. (1966b). *Human brain and psychological processes*. New York: Harper and Row.

Malim, T. & Birch A. (1998). *Introductory psychology*. New York : Palmgrave

Magnuson, D.(1996).Interactionism and the person approach in developmental psychology.*European child and adolescent psychiatry*, 5,1,18-22.

Mayer, J. D., & Geher, G. (1996). Emotional intelligence and the identification of emotion. *Intelligence,* 22, 89-113.

Mayer, J. D., & Saslovey, P. (1993). The intelligence of emotional intelligence. *Intelligence*, 17, (4), 433-442.

Mayer, J. D., Caruso, D. R., & Salovey, P. (2000). Emotional intelligence meets traditional standards for an intelligence. *Intelligence,* 27, 276-298.

Moore, K. (1995) *Classroom Teaching Skills.* (3rd Ed.). London: McGraw-Hill, Inc.

Naglieri J, Das JP. (1997). *Das-Naglieri Cognitive Assessment System (CAS).*
Itasca, IL: Riverside.

Piaget, J. (1960). *The psychology of intelligence.* Patterson, NJ: Littlefield, Adams, & Co.

Piaget, J. (1970). *Piaget's theory: In child's conception of space*. New York: Norton.

Pool, C. (1997). Maximizing learning: a conversation with Renata Caine. *Educational Leadership*, 11-15.

Palmer, P. J. (1998). *The courage to teach: Exploring the inner landscape of a teacher's life.* San Francisco: Jossey-Bass.

Perkins D.N & Tishman S. (1998). *Dispositional Aspects of Intelligence.*

Rushford, H. & Ireland, H. (1997). Fit for whose purpose? The contextual forces underpinning the provision of nurse education in the U.K. *Nurse Education Today,* 17,437-41.

Senge, P. (1990). *The fifth discipline: The art and practice of the learning organization.* New York: Doubleday.

Schlinger H.D. (2003). The myth of intelligence. *The Psychological Record*, 53, 1, 15-18. Availabele: Infotrac

Schofield, H. (1972). *The Philosophy of education, An introduction.* London: George Allen and Unwin Ltd.

Skinner, B.F. (1953*). Science and human behavior.* New York: Macmillan.

Slater, A. & Bremner, G. (2003). *An introduction to Developmental psychology.* Oxford : Blackwell publishing

Slater, A. & Bremner, G. (2006). *Developmental psychology.* Oxford . Blackwell publishing.

Smith, J. & Baltes, P. B.(1997). Profiles of psychological functioning in the old and oldest old. *Psychology and Aging,* 12,34,58-72

Spearman, C.(1904).General Intelligence, Objectively Determined And Measured. American Journal Of Psychology, 15,201-293

Spearman, C. (1927). *The abilities of man.* London: MacMillan.

Sternberg, R. J. (1985). *Beyond IQ: A triarchic view of human intelligence.* Cambridge, England: Cambridge University Press.

Sternberg, R. J. (1994). Commentary: Reforming school reform: Comments on Multiple intelligences: The theory in practice. *Teachers College Board Record, 95*, 561-569.

Stones, E. (1968). *Learning and teaching – A programmed instruction.* London: John Wiley & Sons.

Tennant, M. (1997) *Psychology and Adult Learning* (2ed). London: Routledge.

Thorndike, E.L. (1927). The law of effect. *American Journal of Psychology,* 39, 212-222.

Toga, A.W. & Thompson, P.M. (2005).Brain atlases of normal and diseased populations. *Interbational review of neurobiology,* 66,1-54.

Turkheimer, E. (1991). Individual and group differences in adoption studies of IQ. *Psychological Bulletin,* 110, 392–405.

Turkheimer, E., Haley, A., Waldron, M., D'Onofrio, B. & Gottesman, I. (2003). Socioeconomic status modifies heritability of IQ in young children. *Psychological Science,* 14,623–628.

von Glasersfeld, E. (1995).*Radical constructivism: a way of knowing and learning.* Washington, DC: The Falmer Press.

Vygotsky, L.S. (1978). *Mind and society: the development of higher mental processes.* Cambridge, MA: Harvard University Press.

Weber, E. (1995). *Creative learning from inside out.* Vancouver, British Columbia: EduServ Inc.

Weber, E.(1997). *Roundtable Learning: Building understanding through enhanced MI strategies,* Tucson, Arizona: Zephyr Press.

Weber, E. (1999). *Student Assessment that Works: A practical approach.* Needham Heights, MA: Allyn & Bacon.

Weber, E. (2000). *Five-phases to PBL: MITA model for redesigned higher education classes. Problem-based learning: educational innovation across disciplines* Singapore:Tamasek Center for Problem Based Learning:

Weber, E. (2005). *MI strategies in the classroom and beyond: using roundtable learning.* New York: Pearson Publishers.

Wechsler, D. (1939). *The measurement of adult intelligence.* Baltimore, MD: Williams & Wilkins.

Weinberg , R. (1989). Intelligence and IQ. *American Psychologist*, 44, 98-104.

Yekovich, F. R. (1994). *Current Issues in Research on Intelligence.* Available: ERIC Clearinghouse on Assessment and Evaluation, The Catholic University of America, Department of Education, O'Boyle Hall, Washington, DC 20064 .York: Harper & Row.

In: Nursing Education Challenges in the 21st Century   ISBN 1-60021-661-7
Editor: Leana E. Callara, pp. 49-113   © 2008 Nova Science Publishers, Inc.

Chapter 3

THE ROLE OF THE CLINICAL NURSE SPECIALIST, LECTURER PRACTITIONER AND PRACTICE EDUCATOR IN THE EDUCATION OF CLINICAL STAFF

Andrea J Graham[1] and Carol Bond[2]
[1] Poole Hospital NHS Trust England
[2] Bournemouth University, England

ABSTRACT

Central government has placed an emphasis on providing education within the National Health Service (NHS) close to the employees' workplace, which is clinical practice (United Kingdom Central Council - UKCC 1999, Department of Health - DOH 2001a). Subsequently, there has been an emergence of new roles defined as 'educators in practice' in particular the roles of lecturer practitioner and practice educator have been promoted as being the most noteworthy (Jowett and McMullan 2003, Elcock 1998). Despite this there is evidence of an earlier role advocated as providing education within practice that of the clinical nurse specialist (Hamric and Spross 1983). With the drive to meet central government policy it is possible the newer roles of the lecturer practitioner and practice educator have led to the demise of the clinical nurse specialist as a 'recognised' educator in clinical practice. The purpose of this research therefore was to measure, describe and compare the activity and experiences of clinical nurse specialists, lecturer practitioners and practice educators in providing education within an acute NHS trust hospital.

A non-experimental design using mixed methods was adopted. A questionnaire generated both the quantitative and the qualitative data. The mixed methods approach was used in order to capture the 'complete' view of both educational activity and personal experiences of the participants. Voluntary participants were obtained by postage of the questionnaire to the study population. A response rate of 70.5% provided 60 research participants. Because a small number of practice educators and large group called 'trainers' contributed to the study these were combined to form a group of 'educators in practice'. This group was used in the comparative analysis.

The results of this research found similarities between all the roles identified including their biographical profile and teaching activity. However, a small number of differences were found, these focused mainly on activity relating to a local university. Lecturer practitioners were found to be more involved with constructing and marking educational assessments and clinical nurse specialists in particular identified they would like to have been given the opportunity to contribute to university curriculum. Within clinical practice the clinical nurse specialists were found to be more involved in providing education for patients and carers.

It has been shown that the clinical nurse specialists within this research were motivated educationalists within clinical practice alongside the roles of lecturer practitioners and other educators in practice. Therefore one of the recommendations of this study has been that the educative aspect of the clinical nurse specialist role is formally recognised and subsequently valued.

INTRODUCTION

Political change has had an impact on the delivery and expectations of education within the National Health Service (NHS). To meet the targets set in 'The NHS Plan' (Department of Health - DOH 2000) and the white paper 'Working together, learning together' (DOH 2001a) a wide range of education, training and support strategies will be required to meet the professional development needs of staff working in the 'new' NHS.

The Department of Health states, "Planning and evaluation of life-long learning should be central to organisational development and service improvement" and "The infrastructure to support learning should be as close to the individual's workplace as possible" (DOH 2001a p6). In addition it is recommended pre-registration nurse education becomes more competency based with an emphasis on acquiring clinical skills (UKCC 1999). Central to achieving this will be the promotion of education in practice. Within nurse education alongside the role of the lecturer at university there are roles based in practice which are promoted as being educative, these are the lecturer practitioner, the clinical nurse specialist and more recently the practice educator (Day et al 1998, Nursing Midwifery Council- NMC 2002).

Unfortunately as much as these roles are promoted as educative, the role of the clinical nurse specialist in particular has been associated with the potential to 'de-skill' the workforce rather than increase their knowledge and clinical skills (Marshall and Luffingham 1998, Jack 2002 and Mytton and Adams 2003). This research therefore has the potential to inform locally to a university in the South of England, a hospital in the South of England and key stakeholders the scope of activity the roles, lecturer practitioner, clinical nurse specialist and practice educator have in education. This has not been measured previously within the local NHS Acute Trust.

In addition, with an increasing workload and diversity of roles and responsibilities within the NHS there are perhaps possible barriers in providing education locally, these barriers could potentially impact on the scope of activities the lecturer practitioner, clinical nurse specialist and practice educators are able to undertake. This research sought to identify and describe those possible barriers. Alongside this an exploration and description of the attitudes, beliefs and experience of the participants places this research in the current context and provides a richness and depth to the data. Again this will provide information on which the hospital, university and key stakeholders can base future service development.

Study Aims

This study aims to provide the reader with a systematic description, measurement, comparison and analysis on the educational activity of the clinical nurse specialist, lecturer practitioner and practice educator roles within practice. In addition, this study aims to explore the participant's attitudes towards education in practice as well as the concept of 'deskilling' and aims to demonstrate the perceived barriers or difficulties to providing education in practice for the participants within this study.

LITERATURE REVIEW

Adult Learning

Understanding how adults learn is pivotal to the implementation of education within the workplace, from learning styles to constructivist theory many authors have sought to characterise the most appropriate teaching method for adult learners (Quinn 1992, Benner 1984 and Gibbs and Habeshaw 1989). The premise is that an adult's learning is an individual experience and that each adult will learn in a unique way. Wilson (2000) proposes that when designing and developing learning experiences a varied approach to teaching methods will optimise the learning outcomes for the adult. Adult learners need to be able to assimilate new knowledge with prior learning or experience this is known as constructivist theory (Cottrell 2001).

The foundations of constructivist theory accompanied by experiential learning are established by the contributions of John Dewey, Kurt Lewin and Jean Piaget. These three theorists pioneered the concept of learning as a life long process (Kolb 1984). Constructivist theorists believe that understanding is developed by interaction between new information and prior knowledge (Daley 2001). Learning therefore becomes unique to the individual, as each person has unique life or professional experience (Gibbs and Habeshaw 1989). Kolb (1984) advocates that constructivism should acknowledge the experience of the student and should use that experience to form new learning. In comparison, Lave and Wenger (1991) propose that learning is an integral part of society which occurs culturally with or without an educational construct, learning is considered to be situational socialisation.

The work of Kolb (1984) and later Honey and Mumford (1992) have pioneered the concept of learning from experience and using previous experience to assimilate new knowledge. In Kolb's experiential learning cycle experience is converted into learning through a process of observation, conceptualisation and activity. Kolb (1984) recognised that each student would experience situations differently therefore each would have an individual learning style. Kolb (1984) defines four generic types of learning style, Diverger, Assimilator, Converger and Accommodator. Honey and Mumford (1992) expanded on the work of Kolb

(1984) and also identified a learning cycle acknowledging that adults will have individual learning styles.

The learning cycle devised by Honey and Mumford (1992) is comparable to Kolb's in that the experience is the trigger for learning. Despite being proposed as an opposing view Lave and Wenger (1991) show similarity in that social integration is the catalyst to learning in any given situation. Similarly, the role of reflection in professional practice is well documented (Williams 2001) and can be defined as a process of making oneself aware of personal behaviour and wisdom it is usually a process that is triggered by an incident or experience (Jones 1995). In terms of education, reflection can be used to provide a vehicle for discussion and interpretation of new knowledge into practice. Schon (1987) denotes this as "reflection-on-action", the aim of which is to generate knowledge for future practice.

Mumford (1995a) highlights that learning can fail if a lecture or activity focuses only on one part of the learning cycle. Lectures for example can be formulated as a means of delivering information and this can be done at the cost of providing time to act on that information. Honey and Mumford (1992) devised a questionnaire to help identify which learning style a person may have. As in Kolb (1984), Honey and Mumford (1992) also promoted four learning styles, that of Activist, Reflector, Pragmatist and Theorist. When compared to Kolb (1984), the Activist shows similar qualities to that of the Converger in that both types are perceived to appreciate the action of learning for example active experiment and discussion. Reflectors and Assimilators are comparable in that they like to observe and listen whereas Accommodators and Theorists are more systematic in their approach to learning and prefer well-structured activity and course work. The Pragmatist and Diverger seem less comparable with the Pragmatist linking the subject matter to a job related problem and the Diverger enjoying brainstorming activities and reflective activities (Mumford 1995a, Kolb 1984, Buch and Bartley 2002). The learning styles identified in theory highlights the need for the assessment and recognition of a student's learning style; within a long-term relationship such as mentoring identification of the student learning style can be seen to be invaluable (Mumford 1995a).

The Context of Education in Clinical Practice

The provision and facilitation of education in practice is promoted as balancing the perceived theory-practice gap in nursing (Field 2004). The premise of the theory-practice gap has perhaps left behind the negative perspective initially suggested within the nursing literature instead receiving more positive connotations in which the gap exists between the two to provide opportunities for new research and to provide a stimulus on which to challenge current nursing practice (Hewison and Wildman 1996, Williamson and Webb 2001). Vaughan (1990 p106) highlights "integrating theory in a turbulent and unpredictable environment was in many ways more difficult than teaching in the relatively safe classroom environment."

Within this context Dearmun (2000) argues that the creation of new nursing posts whose remit is clearly both practice and education is the solution to bridging the theory practice gap. Hewison and Wildman (1996 p755) obviously support this concept of developing nursing posts as they state these posts "could work to ensure the fusion of theoretical knowledge and practical experience for students". In the context of Lave and Wengers' (1991) socio/cultural learning theory Field (2004) argues for the adoption of educators in practice who could provide the wisdom to prevent the formation of a 'hidden curriculum' one which is based within ritualistic practice rather than a theoretical framework. In comparison, defined as practical knowledge McCormick (1999 p133) highlights the importance of combining scientific theory with humanistic knowledge, "we should teach students how to reason qualitatively about the world, using ideas that come from their everyday life and that of experts who deal with the practicalities of that world."

Central government (DOH 2000, 2001a Audit Commission 2001) encourages the provision of education within the workplace; in particular the documents 'Working together – learning together' (DOH 2001a) and 'Hidden Talents' (Audit Commission 2001) propose methods of increasing education and training in order to support the expansion of practitioners' roles to meet the needs of the NHS patient. Carnwell (2000) and (Wilson-Barnett 1997) argue that because nursing roles are expanding and that professional boundaries are becoming blurred training within the workplace and perhaps more importantly support will be needed for the professionals learning and practising new skills. The Department of Health (2002) developed a virtual educational organisation based within and for the NHS. Called the NHSU and described as a 'corporate university with a difference' this vision of educational provision despite early promise has not been realised with its abolishment in 2005 (*NHSU Abolition order.* 2005).

In contrast other projects whose aim was to support education of staff in practice have continued to develop, the Higher Education Funding Council for England alongside the Department of Employment and Learning for Northern Ireland have in 2003 collaborated with local universities in a project 'Making Practice Based Learning' the aim of this project is stated as being "to make practice educators". The project supported by a website (www.practicebasedlearning.org) provides a wide range of practice education guidance and resources (Mulholland 2005). The project appears to take a top down information giving approach and the involvement of those 'practice educators' to which the project is aimed appears limited, there was a discussion board but this showed no participation however further engagement with educators is being sought through locally held workshops. In contrast another project 'Centre for Excellence in Healthcare Professional Education' led by the universities for the North East appears to actively seek user involvement and describes this group as 'people with experience' Their website www.cetl4healthne.ac.uk however contains only information on the project and this suggests their project is to focus more of interaction in practice with local service providers and appears to be very much a bottom up approach (Hammond and Pearson 2004. The Audit Commission (2001 pg 73) concludes, "staff at all levels have an important part to play in training and development," and recommend that in order to identify training and educational needs a 'bottom up' approach is adopted.

Pre-registration nurse education has also been influenced by central government; the report 'Fitness to Practice' changed the curriculum of pre-registration nurse training and placed an emphasis on developing practical skills earlier in training with more importance on longer clinical placements for attainment of clinical knowledge (UKCC 1999). The accomplishment of these changes in terms of student nurses being prepared for practice is reported by Fulbrook et al (2000 pg 356) as having some modest success however they report there is "still clearly room for improvement".

As previously highlighted (Lave and Wenger 1991, McCormick 1999) the role the practice environment plays in supporting learning cannot be underestimated. In addition, Ward and McCormack (2000) found in an action research study that key qualities of a learning environment are a flexible workforce, good communication and clear problem solving strategies. In addition, Garcarz and Chambers (2003) propose factors necessary for learning in a NHS organisation including the need for a shared vision, leadership, empowerment of the workforce, time for learning and reflection and an identified and protected education and training budget. The emphasis for the Audit Commission (2001) is for organisations to develop a culture that values and expects training and learning by all staff; to achieve this it is recommended that an organisation makes every employee aware of their educational role and responsibilities. Hutchings and Sanders (2001) also stress the importance of preparing staff and the clinical area in terms of identifying learning opportunities and ensuring staff are up to date with teaching strategies and educational policy, this is also a reflection of government and professional policy (English National Board-ENB/DOH 2001a, UKCC 2001).

The guidance paper 'Placements in Focus' (ENB/DOH 2001a) outlines the requirements of clinical environments to provide a well prepared and supportive learning environment for the learner. Key to this provision is identified as the workforce, the paper recommends, "There should be clinical staff with appropriate qualifications and experience to support the student's achievement of the learning outcomes" (ENB/DOH 2001a pg13). In comparison a minimum requirement of the NMC (2004 pg10) is that as a registered nurse, midwife or community public health nurse, "You have a duty to facilitate students of nursing, midwifery and specialist community public health nursing and others to develop their competence". Likewise, the UKCC (2002) highlights the requirement for nurses in higher practice to create an environment in which clinical practice development is fostered alongside the identification of learning activities which will contribute to clinical teaching.

Conversely, the clinical environment also has the potential to obstruct learning in practice (Gopee 2001, Flanagan et al 2000 and Belling et al 2003). In particular organisational factors contributing to a reduction of learning in practice are proposed as,

- Pressure to give priority to short term financial targets
- Day to day pressures of work
- Lack of time
- Lack of interest and support from senior management
- Too many changes in workforce
- Poor motivation of self and others

[Belling et al 2003 pg 244].

In addition it is highlighted by the Audit Commission (2001) that lack of funding, inability to release staff for training, inappropriateness of training and poor provision of mentors will have an adverse effect on the provision of education in practice. Consequently it has been shown a supportive clinical setting has the enormous potential to provide a student with a rich resource on which to assimilate the theoretic base of learning and indeed to provide the trigger for theoretical learning.

Competency in Practice

Alongside theoretical knowledge and developments in research clinicians working within the NHS are as part of improvements in patient care, treatment and diagnosis increasingly exposed to new healthcare technologies. Keeping up to date with new technology is an essential role of all healthcare professionals and nursing in particular has been at the forefront of using new equipment in the monitoring and treatment of patients (Medical Devices Agency 2000). The Department of Health (1999, 2001a) clearly highlights the requirement of nurses to acquire new skills and update clinical skills to utilise the new technologies in patient care. In terms of continuing professional development, "education will increasingly be work based. The acid test must be competence in doing" (DOH 2001 pg 40). The assessment therefore of practitioners within the clinical setting is important both in terms of staff development and patient safety.

The growing trend for the increased use of sophisticated medical equipment to support patient care has led hospital and primary health care trusts to place an emphasis on providing documented evidence of a practitioner's competence to perform a specific clinical skill or the ability of a practitioner to use certain types of equipment (Douglas et al 2001). The purpose and motivation for the trust is the protection of patient safety and ultimately to safeguard trust liability. However, in terms of staff development this could be an ideal opportunity to benchmark best practice and to provide a framework for skills acquisition and progression, the premise being that the purpose of assessment should be central to learning and not just a measure of performance (Quinn 2000, Brown and Knight 1994).

Importantly Ramritu and Barnard (2001) found that competence was an evolving concept. Similarly Benner's (1984) work supports a continuing ongoing process of skills acquisition leading to competence. Benner (1984 pg 26) describes the characteristics of the competent practitioner are that of "an increased level of efficiency, have an ability to cope with and manage the many contingencies of clinical nursing". Within Benner's model a competent practitioner can become a novice in a new clinical situation for that reason competency can be seen to be transitional and reliant on experience. Providing reliable and valid evidence of a clinician's competence of a practical skill can be burdened with difficulty (Norman et al 2002) and the supporting role of educators within practice could be critical in affecting the reliability and value of that assessment.

Role of the Educator in Practice

The impact the teacher has both in terms of effectiveness and student motivation should not be underestimated (Gibbs and Habeshaw 1994). Simplistically the ultimate role of the teacher is to enable the student to understand new knowledge or experience in order to change behaviour (Walkin 1990). Lam et al (2002) found that a teacher's performance and attitude will directly affect the curriculum by influencing content, structure and teaching strategy; it is implied that the teacher has the power to choose those aspects of education in which they are most comfortable or confident. This is supported by Thornton (1997) who proposes that the ideals of the tutor will direct the selection and depth of subject content to be presented to the learner. In contrast Lave and Wenger (1991 pg 97) support the view that the student constructs their own curriculum of learning through interaction with the clinical environment, in contrast to a teaching curriculum it is proposed " a learning curriculum consists of situated opportunities evolved out of participation in a specific community." Similarly, inquiry-based learning places the student in the 'driving seat' and at the centre of learning but balances the 'student as teacher' approach with 'expert' facilitation (Morris and Turnbull 2004). In ensuring that learning opportunities for the student are not biased or extreme the role of the educator in practice can be seen as critical (Sadler-Smith 1996).

Equally the learner and the tutor are central to the success or failure to attain learning (Quinn 2000). The provision of student support is acknowledged as being essential for maintaining and improving the quality of the learning experience (Cottrell 2001). More than ever there will be an increasing demand for a range of strategies to support learners as information technology and government policy increases accessibility to higher education by encouraging more flexible ways to learn (Department for Education and Skills - DFES 2003). The accepted strategy that prevails to supporting learners in the workplace is provision of effective mentorship (Mumford 1995b, Spouse 2001, Johnston and Boohan 2000, Cope et al 2000).

Spouse (2001) found that mentorship was the most significant influence on a learner in practice; one critical finding was that the role facilitated the learner to become accepted in a new setting this is defined this as 'sponsorship'. Similarly Lave and Wenger (1991 pg 68) support this concept and view models of apprenticeship in terms of legitimising the students' participation in practice and providing a model of practice which is absorbed by the student in the context of socialisation; this may be on a formal or informal level, "apprenticeship happens as a way of, and in the course of daily life. It may not be recognised as a teaching effort at all."

In comparison Cope et al (2000) highlight that the strategy of mentorship employs methods of modelling, coaching, articulation, reflection and exploration and is in essence providing the learner with a 'cognitive apprenticeship'. Important roles within the practice setting could hold the potential to support and promote education within practice. However Cahill (1996) found that the hospital culture and hierarchy separated those who had knowledge from those who needed to learn it. It is proposed that clinicians acting as role models should be the providers of coaching, formal education and facilitators of critical reflection enabling the direct application of theory into practice (Hewison and Wildman 1996, Dearmun 2000, Cope et al 2000 and Field 2004). A review of the literature promotes three main nursing roles as clinicians in practice who have both a clinical and educational role, that of the clinical nurse specialist, lecturer practitioner and practice educator (Humphris 1994, Elcock 1998, Jowett and McMullan 2003).

Clinical Nurse Specialist Role

There is ambiguity amongst the current accumulation of titles and roles of nurses considered to be in specialist practice (Ormond-Walshe 2001) this perceived identity crisis can lead employers and post holders to struggle to define accurately the attributes and therefore value of their role (Daly and Carnell 2003). For this reason there is a growing amount of literature seeking to clarify and quantify the roles of nurses in specialist practice (Ibbotson 1999 and McGee et al 1996).

Since the 1970's the earliest established role and therefore title of a nurse in specialist practice is that of the clinical nurse specialist. The remit for the role of clinical nurse specialist is diverse and as such several authors have sought to conceptualise the role into a framework of sub-roles (Humphris 1994). Prevalent within nursing literature the works of Hamric and Spross (1983) and Ryan-Merrit et al (1988) are acknowledged to be the foundation on which to base practice and evaluation, the sub-roles promoted are, expert practice, consultation, education, research and management. Humphris (1994) emphasises a fundamental part in the role of the clinical nurse specialist is the provision of education and likewise Cattini and Knowles (1999) highlight that the core competences for a nurse specialist are to provide professional support for staff by acting as role model, delivering and facilitating training and education. It is therefore suggested that the role of the clinical nurse specialist is educational; however to what extent the role of clinical nurse specialist integrates education into practice is not made explicit (Hamric and Spross 1983 and Ryan-Merrit et al 1988).

An evaluation of the clinical nurse specialist role by Martin (1997) found eight observable services carried out by the clinical nurse specialist two of which were education and practice development. In this study Martin (1997 p152) quotes a patient who states, "she teaches the others which is important as she can't see every one". In comparison, Hurlimann et al (2001) and Gibson (2001) recognise methods adopted by clinical nurse specialists in delivering education as conducting bedside teaching, working with and mentoring new nurses and the provision of formal lectures. Interestingly Bamford and Gibson (2000) found although education and training was identified by practising clinical nurse specialists as one of six key components of their role, the amount of time spent on this activity varied, with clinical work identified as absorbing the majority of time. Similarly, Chang and Wong (2001) identified nurse specialists and general nurses placed more importance in the clinical aspect of the nurse specialist role compared to nursing officers and doctors who ranked provision of education as the most important. Interestingly ward managers within this study viewed education as the least valuable ranking research as the main function of the nurse specialist role. Bousfield (1997 p 253) concludes, "while patient care is the overriding priority additional role components of consultation, education and research must be developed and fully integrated."

Although the role of the clinical nurse specialist is limited in terms of funding educational placements acting as a resource for information is seen a fundamental role (Bale 1995). The basis for being a resource for information is the ability to link theory into practice in a way that will have significance for the staff providing patient care, although this is seen to be a challenge for all nurse specialists (Martin 1997, Bousfield 1997).

In the acquisition of a new skill as a result of the advancement in healthcare technology the nurse specialist is in the position to enhance the transition from theory into practice. The nurse specialist will already possess the necessary cognitive and psychomotor skills to optimise specialist technology for patient care and is consequently the ideal person to provide the education and act as a role model in using that particular device (Graham 2005). Fundamental to skills acquisition is the process of assessment (Benner 1984, Knight et al 2000, Brown and Knight 1994) it follows therefore that the clinical nurse specialist should be involved in the assessment of clinical skills. Although there is general agreement within the literature that the educative role of the nurse specialist is important there appears to be no reference to the involvement of the nurse specialist in clinical skills assessment (Hurlimann et al 2001, Cattini and Knolwes 1999, Gibson 2001, Bousfield 1997 and Martin 1997).

It therefore emerges that the role of the clinical nurse specialist is inextricably linked with education nevertheless; it appears the role of the clinical nurse specialist is one of provider rather than leader in education. Hamric et al (1996) supports the view that having reached the status of clinical nurse specialist there is an intrinsic obligation to lead. The role of the clinical nurse specialist is generally accepted as the lead for nursing practice within their sphere of speciality (Humphris 1984). In promoting practice and organisational development Cattini and Knowles (1999) highlight the clinical nurse specialist contributes to the establishment of systems of work and defining best practice.

Alongside defining best practice the clinical nurse specialist role in terms of education is seen as one which challenges practices and attitudes whilst being tolerant and accepting, "if a nurse specialist was the kind of person who made you feel stupid you wouldn't ask for their help again." (Martin 1997 p153). Petty (1998) sees questioning as a key part of reinforcement in education and assessment. Expanding on this Rolfe and Fulbrook (1998 p156) promote the role of clinical nurse specialist as "a visionary leader who generates and has the managerial skills to create an evaluative culture that advances local and national practice." In considering the role of the clinical nurse specialist to be part educator and part leader it appears justified to hypothesise that the two components of the role should not be separate but as one; leading education within the sphere of clinical practice the nurse is considered to be the specialist.

In contrast not all nurse specialists chose to exercise the responsibility to lead education in practice, perhaps this is because specialist posts have been developed in light of different healthcare needs or the precedence for education can be dependant on both the clinical demands upon workload and the differing emphasis placed on these roles by the nurse specialist (Chang and Wong 2001). As Hunt (1999) argues the role performed by the nurse specialist is diverse purely because of the personal agenda of the person in post. The lack of opportunity to lead education in practice may also have an influence on the educational activity of the clinical nurse specialist; the curriculum for education in practice may be driven centrally by the university, the healthcare trust or indeed central government (DOH 2001a, UKCC 1999, Burke 1997).

Strohschein et al (2002) highlight there is a need for a shared vision amongst practitioners when developing and providing practice-based education in order to place an emphasis on the connection between theory and practice in the clinical education setting. It is argued that clinical nurse specialist input into education and teaching is essential (Gibson 2001) whilst Burke (1997) emphasises that an educator should be clinically credible it is therefore suggested the clinical nurse specialist potentially possesses the skills and knowledge for this to be true. In contrast, however, academic credibility is also currently being emphasised by professional bodies (NMC 2002, NMC 2005). In this context Bousfield (1997) recommends a theoretical and academic framework for the development of clinical nurse specialists. Likewise, Bamford and Gibson (2000) propose a continuum of role development for nurse specialists based on Benner's (1984) process of skills acquisition that incorporates academic progression. In contrast however, Flanagan's (1997) study found 34% of tissue viability nurse specialists in post within the UK had no academic qualifications.

In contrast to being educative, the role of the clinical nurse specialist has been associated with 'deskilling' (Mytton and Adams 2003, Marshall and Luffingham 1998 and McGee et al 1996). No accepted definition of the term to 'de-skill' can be found (Jack 2002) however it is suggested that 'de-skilling' is the steady reduction of experience, knowledge and clinical skills. McGee et al (1996) suggest that the general nurse readily relinquishes aspects of patient care to the clinical nurse specialist, which in turn leads to a loss of skills for the general nurse. Jack (2002) however found it was the most senior members of the healthcare team who felt threatened by the potential of a clinical nurse specialist to 'deskill' others.

So far it has been argued a nurse specialist should already possess the necessary cognitive and psychomotor skills to optimise clinical advances for patient care and is consequently the ideal person to lead specialist education and act as a role model in clinical practice (Hamric et al 1996, Gibson 2001, Graham 2005). Perhaps for this reason the clinical nurse specialist must take the lead in developing and providing education in practice for their sphere of specialty in order to directly influence the content of what is taught. Similarly, early literature supports this view, as Adderley and Hunter-Hill Hill (1979 p 329) state "of the many roles in which the clinical nurse specialist may function, one of the most important, most rewarding and potentially with the most lasting results is that of educator."

Lecturer Practitioner Role

In comparison to the role of the clinical nurse specialist more recently in the 1980's the role of the lecturer practitioner has materialised, primarily developed in nursing within Oxford England, an obvious observation is that in the role can be any professional for example physiotherapist, dietitian, solicitor or social worker (Elcock 1998, Fairbrother and Mathers 2004). The role by suggestion of the title is visibly embedded within education however it is comparable with that of the clinical nurse specialist in that there is an expectation for the role to provide clinical expertise in a specific field of practice, have direct patient contact, an ability to change and influence practice and to be involved in research (Fairbrother and Ford 1998). Indeed far from being distinct Lathlean (1997) proposes the lecturer practitioner role would fit a model of 'specialist nurse practitioner'. However, Vaughan (1990) proposes the primary aim of the lecturer practitioner is to maintain standards of practice whilst preparing and contributing to programmes of education. In comparison Lathlean (1997) identifies the functions of the lecturer practitioner role include, preceptorship, mentorship, teaching and assessment both within practice and within the university alongside holding a responsibility for programs of education. The main purpose of the role however is seen as, "an appropriate way of resolving the tension inherent in the desire to combine the academic status with a clinical base" (Lathlean 1997 pg 154) and as "finding a match between what was done in practice and what was being taught in theory" (Vaughan 1990 pg 106). Interestingly Lathlean (1997) found an unsolved theory-practice problem despite the introduction of lecturer practitioners.

Richardson and Turnock (2003) found within a critical care setting lecturer practitioners were viewed as having an educational and clinical impact, the lecturer practitioner was viewed as valuable in giving expert clinical advice and guidance. Similarly Jones (1996 pg 340) found lecturer practitioners defined their role as "a senior nurse with educational responsibilities"

In contrast to the clinical nurse specialist, the lecturer practitioner is usually employed by both the university and the clinical organisation in which they practice this therefore provides a formal association between the university and the clinical setting (Fairbrother and Ford

1998). Described as 'living a dual role' (Fairbrother and Manther 2004) this aspect is thought to have disadvantages in addition to benefits (Jones 1996, Dearmun 2000 and Williamson et al 2004). The obvious benefits cited are the improvement in communication between the service provider and the educational organisation (Jones 1996) and the ability to reinforce the integration of theory into practice (Dearmun 2000, Elcock 1998, Camkooski 2002 and Hope 2003). In contrast it is proposed by Fairbrother and Mathers (2004) by having two roles and subsequently two different employers the lecturer practitioner suffers stress, possible burnout and low levels of job satisfaction. Williamson et al (2004) however found this not to be true and described lecturer practitioners with a high levels of job satisfaction who 'thrived rather than just surviving'. A source of stress may also be the theory practice gap itself as Fairbrother and Manthers (2004 p545) highlight some lecturer practitioners "expressed their concern about their ability to combine both theory and practice when teaching their students."

Although the lecturer practitioner role appears to have a planned structure from its concept towards models of practice unlike that of the clinical nurse specialist which appears to of evolved (Vaughn 1990, Hamric et al 1996) practitioners in post appear to place more emphasis on the clinical aspect of the role rather than the educational. Jones (1996) found that lecturer practitioners recognised their key role as a practitioner rather than a university tutor and stressed the importance of maintaining their clinical practice. Similarly Jones (1996 pg 344) strongly recommends that the role of the lecturer practitioner is "as much service driven as it is educational."

Credibility in terms of clinical and academic levels has also been identified as an issue for the lecturer practitioner the role (Fairbrother and Ford 1998, Lathlean 1997). Lecturer practitioners identified that they should be at least educated to diploma level and hold a nationally recognised teaching certificate (Jones 1996 Lathlean 1997). Across professions Fairbrother and Mathers (2004) also highlighted the value of being credible as a practitioner alongside academic credibility as a tutor. Prevalent within literature is the recommendation that the lecturer practitioner post should have an infrastructure to support both the clinical and the academic aspects of professional development (Jones 1996, Fairbrother and Mathers 2004, Williamson et al 2004).

Their appears to be similarities in role and practice between the lecturer practitioner and the clinical nurse specialist, Jones (1996 pg 343) states within nursing, "the purpose of the lecturer practitioner role is to improve the care of patients and link the education of nursing more closely to its clinical practice" this is not too dissimilar to the literature pertaining to the role of the clinical nurse specialist (Hamric and Spross 1983 and Ryan-Merrit et al 1988, Humphris 1994). However within the current literature there is no reference to the role of lecturer practitioner as one which has the potential to 'deskill' the workforce.

Practice Educator Role

Practice educators are the most recent development for nurse education in practice (Jowett and McMullan 2003) and as such published literature regarding the role is limited. Clay and Wade (2001) report the demise of the community practice teacher role which is to be superseded by mentorship and education in practice supported by the new role of practice educator. This report is based upon the NMC (2002) *Standards for the Preparation of Teachers of Nursing, Midwifery and Health Visiting* and the ENB/DOH (2001) *Preparation of Mentors and Teachers; a new framework of guidance* which highlights that practice educators would take a lead in supporting mentors and students in practice. Clay and Wade (2001 pg 215) perceive the role of practice educators to be, "the prime educators in practice."

Brennan and Hutt (2001) offer a personal perspective on their own roles as practice educators within a large NHS trust; the proposed role is one of a clinically competent practitioner who works alongside under-graduate nurses and newly qualified nurses to provide education, but also one which teaches in a classroom setting. Hudson (2000) supports this view and sees the role as a practitioner/teacher within the community setting and in her description emphasises a need for practice educators to be both expert practitioner and educator. Additionally Jowett and McMullan (2003) concluded that the practice educator role is pivotal to the link between university and practice for the student nurse.

Alongside this Hudson (2000 pg2) promotes the role of practice educator as; "required to integrate theory into practice, teach theory at degree level, plan and run entire practice placement programmes, tailor make programmes of teaching and learning and develop learning contracts and assessment tools." In addition to this in a wider context Hudson (2000) recommends practice educators need to be able to maintain and develop their role as 'expert practitioners.' In contrast Brennan and Hutt (2001) found difficulty in demonstrating 'clinical competence and credibility' this may be attributed to the diversity of clinical settings in which they worked, they described themselves clinically as 'jacks of all trades, masters of none' (pg 184).

A common theme from the literature is the need for practice educators to promote and support mentorship (Clay and Wade 2001, Jowett and McMullan 2003, ENB/DOH 2001b and NMC 2002). In supporting mentorship for nurse learners in practice the roles of practice educator and lecturer practitioner are comparable, both roles are promoted as acting as a role model, facilitating reflection and providing learners with opportunities for practice and assessment in key clinical skills (Fairbrother and Ford 1998, Brennan and Hutt 2001). It is thought that because these roles are independent of the clinical workload there is more opportunity for direct supervision and support of the learner.

In summary there is a significant importance placed on the provision of education within practice (DOH 2000, 2001a, UKCC 1999, NMC 2002) alongside this the emphasis on providing new 'clinical educator' roles has increased the ambiguity and diversity of clinical role titles; this in turn has potentially lead to the devaluing of existing clinical roles who provide practice education in particular the clinical nurse specialist. Undoubtedly there is a need for nurse education to supply credible and knowledgeable champions and providers of education within the practice environment however, in the implementation of central government policy the opportunity to recognise, enhance and support what already exists within practice may have been missed. This research therefore seeks to describe the current context and activity within a clinical practice education setting of the roles clinical nurse specialist, lecturer practitioner and practice educator. The aim of the research is to recognise the similarities and to highlight the differences between the roles, if a large quantity of differences are found then perhaps the need for new 'education roles' within practice appears justified.

Research Questions

The aim of the research was to measure and reveal the possible activities utilised by the roles of clinical nurse specialist, lecturer practitioner and practice educator in education and to appraise and define the views and potential barriers for these roles in providing education in the practice setting. To help structure the research the aim was expressed as a question - what was the role of the clinical nurse specialist, lecturer practitioner and practice educator in clinical education? In answering this question the study collected data on the following:

- What was the biographical profile of each role?
- How were the roles involved in providing clinical education?
- What were the views and perceived difficulties of providing clinical education?
- Were there similarities/differences in the roles?

To reach a greater appreciation and understanding of education in practice the study sought to describe similarities or differences in the context and educational activities of the clinical nurse specialist, lecturer practitioner and practice educator. Walliman (2001 p91) argues that descriptive research "attempts to examine situations in order to establish what was happening, the data collected is organised and presented in a clear and systematic way so that analysis can result in valid and accurate conclusions."

Methodological Approach

The body of research regarding the attributes of the role clinical nurse specialist is established and growing (McGee et al 1996, Martin 1997 and Ibbotson 1999), therefore it is important to test the accuracy of the assertion that the clinical nurse specialist role is one concurrent with education. Alongside this, the role of the lecturer practitioner and practice educator needs to be measured in order for comparisons to be made. The need to test existing knowledge and theory is promoted as a positivist view, with a positivist approach seeking to uncover or reveal a single reality through careful measurement (Tarling and Crofts 2002).

The strength of this approach lies in producing numbers that can be ordered to describe phenomena in terms of statistics (Paniagua 2002). Walliman (2001 p 166) highlights that the positivist approach is adopted by "a social scientist to achieve a clear, well founded analysis and interpretation of social phenomena, based on testable and verifiable data." However Ratcliffe (1998) suggests a weakness to this approach is that the analysis of data by statistics looses the richness of meaning. In recognition that one single reality may not truly exist, a post-positivism paradigm evolved. The post-positivist view argues that one cannot be absolute about a singular view when studying the behaviour and actions of humans and that knowledge develops from careful observation and measurement of the reality that exists in the 'real' world which may contain several perspectives that can be measured in research (Creswell 2003). This study is underpinned by a post-positivist methodology as it sought to measure a variety of activities undertaken by an individual's educative role within practice.

In contrast to positivism and post-positivism a humanistic approach acknowledges that reality varies for each person in differing contexts (Tarling and Crofts 2002). Also defined as interpretivism Parahoo (1997 pg 41) highlights, "that human behaviour can only be understood when the context in which it takes place and the thinking processes that give rise to it are studied." In order to explore the potential barriers to the provision of education by the participants in the research a more humanistic approach was needed as the barriers of providing education would potentially have a personal bearing. For this reason a post-positivist approach with a humanistic element was adopted to gain accurate information to affectively describe the current context of the educational activity by the roles of clinical nurse specialist, lecturer practitioner and practice educator.

RESEARCH DESIGN AND METHODS

Clarke (1998) highlights that both qualitative and quantitative methods of research can be utilised from a humanistic or positivist perspective. In appreciating the need for both paradigms Buchanan (1998 p447) concludes that "most scholars acknowledge today the necessity of establishing a third option: something in-between." This is further supported by Roe and Webb (1998) who argue that the research questions should determine the methods used rather than being fixed by or arguing for a humanistic or positivist stance.

As this study was constructed around the philosophy of both a post-positivist and humanistic perspective in order to generate the appropriate data on the role of the clinical nurse specialist, lecturer practitioner and practice educator both quantitative and qualitative methods were used. Similar to the positivist and humanistic paradigms the philosophical underpinnings of quantitative and qualitative research also differ, whilst qualitative research seeks to interpret the attitudes, beliefs and motivations within a subject quantitative research collects hard and reliable data which can be tested (Cutcliffe and Ward 2003). Because of this qualitative data collection tends to be unstructured allowing themes to emerge whilst the quantitative method of data collection is more robust and structured (Walliman 2001). Defined as mixed methods research Hanson et al (2005) describe the collection, analysis and integration of quantitative and qualitative data in a single or multiphase study. Although several authors (Punch 1998, Creswell 1994, Denzin 1989 and Morse 1991) support the use of mixed methods in research this study was constructed on the concept of mixed methods as described by Creswell (2003), the approach of combining quantitative and qualitative methods to provide a general picture of phenomena. Also described as methodological triangulation Denzin and Lincoln (1998) define this as a method of research, which utilises multiple methods to study a single problem. Promoted by Creswell (1994) as a dominant/less-dominant design this study has a dominant quantitative design that also draws data from a qualitative paradigm. A concurrent nested strategy has been used which simultaneously collects the quantitative and qualitative data; the qualitative data is embedded within the quantitative data and addresses a different research question (Creswell 2003).

Two authors in particular have successfully combined research methods to examine the role of the nurse specialists. Ibbotson (1999) in a local study uses a quantitative questionnaire followed by in-depth interviews to obtain qualitative data. Whereas Williams et al (2001) used focus groups to obtain both qualitative data on perceptions and feelings and to provide information on which to base a quantitative questionnaire.

Creswell (2003) argues that a mixed method approach has the ability to collect diverse types of data to provide a holistic understanding of a research problem. In comparison, Parahoo (1997) contends that it is naïve to consider that a researcher using both approaches will find a constant view. Conflict within the research findings may contradict the research purpose, for instance what may appear from qualitative interviews as a positive aspect of nursing care may not in quantitative data collection be shown as occurring in practice. However, this argument also supports the view of Creswell (2003) in that by adopting a mixed method approach the research has the potential to reveal the whole picture of a phenomenon. Creswell (2003 pg 21) highlights that "the study may begin with a broad survey in order to generalize results to a population and then focuses in a second phase on detailed qualitative, open-ended interviews to collect detailed views from participants."

In returning to the research questions, the purpose of the biographical information was to generate quantitative data, which would build the context on which the research has been undertaken. This provides the reader with a greater appreciation on the attributes of the research participants in terms of educational qualifications and nursing experience.

How the research participants were involved in the education of others was demonstrated in the research by analysing and defining the specific activities and methods the participants adopted to facilitate or provide education. The purpose of this quantitative data was to determine the types of teaching and learning strategies in use within the clinical setting and to compare this to the theory of the adult learner.

In the final research question, the views and perceived barriers of providing education by the research participants was uncovered; the qualitative data generated was used to describe the potential difficulties the clinical nurse specialist, lecturer practitioner and practice educator had in fulfilling their roles as an educationalists. In further exploration of the context in terms of participant experience and feelings additional qualitative questions were included which linked to the theory of education in practice and the role of the clinical nurse specialist.

Consequently, as the research questions required an evaluation of both quantitative and qualitative aspects of the educational role the use of mixed methods in researching the role of the nurse specialist, lecturer practitioner and practice educator was appropriate.

DATA COLLECTION

For the purposes of this study a small-scale survey was constructed in the form of a postal questionnaire (Appendix A1) which generated both quantitative descriptive statistics and qualitative descriptive data. The advantage of this method was the ability to access a large sample group and to offer the respondent the convenience of when and where to complete the questionnaire (Punch 2003). One of the possible disadvantages with a questionnaire is a low response rate. Oppenheim (1992) and Cohen et al (2003) identify numerous ways in which to increase response rates including the design of the questionnaire in terms of length, presentation, assured anonymity and the provision of return envelopes; in addition it was highlighted that advanced warning, explanation and publicity help to increase the response rate. Traditionally, clinical nurse specialists have been shown to be motivated to participate in research by the completion of questionnaires (Ibbotson 1999, McCreaddie 2003). However, in order to maximise response rates an unbiased description of the research was given to each participant in the form of a covering letter and participant information sheet (Cohen et al 2003 and Oppenheim 1992).

A survey approach to the design of the study was pertinent as Caulder (1998) argues the purpose of a survey is to gather data from a population which is currently not collected, as previously stated the data on the role of the clinical nurse specialist, lecturer practitioner and practice educator in education has not been previously collected at the hospital studied within this research. In addition the survey approach to data collection is seen to be important as it provides an organisation with information on which to act (Oppenheim 1992).

Secondary Data

Secondary data was obtained from the centrally held list of clinical nurse specialists, lecturer practitioners and practice educators held by the Assistant Director of Nursing. In addition this list was compared to the directory of the hospital e-mail addresses. This data provided supplementary information to the study on the number of staff employed within the roles studied.

Questionnaire Design

The questionnaire was constructed using the theory of questionnaire construction and design as cited by several authors (Oppenheim 1992, Parahoo 1997, Bell 1999, and Gendall 1998). The purpose of any questionnaire is to collect information on a given subject, within the research paradigm this must be a rigorous process which is capable of producing reliable and valid data (Parahoo 1997). The questionnaire content was constructed from the literature review in order to answer the research questions; content domains of teaching strategies, students, assessment strategies and curriculum development were developed alongside biographical and qualitative questions.

A closed question structure was used being specific as possible, simply worded and not double-barrelled whilst ensuring the questions were not leading. Most questions offered a three way response e.g. yes, no or don't know. Parahoo (1997) recommends use of the 'other (please specify)' option prevents what is described as 'forced choice'. Therefore where a checklist format was used (the respondent could select from a large range of possibilities) the term 'other (please specify)' was also used to allow the respondent the opportunity to offer an alternative answer consequently this prevented the respondent being lead. The use of closed questions to examine existing theory was considered appropriate for this research. Parahoo (1997) and Oppenheim (1992) advocate the use of closed questions for answers which are predictable.

The use of open questions allowed the respondents to interact with the questionnaire giving the respondents a freedom and naturalness in answering; they used their own language to describe the phenomena or express their feelings, in comparison to interviews open written answers could be more considered instead of replying with what was at the forefront of the mind at the time (Oppenheim 1992). The trigger for responding to the open questions was a simplified rating scale this enabled the strength of feeling to be considered. Oppenheim (1992 pg 236) highlights that, "a scale of subjective importance can be applied to many kinds of situations, they yield attitudes rather than objective assessments". The sequence of the questions followed a logical progression and culminated with the qualitative open questions, Gendall (1998) defines this as a 'downward funnel' in which general or non-threatening questions are asked first following with the more personal ones towards the end of the questionnaire.

The questionnaire was designed to be anonymous; as previously highlighted respondent anonymity is cited as improving response rates however in contrast the ability to follow up non-respondents is negated thereby potentially lowering the response rate (Oppenheim 1992). Anonymity was assured by non-encryption and by the content of the questions to ensure that no respondent could be identified.

The questionnaire was piloted, looking at length of time to complete, clarity of instructions and questions, layout and whether the respondents found any question difficult or uncomfortable to answer (Bell 1999). The questionnaire was sent to 20 senior nurses who would not be included in the research, i.e. they were not employed within the setting which was studied. The result of the pilot questionnaire showed 16 senior nurses responded and was reported to take twenty minutes to complete. There was no question with which the pilot group felt uncomfortable in answering although consideration of the pilot results indicated a potential ambiguity in three questions this was adjusted by incorporating further explanation and simplification of terminology to increase reliability in answering.

THE SAMPLE

The target population of the study was all qualified nurses employed as a clinical nurse specialists, lecturer practitioners and practice educators in a local NHS trust hospital. Parahoo (1997 pg 218) defines a population as "the total number of units from which data could be potentially collected" whereas Fink (2003) highlights the population is the 'universe' to be sampled. In light of this and because the target population was potentially small and accessible it was decided to survey the entire target population. The secondary data provided two lists of staff employed in the roles to be studied and provided the names of the staff which were approached to be part of the study. A total of eight-five staff members were identified from the secondary data this was the population of known employees within specialist practice at the time of the study. These were then approached to become participants in the study. By using the target population as the survey sample it provided results which were applicable and generalisable to the organisation. It also reduced the potential for researcher bias as each member of the population had equal opportunity to participate in the research (Fink 2003).

As Ormond-Walshe (2001) has suggested and this research has also confirmed there was an ambiguity of nursing titles in use perhaps especially within the context of clinical education. Secondary data from the hospital held list of nurse specialists and educators identified a range of titles in use including the terms facilitator and practice developer. In addition the results of the research highlighted a further range of titles including clinical trainer, trainer, clinical skills trainer, educational facilitator, practice education facilitator and practice developer.

In order to analyse and compare the roles the following categories were developed; firstly the category called clinical nurse specialists included all the respondents who identified themselves as clinical nurse specialists and the second category developed included all the respondents who identified themselves as lecturer practitioners. A third category was developed by grouping together the respondents who identified themselves as a clinical trainer, trainer, clinical skills trainer, educational facilitator, practice education facilitator and practice developer. In addition as only one practice educator participated in the research they were also included in this category. This category was entitled 'educators in practice' it was felt this reflected the common occupation and purpose the participants had in terms of providing education. The final category to be developed was entitled 'other' and this included participants holding the title, clinical leader, research nurse, counsellor in addition to any respondent who did not specify their role title.

DATA ANALYSIS

Punch (2003) proposes quantitative research sees the world as made up of variables and that a survey method of data collection provides the researcher with an extensive volume of data on which to answer the research questions enabling the comparison or measurement of variables to be made.

This was non-experimental study as the variables under investigation were naturally occurring phenomena. In terms of data analysis although the importance of variables could not be underestimated within a descriptive survey as Roe and Webb (1998 p 130) highlight "the goal of the descriptive survey was to provide as complete a description as possible with identification of variables of interest and the frequency of their occurrence." This research sought to describe the variables in terms of nominal data Miller et al (2002 pg 59) describe this as; categorical data which does not have a liner order and was used to "differentiate between the categories." The questionnaire was coded and analysed to produce the nominal data variables which were then entered into a spreadsheet. A statistical computer package called Statistical Package for Social Sciences (SPSS) was used to process the nominal data into descriptive statistics.

The nominal data was then analysed and compared in terms of frequency distribution which was a method of tallying and representing how often certain results occurred (Salkind 2000, Miller et al 2002). In addition cross tabulation tables were used to examine the frequency distributions and compare in terms of percentages the sub-samples of lecturer practitioner, clinical nurse specialist and educators in practice in addition to the 'other' category (Oppenheim 1992). Because the research and survey population was small a non-parametric test for the determination of statistical significance was inappropriate and therefore not used (Miller et al 2002).

Qualitative data was also generated in the questionnaire by using open questions encouraging reflection on practice to allow the exploration of attitudes, beliefs, motivation and feeling (Polit and Hungler 1989). Previous authors have used these techniques to successfully examine the perceptions surrounding roles in both nursing and education (McSherry 1997, Clifford 1993, Sloan 1999). Creswell (2003) describes a generic process to apply in the analysis of qualitative data and this was used to start the process of analysis for this study. The process involved the organisation and preparation of data by transcribing the data, reading all of the data to obtain a general meaning of the data followed by analysis of the data to expose categories of meaning. The data was then conceptualised into themes using an approach described as content analysis (Polit and Hungler 1989, Graneheim and Lundman 2004) this was a rigorous method to ensure objectivity by coding the written data to produce systematic information.

Content Analysis

The framework for content analysis as defined by Lutz et al (1992 pg 227) was used to analyse the written responses to the open ended questions. A sub-sample of 25 questionnaires (the first 25 returned questionnaires) was selected and the responses to the open questions typed onto separate sheets. These were then analysed to see whether any recurring themes emerged. The recurring themes were then generically categorised, described and coded. A code (0) was given for the category of no response/answer and another code number (e.g. 9 if there were 8 generic categories) was allocated for any response/answer that did not fit the generic category; this category was often called 'other'. As a check a further 10 questionnaires were then analysed using this coding system, if the coding system was not easy to work with or it became too complex then the wording and content of the generic categories were revised. When the coding system was satisfactory the remaining questionnaires were then analysed. If the 'other' category became too large this category was further analysed and categorised (Lutz et al 1992). The emerging themes were then described and compared. Direct quotes from the responses were also used to add literary richness to the research report and to as Creswell (2003) highlights convey to the reader the findings of the analysis by use of narrative passage. In the final step of analysis the data was interpreted against the context of educational theory, Creswell (2003) suggests that the interpretation of qualitative data can be made from a personal context or as a means of identifying if the data confirms or diverges from existing theory.

RELIABILITY AND VALIDITY

Quantitative Paradigm

A questionnaire lends itself to controlling researcher bias and maintaining objectivity (Punch 2003). Oppenheim (1992) recommends by using the questionnaire method of data collection the researcher is not directly influencing or encouraging the answers from the respondents As Polit and Hungler (1989 p187) highlight the "successful collection of interview data in contrast to questionnaire data is strongly dependant on interpersonal skills and the ability of the interviewer to probe in a neutral manner." Conversely as Oppenheim (1992) suggests if the respondents know the origins of the questionnaire they may interact and give answers to the person who designed it. This was where the design of the questionnaire in terms of question structure became critical to ensuring reliability and validity.

Validity of research is reliant on the use of appropriate methods and the use of those methods appropriately (Parahoo 1997). Cohen et al (2005 pg 105) recommend quantitative research validity is improved through, "careful sampling, appropriate instrumentation and appropriate statistical treatments of the data". Validity within this research has been increased in several ways firstly the sample was the potential population and was therefore representative. The sample was also unbiased as each potential participant was given the opportunity to contribute to the study (Parahoo 1997). In addition the quantitative nominal data was analysed and described appropriately using a statistical software package, as Creswell (2003 pg 172) highlights, "tell the reader about the types of statistical analysis used" in order to reduce the threat to validity.

Finally the research has used appropriate methods and instrumentation, questionnaire validity relates to the content and the method of administration, the content must remain relevant to the overall research question and aims; in essence the questionnaire must measure what it was designed to (Roe and Webb 1998). The content validity of this questionnaire was qualitatively tested twice, initially through the hospital audit department and 'questionnaire surgery' and secondly by circulation to a group of 'expert' nurses involved with providing education in practice but who were not part of the research study group. Similar to the method of assessing content validity as described by Wallace et al (2003) the 'expert' nurses were asked to review the content of the questionnaire in terms of appropriateness in relation to the research questions and method of dispensation. Parahoo (1997) highlights that content validity of a questionnaire can be assessed by the submission of the questionnaire to a panel of judges with experience and knowledge. There is no statistical test for qualitative content validity assessment however it is recommended that amendment of the questionnaire in light of reviewers comments can improve the overall quality of the questionnaire (Wallace et al 2003). Within this study the questionnaire was formally reviewed and approved by the audit department, in addition the group of 'expert' nurses considered the questionnaire was a suitable method and tool to answer the research questions. The method of circulation to the participants was also considered appropriate for the study.

Reliability in quantitative research relates to the replicability and consistency over time of the research in relation to groups of respondents (Cohen et al 2005). This research if repeated in the same context with a similar population would generate comparable results; the fact that the research produced comparable results in the pilot study also showed the methods used were reliable. The reliability of the questionnaire and therefore research related to the stability of the response, therefore rigorous design and testing of the questionnaire increased reliability by the removal and control of ambiguity in the questions (Punch 2003). A pilot study of the questionnaire revealed two areas of ambiguity; these were corrected by altering the wording and giving an explanation to the terminology, the format of one question was also amended to increase clarity.

Unfortunately, reliability and validity can be adversely affected by the respondent in terms of their frame of mind when answering but also in terms of the researcher's involuntary influence on the respondent who may wish to respond in a way to please the researcher. Again the design of the questionnaire and the numbers of participants involved limited this amount of influence over the research results. In addition, by using a questionnaire respondent anonymity was guaranteed this therefore also increased the freedom of the respondent in answering and in turn enhanced reliability (Punch 2003, Polit and Hungler 1989).

Qualitative Paradigm

Within qualitative research, reliability and validity as Creswell (2003 pg 195) argues "does not carry the same connotations" as they do within quantitative research, validity in particular is seen as the strength of qualitative research but was viewed from the standpoint of achieving accuracy in the findings from the perspective of the researcher and/or participant (Creswell 2003). Emden and Sandelowski (1998) show qualitative researchers have used several alternative words for example 'credibility', 'trustworthiness' and 'authenticity' in an attempt to define validity and reliability in qualitative research. Despite this the construct of reliability and validity within the paradigm of qualitative research remains applicable regardless of the variations in terminology (Emden and Sandelowski 1999)

Validity in qualitative research much like quantitative research has been defined as the ability of the data collecting method to measure what it was suppose to measure (Cohen et al 2005) and within the context of this research this was the perceptions, experiences and feelings of the participants. Defined as the extent to which an account accurately represents the social phenomena studied; validity embodies honesty, depth, richness and truth in the collection and presentation of results, what participants report should be considered fact and remain undisputed and sincerely reported (Silverman 2001). Therefore in analysis of the qualitative data it was important to report literally the feelings and perceptions of the respondents as they have expressed them. Creswell (2003) highlights that accuracy of findings is increased by using rich, thick descriptions of the data to convey the findings; these 'rich, thick descriptions' allow the reader to decide upon their own interpretation of the findings (Lincoln & Guba 1985).

Also described as 'fairness' in reporting Cohen et al (2005) support the need for qualitative interpretation to stay true to the participants' narrative thereby increasing validity in the research. A specific example of validity within this research was the truthful reporting of the written text generated from the questionnaire and the development of 'open coding categories' to represent an authentic interpretation (Creswell 1994, Silverman 2001). Another process of establishing the validity of the findings was to relate them to the existing literature (Strauss and Corbin 1990).

Unlike reliability in quantitative research where results should be replicable and therefore generalisable, qualitative research reliability relates to the degree of consistency with which the raw data is analysed and coded to form categories (Silverman 2001). From the humanistic perspective some traditionalist researchers argue that qualitative research can not be reliable as individuals and social phenomena are by their nature very different and consequently unable to offer uniform results (Creswell 2003). As previously highlighted a consistent and uniform approach in the management of the qualitative data has been used; defined as content analysis (Lutz et al 1992) this framework enabled the systematic analysis and interpretation of a large volume of qualitative data which in turn increased reliability. In addition the explicit narratives on the process of qualitative data analysis, described as a 'decision trail' (Lincoln & Guba 1985) has enabled the reader to achieve a greater understanding which in turn has increased the reliability of the research. There has also been a consistent approach to the presentation of the results again this not only enhanced the validity of the research it also improved the reliability (Silverman 2001).

The use of triangulation and mixed methods in research has also been reported to increase the validity and reliability of research (Cohen et al 2005, Creswell 2003), described as 'completeness' or 'crystallisation' (Tobin and Begley 2004) the use of mixed methods within this study has provided additional information on which the reader gained a more all-encompassing view of the study participants world.

RESEARCHER BIAS

Another means of increasing accuracy within the analysis of qualitative data was to acknowledge and clarify researcher bias (Creswell 2003). Qualitative research in particular has received negative critique as it has been the researcher alone who has been the instrument for analysis, as a consequence of this bias could have been high (Reid 1991). Bias in this research was potentially high because the researcher was a clinical nurse specialist with a particular interest in education within practice. Clarifying research bias from the outset of the study demonstrates that the researcher understands their position and 'any biases or assumptions that impact on the inquiry' (Creswell 2003). In this study it could be claimed that there was the possibility of research bias by the very nature of the researcher's position as a clinical nurse specialist, implying the respondents could have been telling the researcher what they felt they wanted to hear. Despite this it was believed that during this study the respondents had been able as Melia (1982) describes to "tell it as it was". Hill-Bailey and Tilley (2002) highlighted that to 'tell the story' from the perspective of the participant established meaning however in doing so the researcher had to rely on what the participants said. It was anticipated that by staying aware of and reflecting upon the analysis of the qualitative data researcher bias has been reduced.

ETHICAL CONSIDERATIONS

The Research Governance Framework for health and social care (DOH 2001b) defines the broad principles of good research governance and is the key to ensuring that the health and social care research is conducted to high scientific and ethical standards. Therefore prior to commencing the study the research proposal was submitted to the Local Research and Ethics Committee (LREC) and approval to proceed obtained . The study complies with and was conducted within the LREC ethical framework and the code of practice for research governance and ethics in post graduate research (Bournemouth University 2004).

The underlying principle of ethical research is that the research participants should not come to any harm (Oppenheim 1992). Although this study involved nurses and not 'vulnerable subjects' (Couchman and Dawson 1990) in terms of physical danger consideration needs to given to the nurses within this study who may become vulnerable because they were employees of the organisation in which the research was conducted although the researcher held no position of power over the research participants. With this in mind the ethical considerations of non-maleficence and beneficence focused upon confidentiality, privacy, veracity, fidelity and informed voluntary participation.

Anonymity promotes confidentiality, as Parahoo (1997) identifies a self-administered questionnaire has the potential to be totally anonymous as long as the each questionnaire is not numbered to facilitate follow up of non-respondents. Although the questionnaire within this study was not encrypted there was however a potential that the participants may have become identifiable; for instance the uniqueness of nursing specialism lends itself to identification of the individual employed. The construction of the questionnaire ensured no information which could identify the individual was gathered, however it was still imperative that the research participants were also assured of confidentiality and that they would not be disadvantaged or judged by their responses. Alongside anonymity, privacy was assured by secure storage of the data.

In analysis of the data the study must protect the identity of the participants (Creswell 2003) both quantitative and qualitative data analysis within this study protected the identity of the participants. Quantitative data and questionnaires were coded after completion by the participants therefore ensuring anonymity. The qualitative data was analysed by assigning the terms clinical nurse specialist, lecturer practitioner, educator in practice or other to the written quotes this was then also used for the written report.

Respect for autonomy, the study respected the rights of individuals to not participate in the research with participation being entirely voluntary with no method of persuasion or coercion used. As the questionnaire was not coded follow up of non-respondents did not take place.

In terms of beneficence, an indirect benefit of participation would have been the ability to further define the role of the nurse specialist, lecturer practitioner and practice educator to the local university and hospital and add to the pool of nursing knowledge (Parahoo 1998). In defining the possible barriers and difficulties in providing education in practice opportunity for further discussions may arise after the research has been reported. There was no financial benefit to the research participants the only potential benefit for the research participants was a greater insight into their role as an educationalist.

Justice, all the potential and actual research participants were treated equally without judgement. Veracity and Fidelity reflected the need to honour promises and to be truthful and honest throughout the research with respect to the research participants and interpretation and presentation of the research findings.

QUANTITATIVE FINDINGS

Cohen et al (2003) report an acceptable response rate from a questionnaire is 50%; a response rate of 70.5% was achieved in this research with a total of 60 respondents participating in the research. As previously stated 4 research participant groups were formed from the data that of clinical nurse specialists, lecturer practitioners, 'educators in practice' and others. The biographical profile of each role group was built upon the analysis of the study participant's clinical experience and educational achievement. In addition the number of clinical nurse specialists, lecturer practitioners and educators in practice was established, Figure 1 shows the frequency and distribution of roles identified and studied within this research. It was found that there was a greater amount of clinical nurse specialists (n=37) contributing to the study this was supported by the secondary data which also indicated that more clinical nurse specialists were employed within the hospital.

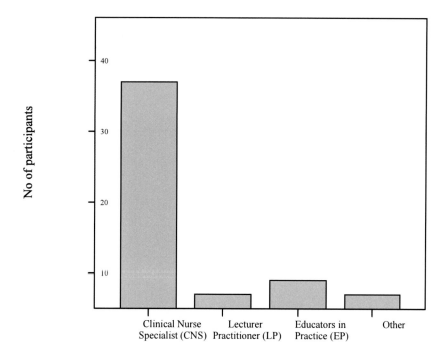

Figure 1. Roles identified within the study.

The proportion of the research participants employed on a full-time basis was 63% (n=38) Figure 2 shows the comparison between the roles reporting to be employed on a full-time and part-time basis. A majority (70% n=5) of lecturer practitioners defined themselves as being employed part-time.

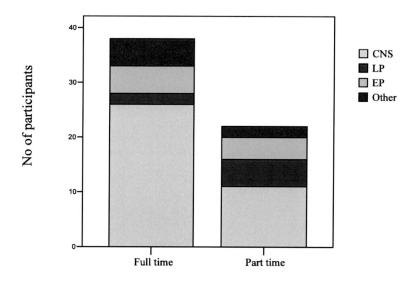

Figure 2. The research participants were employed.

The amount of time the research participants had been qualified as registered practitioners was shown in Figure 3, 92% (n=55) of the participants had been qualified over 11 years.

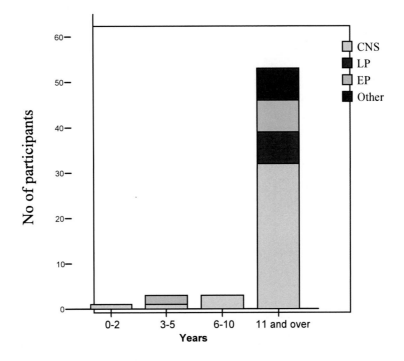

Figure 3. How long participants had been qualified?

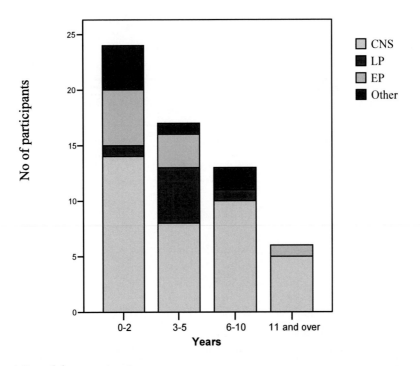

Figure 4. Length in current post.

The length of time participants have been employed in their current role within the studied organisation was shown in Figure 4, 40% (n=24) of the participants were relatively new to their role being in post less than 2 years.

All research participants were found to possess a variety of educational achievements, Figure 5 shows the frequency and type of educational attainment held amongst the four participant research groups. When answering this question the participants were allowed to choose more than one answer. The study of education refers to further courses on education (e.g. City and Guilds 7307, ENB 998) participants had studied.

The following research findings in the quantitative paradigm relate to the 59 research participants who stated they were involved in providing education. In terms of teaching activity all research participants were found to engage in a variety of teaching strategies and methods Figure 6 illustrates the methods which the research participants reported using whilst providing education. Predominately informal and practical strategies were used.

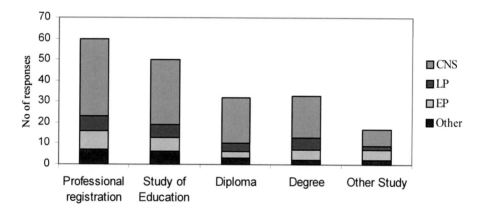

Figure 5. Educational profile of the study participants.

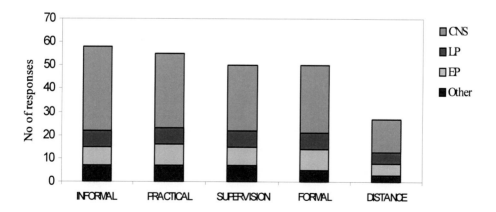

Figure 6. Teaching methods.

All the research participants were found to provide education in a variety of settings; Figure 7 shows the venues in which education was provided and the number of participants who indicated they provided education within that venue. 100% (n=59) participants provided education within their own clinical setting. A minority of participants (n=8) were found to provide education to commercial and private organisations in addition to national and international conferences this data was classified as 'other'.

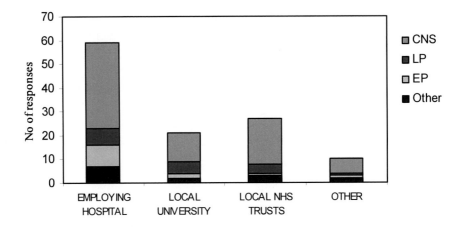

Figure 7. Where education was provided.

The research also found all the research participant groups provided education for a wide range of students Figure 8 demonstrates the personnel the participants identified as their students. In particular the educators in practice did not provide education for patients and carers in addition along with the lecturer practitioners (n=2) they also showed limited involvement with doctors (n=2).

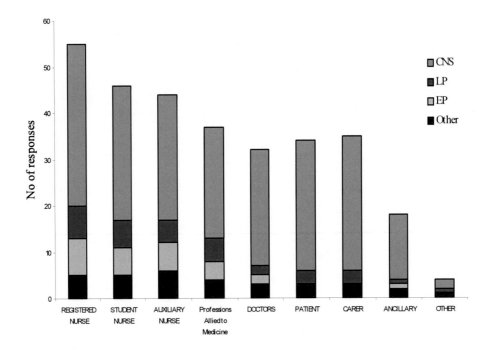

Figure 8. Research participant's students.

Student learning styles were assessed by 35 research participants in comparison to 24 research participants who responded that they did not assess the learning style of their students the distribution of research participant group responses has been shown in Figure 9 no differences were found between the roles.

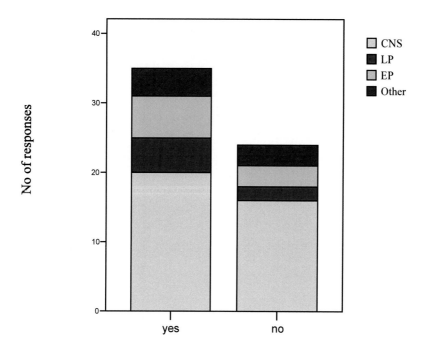

Figure 9. Do you assess learning styles?

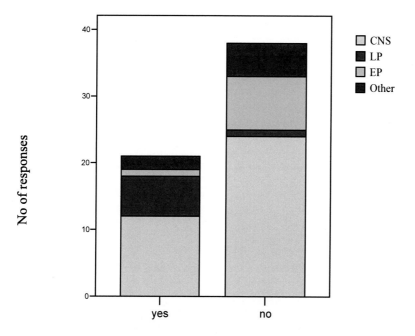

Figure 10. Do you provide formal teaching for post registration university courses?

Figure 10 illustrates the frequency and distribution of research participants involved with providing education for post-registration university students. 64% (n=38) participants stated they did not provide education for university courses this included one lecturer practitioner. Figure 11 shows a similar picture for pre-registration university students with 68% (n=40) of participants not providing education for pre-registration university course the distribution of roles however was equal.

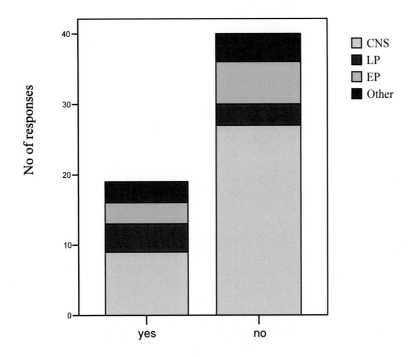

Figure 11. Do you provide formal teaching for pre registration university courses?

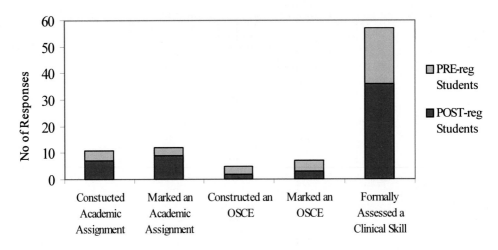

(OSCE = Objective Structured Clinical Examination)

Figure 12. Methods of Formal Assessment.

In terms of student assessment the participants were asked to select from a list the methods they used, the participants were able to choose more than one answer Figure 12 and Figure 13 shows the number of responses the research participants gave. A total of 92 positive responses were obtained for methods of formal assessment (Figure 12) whilst Figure 13 shows the 116 positive responses for informal assessment. Assessment of clinical skills both formally (62% n=57) and informally (56% n=65) was the most prevalent.

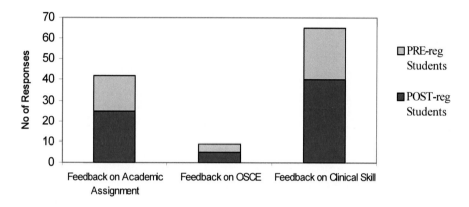

Figure 13. Methods of Informal Assessment.

When looking at how the research participants were involved in curriculum development the majority of participants stated they developed study days related to their specialty (Figure 14).

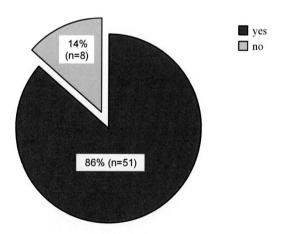

Figure 14. Do you develop study days?

With regard to university courses Figures 15 and 16 shows the frequency of research participants who reported being involved in the development of curriculum for Pre and Post registration courses. Only 20% (n=12) of participants within this study contributed to the curriculum of any post registration university course and even fewer 13% (n=8) contributed to any pre-registration university course.

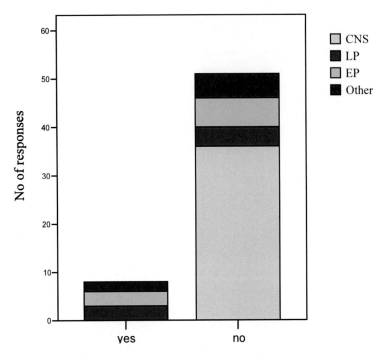

Figure 15. Are you involved in curriculum development for pre-registration students?

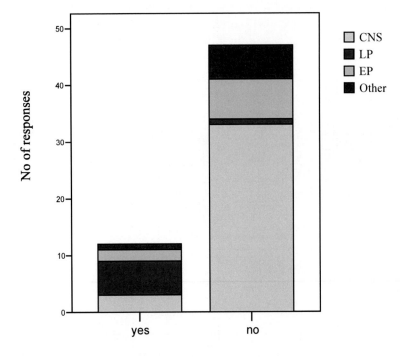

Figure 16. Are you involved in curriculum development for post-registration students?

In terms of contributing to curriculum development within the university, differences between the roles emerged. In comparison to all the research participants a greater proportion of lecturer practitioners contributed to curriculum development for pre-registration university courses 43% (n=3) and post-registration university courses 86% (n=6). No clinical nurse specialists contributed to curriculum development for pre-registration courses and only 3 contributed to post registration curriculum.

Of those participants who did not report involvement (80% n= 47) in university curriculum development Figure 17 illustrates how many participants would like the opportunity to be involved 70% (n=33) indicated they would like to become involved in pre-registration curriculum development with 68% (n=32) participants for post-registration. When asked if participants would like to contribute to university curriculum development of those who said they were not currently involved 66% (n=33) indicated they would like to be involved with pre-registration university curriculum and 69% (n=32) of those participants not currently involved with post-registration university curriculum stated they would like to contribute. Predominately clinical nurse specialists 78% (n=28) stated they wanted to be involved with pre-registration university curriculum development. No difference was found between the roles for post-registration curriculum development however, 24 clinical nurse specialists stated they would like to become involved.

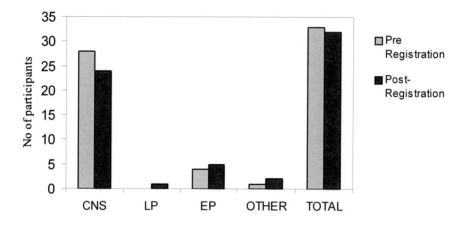

Figure 17. Participants who would like to be involved with curriculum development

Only 42% (n= 25) of participants were found to be the only person employed within their speciality however being the only person within a speciality was not found to have a bearing on the activity of the individual in terms of providing education. It was also found the clinical nurse specialist more frequently (n=30) held the responsibility for a patient caseload in contrast no 'educators in practice' reported having this commitment.

The teaching methods utilised by the participants in this study suggested the setting in which the education was provided influenced the teaching strategy used. Participants within this study most frequently provided informal opportunistic education including the following which was provided on a daily or weekly basis.

One to one training	53%	n=32
Role modelling	45%	n=27
Demonstration of a clinical skill	53%	n=32
Coaching	33%	n=20

Teaching methods used less frequently on a monthly basis included the following.

Formal lectures	40%	n=24
Workshops/seminars	38%	n=23
Clinical supervision	50%	n=30
Group discussion	48%	n=29
Critical incident analysis	38%	n=23

The least utilised teaching strategy within this research was found to be distance learning with 57% (n=34) of participants indicating they never used workbook materials and 77% (n=46) indicating they did not use computer based training programmes.

58% (n=35) of all participants stated they assessed the individual learning styles of their students; of those who did not (n=19) the following reasons were given.

Lack of time and no opportunity	37%	n=7
No opportunity utilise mixed methods	47%	n=9
Don't know why	10%	n=2
Have had no training so wouldn't know how	5%	n=1

The lack of opportunity to assess student learning styles was considered an important contributing factor with the research participants explaining that they rarely met their students prior to interaction or formal training.

The types of students the participants had contact with varied, the clinical nurse specialist role in particular appeared to have the wider student audience, a greater frequency of involvement in providing education for patients (n=28) and their carers (n=29) was found. In contrast the 'educators in practice' were found to have no involvement in providing education for patients and carers. In terms of university students the lecturer practitioner role had greater involvement; the proportion of lecturer practitioner's 86% (n=6) involved with lecturing on post registration university courses was more prevalent in comparison to the proportion of clinical nurse specialists 28% (n=9), educators in practice 12% (n=1) and others 33% (n=2). However, of the participants who said they did not provide formal teaching for university students 72% (n=28) for post registration and 66% (n=27) for pre registration courses identified they would like the opportunity to do so with the majority wishing to use their specialist subject knowledge.

A similar picture was found in terms of mentorship for post registration university students where the proportion of lecturer practitioners 71% (n=5) had greater involvement. However, in contrast only 32% (n=15) of the research participants who were not involved in mentoring pre-registration students volunteered to do so, whereas 67% (n=29) of the research participants not involved in the mentorship of post-registration university students indicated they would like to become involved. All research participant groups were equal in volunteering, no differences between the roles were found.

The majority of participants (n=46) within this study were found to be undertaking students assessments with all roles involved in providing formal and informal assessments for both pre-registration and post-registration students. The most frequent assessment undertaken was for post-registration students relating to the performance of a clinical skill both formally 60% (n=36) and informally 67% (n=40). In terms of constructing practice based assessments all research participants were involved although only 35% (n=21) of participants claimed to be involved with post-registration students and only 10% (n=6) with pre-registration students.

This study found that 85% (n=51) of all participants studied said they were involved in developing education on behalf of the hospital with 70% (n=42) stating they were expected to do so by their employer. All participants expected to provide programmes of education by their employer claimed they fulfilled this obligation however; it was also found that 3 participants who were not expected by their employer to provide education programmes stated they did so. In addition a further 5 participants who claimed they did not know if they were expected to provide education as part of their role, provided education to a variety of students.

QUALITATIVE FINDINGS

The analysis revealed the perceptions of the participants about education within clinical practice. This related specifically to the relationship between theory and practice, the barriers to providing education within practice and the relationship between the participants and the provider of academic education. The emerging data has been discussed within the context of the question however; within each question the qualitative data provides conceptual themes and sub-themes via the process of content analysis (Polit and Hungler 1989, Graneheim and Lundman 2004).

> Question: Do you believe that providing education within the practice setting was important for ensuring staff/students are 'Fit for Practice'?

This study shows that 98% of all participants believed the provision of education within practice was important with 96% of participants expressing the stronger belief of 'Yes a lot'. The overall theme which emerged from the data was entitled 'the real world' and this correlates to the sub-themes of 'theory into practice', 'competence of clinical skills' and 'learning to care'. An emerging thread of meaning for the participants was the concept of embedding academic theory into everyday practice this sub-theme defined as 'theory into practice' drew upon the perceptions of the participants who illustrated the following;

> Once academic knowledge was gained the only way to really use that knowledge was to relate it to practice otherwise it was quickly lost. Practical skills do need a knowledge base but also need to be practiced and put in to context (Clinical Nurse Specialist).

> As health care practice was practice-based, it would be impossible to remove the educational element from the practice setting. Students need to be able to apply theory to practice in a meaningful, realistic, and safe way (Lecturer Practitioner).

> The healthcare setting was a diverse area in which continual education was necessary to maintain knowledge of the ever-changing environment, new developments and treatment/ management strategies. Evidence based practice requires increased levels of knowledge and understanding (Clinical Nurse Specialist).

There was consensus amongst the study group, who believed this concept existed within current practice as the following participants reflect,

> Learning in the practical setting was invaluable in the development of nurses. Education in practice allows theory to relate directly to the practical experience 'makes it real'. Experiences gained in practice are likely to be remembered by students and provide opportunities for reflection –itself another valuable learning tool (Clinical Nurse Specialist).

> The practice environment was an excellent setting for learning; many skills require practice and supervision in order to gain confidence and competence. Education in the practice setting consolidates the theoretical component that the university provides (Lecturer Practitioner).

Another sub-theme to develop from the participants narrative was that of 'competence of clinical skills', this embraces the concept of encouraging practitioners to reach a level of clinical competence in which they could provide a satisfactory level of patient care. One participant reflected,

> Fit for practice relates to being competent within practice so the practice setting in this context makes sense (Lecturer Practitioner)

There was also a view by some participants that a university-based education would lack training on the practical skills of nursing,

> Because they do not get it in the university, more practice better-prepared (Educator in Practice).

> There was too much academia, needs to be more physical (Other).

> The university provides little in the way of clinical skills training (Educator in Practice).

In contrast, other participants reflected more holistically on the concept of practice-based skills and the importance of them in terms of practitioner competence and patient care.

> Whilst theoretical underpinning was important the opportunity to learn practical skills in a supervised environment was essential. The implementation of what has been learned away from the practical environment reinforces that learning and gives opportunity to synthesise what has been learnt. Confidence can also be built by participation in care in the practice setting (Clinical Nurse Specialist).

> To maintain standards, competence and confidence I believe in the value of sitting next to Nellie and learning in the practical/clinical situation. Involving learners/patients/carers together in one session provokes question and discussion. It brings learning 'alive' makes it real (Clinical Nurse Specialist).

Alongside the need for practical skills training the participants within this study also recognised the need for more 'obscure' skills to be learned – 'learning to care' related to the perception that education within practice facilitates the comprehension of the 'softer' clinical skills such as patient communication and empathy alongside the skills of workload management and prioritising care. The following participants illustrate,

> Students need to experience caring for patients with education provided by experienced nurse at the same time. Sometimes it was extremely difficult to link the theory (from UNI) within practice (on the ward) when information was not delivered simultaneously (Clinical Nurse Specialist).

> This was the real world – this was where the student will hopefully work, they should learn to care and be competent, this 'makes theory a reality' (Clinical Nurse Specialist).

> Learning theory suggests the importance of experiential learning 'to develop the cognition, behaviours and effectiveness of the learning process (Lave and Wenger, Palsoon, Guile and Young) (Educator in Practice).

> It enablers people to understand the constraints of a ward whilst providing the care for an individual (Other).

> Question Do you consider the role of the nurse specialist 'deskills' other staff in practice?

This research shows 64% of participants disagreed with this question however, 33% indicated they believed 'a little' that the nurse specialist had the potential to 'deskill' other staff. From the data the emerging theme to develop was identified as 'the clinical nurse specialist as a resource', this symbolised the sub-themes of 'off-loading', 'enhancing skills', 'empowering' and 'expert knowledge'.

'Off-loading' related to the participants believing that the demands and pressure of the clinical workload encouraged clinical staff to unburden some of their workload onto the clinical nurse specialist. Subsequently this lack of performing certain clinical skills was perceived as leading to a loss of expertise by the general clinician.

> Staff are happy to 'offload', the ward environment was so pressured staff are grateful for any assistance with caring for their patients; staff can therefore loose their skills. I am surprised by the lack of knowledge doctors possess they are also keen to off load to a more skilled practitioner (Clinical Nurse Specialist).

> Although I try to ensure it does not happen, the more you do the more they expect you do, especially doctors and outlying wards (Lecturer Practitioner).

> Staff generally feel too pressured (workload) to undertake assessment/intervention when a specialist nurse can be contacted instead (Clinical Nurse Specialist).

Participants also reported the experience of general clinicians having a passive role and saw the willingness of staff to allow the nurse specialist to provide patient care,

> It should not occur however, I believe staff think that if the nurse specialist was carrying out certain skills and passing on knowledge they need not bother to (Educator in Practice).

> In my experience, staff may rely on nurse specialists too much who can inhibit continuity and high stands of care on the wards (Other).

Potentially staff can become reliant on referring patients sometimes inappropriately and ticking it off on their list as done/sorted. But these are opportunities for education of staff e.g. if appropriate giving feedback or inviting someone to sit in whilst you see the patient (Clinical Nurse Specialist).

Nurse specialists are there for advice to ward staff and also teaching, though sometimes it seems that ward staff will just let the nurse specialist get on with it and then they can carry on with other work rather than learn how to do something for the next time (Clinical Nurse Specialist).

The preceding participants' narratives show self-awareness and insight on behalf of the clinical nurse specialists within this study, the following participant encapsulates this,

The role of the specialist nurse should not-deskill others but provide an enhancement for their practice. As a resource on what was current best practice, the specialist nurse has the opportunity to help other staff build their skills and to focus their areas of interest. The existence of a nurse specialist should not be an excuse to for others to be lax in their own skills and knowledge (Clinical Nurse Specialist).

In contrast to 'deskilling', the sub- themes of 'empowering the enhancement of skills' and 'expert knowledge' emerged and this correlates to the participants expectations of their own role and that of others, there was a firm evidence within the data that the participants believed the role of the nurse specialist to be one which facilitates and encourages staff/students to learn new skills within the context of an evolving healthcare environment. One participant comments,

In fact, this role only enhances the skills of staff in practice by maintaining a link with current advances and recommendations for practice. They help us to encourage positive attitudes and enthusiasm for best practice and are pivotal to the process of change in practice (Educator in Practice).

The specialist nurse should be that a specialist in the subject available to educate and give support to general nurses. The word should empower not deskill (Clinical Nurse Specialist). Acts as a learning resource (other)

I think it empowers the nurse to manage their day to day work more effectively, if nurses are deskilled then the specialist nurse was not doing their job properly, the aim was to empower other staff to do their job better (Lecturer Practitioner)

Several participants described the sub-theme of 'expert knowledge' and promoted the nurse specialist role as educational which had a firm foundation within clinical practice,

A CNS should enhance the skills of other staff as nurse specialists are a specialist resource that can be accessed and utilised to improve theory and practical skills of staff (Clinical Nurse Specialist).

You need one or two experts to improve others knowledge (Other).

The role of the nurse specialist involves sharing knowledge and empowering other staff being an advisor in a specialty rather than doing what needs to be done (Clinical Nurse Specialist)

The nurse specialist cannot only use the specialist skills for patients – staff can approach for advice and training (Educator in Practice)

Specialist nurses are highly knowledgeable in their area of practice and are ideally placed to cascade their knowledge to the AHPs GPS and Medics (Clinical Nurse Specialist).

Question Do you think there are difficulties and/or barriers to providing education in practice?

The emerging overall theme which developed was described as 'organisational culture' and depicts the sub-themes of 'time', 'willingness to learn' and 'officialdom'. 96% of all participants felt there were barriers to providing education in practice with 50% who expressed a stronger feeling of 'a lot' in response to the question.

The ability to 'ring fence' time was the overriding sub-theme to emerge and related to the workload and availability of the participant in addition to the workload of the clinical environment,

Time was always difficult to 'protect' for training both mine and the students' (Clinical Nurse Specialist).

It was difficult to gain protected time to spend with learners (Educator in practice).

Despite the perceived lack of time, some participants felt they should still make every effort to support education within practice. This view was further illustrated in the following statements,

It depends on the specialist/practitioners attitudes there can be barriers of time everyone's too busy etc. but you have to be inventive and work around limitations for example making time to go back to an area at a more suitable time (Clinical Nurse Specialist).

Time was a rare commodity, ward based seminars though valuable may not have good numbers attending and staff are called away. The specialist role itself was demanding and my role increasingly has a trust wide remit which can mean spreading oneself a little thin. Producing distance learning package can address this in part (Clinical Nurse Specialist).

With formal training/education the key factor that inhibits this was lack of time and lack of staff. However opportunity to share skills such as demonstration on an informal level are frequent and need to be used as teaching opportunities more often (Clinical Nurse Specialist).

Interestingly alongside lack of time acting as a deterrent to learning within practice, a 'willingness to learn' emerged as a prevalent sub-theme with participants who expressed their view that there appeared a reluctance of hospital staff to engage with learning in practice.

Time constraints of all staff involved. Lack of mutual commitment – some staff like to be 'spoon fed' (Clinical Nurse Specialist).

Lack of time, enthusiasm, and recognition of the importance of education in practice. I think there was not enough emphasis on nurses updating or learning new skills, many can get away without updating on the basics their should be more of a link with appraisal - I know there will be with the knowledge and skills framework of Agenda for Change (Lecturer Practitioner).

Sometimes people feel it disrupts the daily routine of the ward (Other).

Although it was not the scope of this research to construct theory on why barriers to learning occurred and in this instance why there appeared to be a perception of an unwillingness to engage with education in practice, the following comments suggest that the demands of the clinical workload may have a direct impact,

The biggest factor was time, if it was a job one person can do the second person may feel they are wasting time watching and learning (Clinical Nurse Specialist).

I find that what staff say and what they can do vary enormously e, g, they want teaching/developing but can appear so lacking in motivation when it occurs. Ward staffing was horrendous to many unsupervised untrained nurses; lack of communication and poor standards expectations even among trained staff (Clinical Nurse Specialist).

The emergence of the sub-theme defined as 'officialdom' concerned participants who expressed feelings regarding the attitude of the organisation towards learning in practice as the following participants explained,

Attitude towards learning – it was seen as an extra task rather than integral to practice can be the culture of the organisation (Clinical Nurse Specialist).

Ward environment – busy times, political barriers, 'blockers' people who don't see the necessity of it will hinder you (Clinical Nurse Specialist).

Targets demand activity, training was seen as a low priority when activity was threatened training was cancelled (Educator in Practice)

Organisational policy and strategy was predominately concerned with the short-term achievements of targets within a constricted budget. This approach fails to accommodate the proactive approach required to facilitate individual learning and development (Educator in Practice).

There was often little structure in the practice setting as to what was being taught or in fact, what the student hopes to achieve (Clinical Nurse Specialist).

Question Do you feel you have strong educational links with the local university?

'Belonging' emerged as the theme for this question and represents the participants' feelings and experiences of contact with the local university. 57% of the participants stated they felt they had strong links and interestingly being involved in university curriculum development was associated with feeling a strong link with the local university. This was reflected within the two distinct sub-themes which developed that of 'on the outside' and 'within.' In order to have a strong link with the university there was a perceived need to feel part of the organisation, the sub-theme of 'on the outside' developed from the narrative of several participants,

> Although I teach yearly at the university it was only as requested from course organiser although I was involved in planning the course originally (Clinical Nurse Specialist).

> I don't feel the University takes National Vocational Qualifications (NVQ's) seriously – have experiences of a superior attitude if NVQ's are mentioned I fully believe the university should take more advice of what was happening outside of university (Educator in Practice).

> I feel we are 'used' somewhat to do their lecturing (Other).

There appeared from the narrative a negative perception of the university from some participants this was further demonstrated in the following statements,

> I have tried to make links to provide education at the university but have been constantly turned away – "we have our own lecturers who teach that" I therefore do education sessions with the students on placement (Clinical Nurse Specialist).

> In my current role I can find myself being at odds with the university, the approach of an educational institution and service provider are bound to disagree about issues such as time, money and attendance (Other).

> Recently the course involving my specialist area has been removed, more involvement with the university was felt when this was taking place as the lecturer was a colleague. Since then we have no involvement with the university I believe the tutor talks to the students about my specialist area but has had no communication with us in spite of contact from us (Clinical Nurse Specialist).

> I feel quite resentful really, they seem unapproachable – I would like to be involved but don't know how, would like to know what they are teaching about my specialist area and who was doing it – newly qualified staff and students in particular seem to have 'out of date' knowledge. Clinical competencies for student nurses to achieve in practice regarding my specialty are also out of date and do not reflect what was occurring in practice (Clinical Nurse Specialist).

Although for some participants being, 'on the outside' held no issues and almost seemed to be the preferred relationship for the participant with the university,

> It was not an issue I link with students during their secondment at the trust although I'd be interested to know what the UNI teaches about my specialty (Clinical Nurse Specialist).

> The lecturer practitioner in our directorate was the main link and then she feeds back to us. If I want to input anything to the university I tend to go through the lecturer practitioner because of her strong links (Clinical Nurse Specialist).

> I know senior nurses do have links so if I needed to contact they would know whom to ask (Clinical Nurse Specialist).

I personally do not have strong links but appreciate the need and requirement for our hospital education team to translate said information effectively across the hospital network and liaise effectively to enable the translation of theory into practice (Educator in Practice).

Being 'within' had a literal interpretation and feeling a 'belonging' related to the delivery of education within the university, for example,

I am employed two days a week in the university although I feel I belong more to in the trust setting; it has taken a long time to feel part of the university (Lecturer Practitioner).

As I don't have a post-registration course I feel a little isolated (Lecturer Practitioner). Because my role involves working for the university 2 days a week (Lecturer Practitioner).

Because I teach there (Lecturer Practitioner).

Question Do you think the provision of education in practice benefits from having strong links with the local university?

85% of all participants believed this to be true and 46% agreed strongly 'a lot' that links with the local university would benefit education within practice. 'Recognition' emerged as the theme and correlates to the sub-themes of 'theory and practice' 'credibility' and 'sharing of knowledge.' Several participants perceived the linkage between the university and practice setting would facilitate the assimilation of theory with practice and this correlates to the responses given when asked in a previous question about the importance of student to become 'Fit for Practice.

Because this was the way to integrate theory and practice in a safe environment for students. Academic education was really important to enhance clinical/practice based knowledge and skills (Lecturer Practitioner).

If there was good dialogue and appreciation between the university and the hospital then this can illicit the provision of effectively applying theory into practice (Educator in Practice).

Although some participants felt the their own link with the university was poor they still believed the university link should be strong in order to integrate theory and practice as the following participants clarify,

It was important to link theory into the practice setting – they should be integral to each other. Where are the link tutors, perhaps the university tutors are becoming deskilled! Education within practice should be visible and valued (Clinical Nurse Specialist).

At the moment I feel that this relationship was fragmented it can work well when the theory was integrated into practice (Clinical Nurse Specialist).

Yes it would if I had strong links with the university. I think core knowledge from specialists was crucial throughout training linked with skills practice during clinical placements (Clinical Nurse Specialist).

The participants also believed that a link between the university and clinical practice should bring about a communication and dialogue; this was defined as the sub-theme 'sharing of knowledge' the participants' explained,

We should be working as a team (Clinical Nurse Specialist).

Education in practice needs to tie in with course syllabuses and content to ensure clarity and avoid duplication or conflicting advice. However, there was also a large amount of teaching a nurse specialist can do which does not have to directly link to a course or module (Clinical Nurse Specialist).

If links are forged then cross reference development of content gaps identification may occur. I could for example give precise feedback to course tutors and influence the theory to practice integration this needs to be done regularly (Clinical Nurse Specialist).

We all need to be singing form the same hymn sheet (Clinical Nurse Specialist).

The link between the university and the practice setting was also perceived by the participants as having the potential to directly affect the value of education in practice. Defined as 'credibility' this sub-theme encompasses both the positive and negative feelings of the participants,

Nursing was a profession and current developments means that an academic award was justified, always raises the profile of the programme (Lecturer Practitioner).

Unfortunately in our society education and attainment needs to be credible university underpinning support allows learning to be formally recognised (Lecturer Practitioner).

Education can be delivered effectively without university control however in this age accredited courses are seen as most valuable (Lecturer Practitioner).

It gives us credibility (Lecturer Practitioner).

In contrast to the positive perception as described above, some participants viewed the drive to provide education within practice to bolster university education as a potential hindrance to the value of education in practice, the following participants explain,

You do not want to formalise some education that can be taught by knowledgeable practitioners without the bureaucrats of a university – I would feel this would frighten a lot of practitioners away. However self education time needs to be part of weekly working hours (Clinical Nurse Specialist).

There are benefits to having strong links but the provision of education in practice need not be wholly dependant on that. Not all students need or want academic recognition for their work and a lot of students state they prefer the more practical approach of a clinically based teaching team (Educator in Practice).

It was important to have learning in practice recognised with some structure. There was a danger however that practical education can become too centred around academia in order to fulfil university requirements (Clinical Nurse Specialist).

The feelings expressed by these participants mirrors some of the beliefs held around 'officialdom' and the need for organisational recognition in the value of learning within practice as the following participant explains,

Education in practice can be done very informally by the experienced nurse with no direction from the university. A lot of what was needed to be gained by nurses learning new skills and acquiring new knowledge has nothing to do with university but was gained directly from the clinical setting. Experiencing nursing in practice under the direct supervision of expert nurses was extremely valuable and fundamental to the nursing of other good nurses (Clinical Nurse Specialist).

The findings of this research suggested that staff employed within practice were essential to the provision of clinical education indeed central government has recommended the infrastructure to support education in practice should be placed within the learner's workplace (DOH 2000, 2001a and Audit Commission 2001). In terms of personnel who had the potential to support education in practice this research found 98% (n=59) of the participants were involved in training or education only one participant, a nurse specialist/nurse practitioner indicated they were not. The majority of the participants were found to be employed on a full-time basis this compares to the findings of Ibbotson (1999); however within the lecturer practitioner group five participants identified themselves as part-time this may have been because they saw their time spit between the university and the hospital so they did not consider they were employed within the hospital on a full-time basis (Fairbrother and Ford 1998).

A minority of participants (n=5) had been qualified less than 11 years with only one clinical nurse specialist found to have been qualified less than 3 years, this suggested there was a substantial amount of clinical experience held by the participants. Alongside this experience the length of time in their current post highlighted the further speciality experience held amongst the research participants with 32% (n=19) of all participants being in their current post longer than 5 years this also compares to the findings of Ibbotson (1999) who found 38% of respondents had been in post longer than 5 years. The role of the clinical nurse specialist appeared from the results of this study and in comparison with nursing history (Humphris 1994) to have been the earliest established role however, this research could not confirm the assumption that the practice educator role was the most recent development (Jowett and McMullan 2003).

In comparison, the educational profile of the participants also showed that in addition to clinical experience educationally the participants within the research were also experienced with 53% (n=32) holding a qualification of diploma and 55% (n=33) holding a degree. In contrast to the study by Flanagan (1997) this research found 54% (n=20) of clinical nurse specialists held a degree qualification as opposed to 28% (n=24); McCreaddie (2001) also reported a lower prevalence of degree attainment amongst clinical nurse specialists with 45% (n=9). In addition to educational study 83% (n=50) of the participants had also studied educational theory through various post registration courses. In relation to Jones (1996) and Fairbrother and Mathers (2004) it appeared that the majority of all the participants within this study were educationally and clinically credible as educators in practice and no differences between the roles studied were found.

This research also found in the biographical data that the clinical nurse specialist more frequently held the responsibility for a caseload of patients than the other participants. This was of interest as it not only supported the view that the clinical educator should be close to the learners area of work (DOH 2001a) it also began to question the assumption of Fairbrother and Ford (1998) and Brennan and Hutt (2001) that roles independent of clinical workload gave more opportunity for direct supervision of the learner. The participants identified as free of clinical workload within this study were the 'educators in practice' who were found to have no patient caseload and provided no patient and carer education this suggested their involvement with patient care was at a more superficial supervisory level. An association between the responsibilities of clinical caseload and potential barriers to the provision of education was not highlighted by the participants however, within the qualitative data several participants highlighted that the provision of patient/care education and care gave the opportunity to simultaneously provide clinical education for staff one participant described this as 'sitting next to Nellie' the theme of 'the real world' which developed from the qualitative data to also substantiates this perception.

The majority of the teaching activity undertaken by the research participants took place within the clinical setting and predominately within the hospital environment, 100% (n=59) of participants who indicated they provided education did so within the hospital environment this further reflected the central government's vision of lifelong learning within the NHS (DOH 2001a). However, 36% (n=21) of these participants also provided education within the university away from clinical practice, as expected from the work of Fairbrother and Ford (1998) 71% (n=5) of lecturer practitioners were identified as providing education within the university setting however this only represented 23% (n=5) of those participants providing university education with the larger provider found to be the role of clinical nurse specialist, 57% (n=12).

These results therefore confirmed that the role of the clinical nurse specialist was critical to the provision of education alongside the roles of lecturer practitioner and educators in practice (Day et al 1998, NMC 2002 and Humphris 1994). In addition statements from the research participants who also identified 'the clinical nurse specialist as a resource' showed an appreciation and value of the educative role of the clinical nurse specialist and supported the construct of specialist practice proposed by Hamric and Spross (1983) and further reinforced the notion that a clinical nurse specialist role was concurrent with education.

In contrast to 'deskilling' the workforce many participants within this research supported the view that the clinical nurse specialist role enhanced the skills of other staff and this was in keeping with the findings of Mytton and Adams (2003) and Jack (2002). Also comparable to the findings of McGee (1996), Jack (2002) and Mytton and Adams (2003) was the identification of the concept 'off-loading' which related to the participants believing that the demands and pressure of the clinical workload encouraged clinical staff to unburden workload onto the clinical nurse specialist. Subsequently this lack of performing certain clinical skills was perceived as leading to a loss of expertise by the general clinician. The clinical nurse specialists in particular showed within the qualitative data an insight into their potential to 'deskill' and many reported using this self awareness to limit or prevent this possibility. In contrast, several participants throughout the qualitative data talked in terms of 'should' and this suggested that there was a possibility what they were saying was not actually occurring in practice the quantitative descriptive statistics however have clearly shown the engagement of clinical nurse specialist with providing education alongside their clinical responsibilities of patient care.

Participants have also shown within this research an insight into the reality of providing education within the clinical setting of today and they supported the need for themselves to enhance the assimilation of theory into practice for their students. This view was substantiated within the literature concerning the perceived theory-practice gap, which proposed the provision of education within practice was essential in providing the mechanism on which to reconcile theory with practice (Hewison and Wildman 1996, Williamson and Webb 2001 and Field 2004). The conceptual theme of 'the real world' which emerged from the qualitative data also highlighted the view of making learning part of everyday practice this compares to Lave and Wenger's (1991 p35) theory of situated learning, as they stated, "learning was an integral part of generative social practice in the lived in world." Similarly McCormick's (1999) view of practical knowledge proposed that the context in which we live gave a third dimensional perspective to the two-dimension construct of theory.

Likewise the conceptual sub-theme which developed from the qualitative data of 'learning to care' reflects the importance of learning the sensitivity and subtleties of care. As Lave and Wenger (1991) and Cope et al (2000) proposed by living or working in a care environment an individual would 'absorb the essence' of practice through a process of cognitive apprenticeship. Several authors have highlighted the value of an experienced knowledgeable practitioner and educator situated within the practice setting who could integrate practice with theory (Cope et al 2000, Johnston and Boohan 2000, Spouse 2001). In addition, it was promoted that if students were to learn from the clinical and social environment, they should do so from the perspective of a current, competent and evidence-based context not a ritualistic background (Field 2004).

Expanding on the theory of cognitive apprenticeship (Lave and Wenger 1991) the participants in this study have also shown an insight and appreciation for an adult learners need to assimilate new knowledge into acquired knowledge by application (Kolb 1984). The adoption of multiple teaching methods suggests that the research participants were applying constructivist theory (Cottrell 2001) together with adult learning theory (Wilson 2000, Gibbs and Habeshaw 1989). The process of reflection and learning from previous events was also evident with the participants utilising critical incident analysis and clinical supervision (Jones 1995, Williams 2001) this replicates the cycle of 'reflection-on-action' in which learning from previous experience becomes knowledge for future practice (Schon 1987). In contrast and considering the use of distance learning materials has been suggested to have the potential to widen participation in education (DFES 2003) the use of this teaching strategy by the research participants was not found to be highly prevalent within this research. The findings of this research do not elaborate on why this strategy was not utilised however as (DFES 2003 pg 21) highlight "additional resources will be needed if they are to meet the long-term challenge to maintain and improve high standards, expand and widen access." If these resources were not available then perhaps the participants within this research have relied on the existing strategies of informal opportunistic teaching, role modelling, mentorship and clinical supervision to provide and support education in practice (Spouse 2001, Cahill 1996 and Field 2004).

The need to provide a variety of teaching methods has been further highlighted by Honey and Mumford (1992) and Kolb (1984) who identified that failure to meet the needs of individual learning styles alongside failing to complete the learning cycles could have a detrimental affect on the success of teaching. The use of group discussion, simulation and coaching by the research participants exemplifies this as these methods promoted action on new knowledge enabling assimilation of that knowledge into the student's own practice. The adoption of mixed methods to overcome the shortfall in being able to assess a students learning style further supported the proposal that the research participants had an equal working knowledge of adult learning educational theory. However it has not been shown that the participants were aware they were using this educational theory although there was some indication of this knowledge within the qualitative data as the participants discussed the conceptual construct of 'the real world'.

Similar to the teaching strategies adopted predominately opportunistic informal activity was prevalent in terms of assessment strategy with the provision of feedback used to give a formative assessment on student performance (Brown and Knight 1994). These findings corroborate the continuum of clinical practice and competence as an evolving concept where practitioners require and achieve life-long learning through a process of performance evaluation and assessment (Benner 1984, Petty 1998, Ramritu and Barnard 2001). These findings also suggested that competency in practice was valued and supported the theory of Douglas et al (2001) in that the assessment of clinical skills within the healthcare setting was prevalent.

The role of the lecturer practitioner was found to be more frequently involved with constructing and marking academic post registration assignments unsurprisingly this related to the university role and summative assessment performed by the lecturer practitioner. These results maintain the view within literature that the role of the lecturer practitioner was one which accomplished assessment both within practice and the university setting (Vaughan 1990, Lathlean 1997).

In contrast and despite the extensive literature on the role of the clinical nurse specialist where there was no indication that the role was concerned with assessment (Hurlimann 2001, Cattini and Knowles 1999, Gibson 2001, Bousfield 1997, Martin 1999) this research demonstrated there was definite engagement by the clinical nurse specialists in the process of assessment. In contrast it has been recommended the role of the practice educator was required to construct assessment tools (Hudson 2000) although it was not possible to confirm this within this research three participants from the educators in practice group stated they constructed methods of assessment.

In considering the provision of a flexible workforce was an important component of the learning environment (Ward and McCormack 2000) it appeared that the local trust at the time of this research was in a good position to sustain education within the clinical setting. However the research participants within this study reported barriers to the implementation of education within practice. The ability to protect time for the provision of education was the prevailing sub-theme to emerge from the qualitative data and related to the workload and availability of the participant this was also reflected the findings of McCreadddie (2001), Ibbotson (1999) and Gopee (2001) who reported the negative impact the demands of clinical workload had on the ability to sustain education in practice.

Literature surrounding a successful learning environment also suggested student motivation was dependant upon the value placed on work based learning by others within the workplace and by the organisation itself (Flanagan et al 2000, Garcarz and Chambers 2003). This was substantiated within this study by the emergence of the sub-theme defined as 'officialdom' which concerned participants who expressed feelings regarding the negative and passive attitude of the organisation towards learning in practice. The participants here suggested the value of opportunistic work-based learning was under-valued by the organisation. The sub-theme of 'willingness to learn' which was identified as a barrier towards the provision of education also suggested there was an apathy amongst students towards learning in practice. It has been suggested that for learning to be the culture of a NHS organisation, it needed to be integral to practice and patient care (Garcarz and Chambers 2003, DOH 2001a). In contrast the physical presence of educational resources held locally has not yet been achieved as education continues to be housed in separate buildings away from patients i.e. universities, post-graduate centres, hospital libraries and resource centres. Nevertheless, the use of link tutors, lecturer practitioners, practice educators, trainers and distance learning resources have evolved and made progress in addressing this imbalance (Burke 1997, Jones 1996 and Hudson 2000). The findings of this research suggested that the research participants whose role was primarily patient focused felt undervalued as educators and that the organisation had failed to recognise and support education in practice.

A fundamental role for teachers/educators within the workplace was promoted as the provision of learning in terms of content structure and delivery method, in essence the development of curriculum (Lam et al 2002, Thornton 1997). This unfortunately confirmed the view that despite the traits of leadership, clinical expertise and in-depth knowledge of a specialist subject (Cattini and Knowles 1999, Rolfe and Fulbrook 1998) clinical nurse specialists remained providers of education rather than leaders. In contrast it was expected that lecturer practitioners would have a responsibility for programmes of education (Vaughan 1990, Lathlean 1997).

The choice to contribute to curriculum development may have been influenced by the participant's personal preference or motivation to do so (Chang and Wong 2001, Hunt 1999). The findings of this research proposed this was not the case and suggested that despite motivation the clinical nurse specialist had not been given the opportunity to contribute to university curriculum development. Lecturer practitioners however felt a greater 'belonging' and this was understandable given the nature of the 'dual role' (Fairbrother and Manther 2004 and Vaughan 1990) importantly the qualitative research found that clinical nurse specialists did not feel they had strong links with the local university and predominately felt on the 'outside'. In comparison Lathlean (1997) found "some lecturer practitioners felt they did not 'belong' to either institution". The role of the lecturer practitioner within education has been 'celebrated' and has therefore become visible (Vaughan 1990, Lathlean 1997) this was comparable to the findings of this research however in contrast it was found that the role of the clinical nurse specialist as an educator was perceived by themselves to be under valued and therefore not recognised by academia in addition to the organisation in which they worked.

Strohschein et al (2002) promote the 'shared vision' of practice-based education the participants within this research appeared to share this view by considering that a link between clinical practice and academia would produce a relationship on which to share knowledge. In contrast, some research participants held the view that the university could use practice-based education to sustain academic curricula and this was thought to prevent the valuing of learning from within practice without academic accreditation. Gopee (2001) shared this perspective of university education and highlighted the deflective result of academia on the uptake of learning within clinical practice.

There was also a view by some participants that a university-based education would lack training on the practical skills of nursing. This reflects the report from the UKCC (1999) which emphasised there was a lack of practical skills in student nurses. In comparison another sub-theme to develop from the participants narrative was that of 'competence of clinical skills', this embraced the theory of encouraging practitioners to reach a level of clinical competence in which they could provide a satisfactory level of clinical patient care.

It therefore emerged that some participants held views that the value of learning within the clinical setting was not entirely dependant upon the university as McCormick (1999) advocates, practical knowledge is characterised by expertise used outside of academic settings. Indeed, the vision of central government (DOH 2001a) is the development of a workforce of lifelong learners within the NHS; in recognition, learning in practice is promoted as being integral to good employment practice and essential to organisational performance.

The results of this research however support the view that the curriculum for education within healthcare and clinical practice has been centrally driven by universities and central government (DOH 2001a, UKCC 1999, Burke 1997). In addition there appeared from the results of this study to be little involvement of the majority of educator roles from within practice to the development of a shared vision when developing and providing education for the practice setting (Strohschein et al 2002, Garcarz and Chambers 2003).

STUDY LIMITATIONS

The mixed method approach of the research study was an appropriate strategy to answer the research questions and the use of a questionnaire as a data collection method was suitable for the context of a busy healthcare organisation. There was no one 'recipe' book for methods chosen, although Creswell (2003) was the basis for the structure of the research to further guide the research process a multitude of additional sources were used. A successful and valid questionnaire was vital to the achievement of this research and every moment spent on construction and revision proved advantageous (Oppenheim 1992). However, the use of a mixed methods approach to this study had a downside; the large quantity of data produced required analysis by multiple methods, which proved to be time consuming and challenging. Equally, the mixed methods analysis of this study generated interesting results that proved to be both comparable to the existing literature and which produced new information for discussion at a local level.

A major disappointment in this study was the participation of only one practice educator; the research questions therefore had the potential to remain valid for only the roles of the lecturer practitioner and clinical nurse specialist within the trust. Rewardingly a third group of participants emerged from the data, was categorised as 'educators in practice' and provided further opportunity for analysis. The design of this study was to meet the needs of the local target population although the size of the population was too small for statistical significance testing using non-parametric tests. In terms of generalisability, the interpretation of the results to other settings therefore remains limited.

Bias within this research was potentially high; research that relies on voluntary participation has an element of respondent bias and although this study had limited this bias with a high response rate, it was possible those members of staff who participated in the study were motivated to do so by their interest and knowledge in the content of study. Researcher bias has also had an influence, although the questions were constructed from the literature review just by choosing which questions to ask had already influenced the content of the study. However, the assessment of content validity has minimised this bias. The use of the questionnaire to collect qualitative data has also limited researcher bias by allowing the participants a freedom to respond without researcher influence. A weakness of this nonetheless has been that further enquiry and clarity could not be ascertained through further questioning; in particular the reason why certain teaching strategies were used over and above other methods and the verification of the participants awareness, knowledge and application of adult learning theory.

Finally, this study may have been enhanced by seeking views from the students in practice and discovering how they feel the roles of the clinical nurse specialist, lecturer practitioner and practice educator have contributed to their education in practice, this could however be studied subsequently to this study.

CONCLUSION

This study aimed to provide a systematic description, comparison and analysis on the educative roles within practice of the clinical nurse specialist, lecturer practitioner and practice educator in a healthcare setting. With regard to the roles of clinical nurse specialist, lecturer practitioner and 'educator in practice' this has been achieved. Alongside a quantitative description on educational activity; the qualitative data has provided the context and ethos within which the roles identified within this study were practising. This study showed a remarkable resemblance between the roles identified and in particular, the role of the lecturer practitioner and clinical nurse specialist within the practice setting appeared the most equivalent.

The results of this study have answered the research questions and the main findings have shown that all the roles within this study were comparable in terms of biographical profiles, clinical and educational experiences and the provision of a wide variety of education to a variety of students. Slight differences in role activity were found in clinical patient caseload and involvement in academia.

As demonstrated within the literature review the demands upon the NHS to build a culture of 'life long learning' within the workplace have been centrally driven from government policy (DOH 2000, 2001a, Audit commission 2001 and UKCC 1999). Nevertheless, there has also been strong evidence to support the development of education within practice to meet the needs of the clinician and support worker (Ward and McCormack 2000, Lave and Wenger 1991, and McCormick 1999). The benefits for an organisation and the individual are many but focus mainly around the development of a motivated, innovative and efficient workforce who had increased job satisfaction (Garcarz and Chambers 2003, Audit Commission 2001 and Belling et al 2003). The benefits for the NHS also include the development and retainment of competent staff that can adapt and develop their roles to meet the diverse needs of an increasing patient population (Medical Devices Agency 2000, Douglas et al 2001 and UKCC 1999). Within this context this research has highlighted a population of staff within a hospital in the south of England who are able to support education within practice.

In addition, as the NHS strives to provide patient care which is based upon clinical evidence the provision of work-based education becomes essential to the integration of theory and evidence into practice (DOH 2001a). In order to meet the requirements of providing education within practice, 'educator' roles have developed to facilitate clinicians in acquiring new clinical skills and becoming competent, these roles it has been proposed have the ability to assimilate theory into practice that can have a personal bearing for the individual learner (Hewison and Wildman 1996, Dearmun 2000 and Field 2004). All participants within this study appeared to value the integration of theory into practice to enable staff to become competent in clinical practice.

This research has shown that within a local NHS hospital the roles of the clinical nurse specialist, lecturer practitioner and 'educator in practice' were synonymous with providing education within practice. Despite this, as new roles have been developed to specifically provide education in practice the clinical nurse specialist as 'educator' appeared to have been under utilised by both the hospital and the local university. Although there is a perception that the clinical nurse specialist and 'deskill' the workforce (Jack 2002, Mytton and Adams 2003) within this research this was unfounded with the role of clinical nurse specialist described as 'enhancing skill'. However, the clinical nurse specialists within this research were found to feel undervalued and 'on the outside.' Despite this the clinical nurse specialists within this study showed great motivation to becoming involved with both pre and post-registration university courses and students nevertheless, the clinical nurse specialists appeared to need the opportunity to effectively contribute.

Further barriers to the provision of education in practice were identified and included failure to 'ring fence' time for education, 'officialdom' incorporating the perceived lower value of education provided in the clinical setting and the poor willingness of staff to engage in clinical educational opportunities. The central drive from universities and government to provide clinical education (DOH 2001a, UKCC 1999, NMC 2002, Burke 1997) may have prevented the engagement of the educators in practice within this study and the achievement of the 'shared vision' (Strohschein et al 2002) practice-based education was supposed to accomplish.

RECOMMENDATIONS

A series of recommendations for the future have therefore been suggested which should serve to enhance the provision and development of education in practice within a local hospital.

The role of the clinical nurse specialist as an 'educationist' should be formally recognised and valued by both the hospital and the university.

Clinical nurse specialists should continue to make 'visible' the valuable contribution to education they make within practice.

In order to create a feeling of 'belonging' and to promote a 'shared vision',

The curriculum for both pre and post registration university courses should be made 'visible' and accessible for all educators based within practice.

The local university should seek to establish 'links' and begin a dialogue with clinical nurse specialist groups in which the curriculum for both pre-registration and post-registration courses could be discussed alongside mentorship.

A hospital wide portfolio of clinical education should include the contributions made by the clinical nurse specialists, lecturer practitioners and some of the 'educators in practice' who were not currently included.

An 'open' forum is created in which all clinical educators and educational leads have the opportunity to regularly meet and discuss practice education issues.

Research on the views of the learners in practice and academia with regard to the roles of clinical nurse specialist, lecturer practitioner and 'educators in practice' would further contribute to the discussion.

ACKNOWLEDGEMENTS

The participants who contributed to this study; they have shown how motivated and valuable they are as clinical educationalists. They remain anonymous but inspirational.

REFERENCES

Adderley, B.V. And Hunter Hill. M., 1979. The Contribution Of The Clinical Nurse Specialist To The Education Of Student Nurses. *Journal Of Advanced Nursing,* 4, 327-329.

Audit Commission, 2001. *Hidden Talents.* London: Audit Commission Publications.

Bale, S., 1995. The Role Of The Clinical Nurse Specialist Within The Health-Care Team. *Journal Of Wound Care,* 4 (2), 86-87.

Bamford, O. And Gibson, F., 2000. The Clinical Nurse Specialist; Perceptions Of Practising Cnss Of Their Role And Development Needs. *Journal Of Clinical Nursing,* 9 (2), 282-292.

Bell, J., 1999. *Doing Your Research Project.* 3rd Ed. Maidenhead: Open University Press.

Belling, R. James, K. And Ladkin, D., 2003. Back To The Workplace: How Organizations Can Improve Their Support For Management Learning And Development. *Journal Of Management Development* [Online], 23 (3). Available From: Http://Www.Emerald insight.Com/10.1108/02621710410524104 [Accessed April 20th 2005]

Benner, P., 1984. *From Novice To Expert.* California: Addison-Wesley Publishing Company.

Bournemouth University, 2004. *Ihcs Code Of Practice Research Governance And Ethics In Postgraduate Research.* Supervisors And Supervision Working Group.

Bousfield, C., 1997. A Phenomenological Investigation Into The Role Of The Clinical Nurse Specialist, *Journal Of Advanced Nursing,* 25, 245-256.

Brennan, A And Hutt, R., 2001. The Challenges And Conflicts Of Facilitating Learning In Practice: The Experiences Of Two Clinical Nurse Educators, *Nurse Education In Practice,* 1, 181-188.

Brown, S. And Knight, P. 1994. *Assessing Learners In Higher Education.* London. Kogan Page.

Buch, K. And Bartley, S., 2002. Learning Style And Training Delivery Mode Preference. *Journal Of Workplace Learning,* 14 (1), 5-10.

Buchanan, D.R., 1998. Beyond Positivism: Humanistic Perspectives On Theory And Research In Health Education. *Health Education Research Theory And Practice,* 13 (3), 439-450.

Burke, L. M., 1997. Teachers Of Nursing- Presenting A New Model Of Practice. *Journal Of Nursing Management,* 5, 295-300.

Cahill, H.A., 1996. A Qualitative Analysis Of Student Nurses' Experiences Of Mentorship. *Journal Of Advanced Nursing,* 24 (4), 791-799.

Camsooksai, J., 2002. The Role Of The Lecturer Practitioner In Interprofessional Education. *Nurse Education Today,* 22 (6), 466-475.

Carnwell, R., 2000. Pedagogical Implications Of Approaches To Study In Distance Learning: Developing Models Through Qualitative And Quantitative Analysis, *Journal Of Advanced Nursing,* 35, (5), 1018-1028.

Cattini, P. And Knowles, V., 1999. Core Competences For Clinical Nurse Specialists:A Usable Framework. *Journal Of Clinical Nursing,* 8, 505-511.

Caulder, J., 1998. Survey Research Methods. *Medical Education,* 32, 636-652.

Chang, K.K, And Wong, K.S.T., 2001. The Nurse Specialist Role In Hong Kong: Perceptions Of Nurse Specialists, Doctors And Staff Nurses. *Journal Of Advanced Nursing,* 36 (1), 32-40.

Clark, A.M., 1998. The Qualitative-Quantitative Debate: Moving From Positivism And Confrontation To Post-Positivism And Reconciliation. *Journal Of Advanced Nursing,* 27, 1242-1249.

Clay, G. And Wade, M., 2001. Mentors Or Practice Educators? *Community Practitioner,* 74 (6), 213-215.

Clifford, C., 1993. The Clinical Role Of The Nurse Teacher In The United Kingdom. *Journal Of Advanced Nursing,* 18, 281-289.

Cohen, L, Manion, L And Morrison K., 2000. *Research Methods In Education.* 5th Ed. London : Routledge/Falmer,

Cope, P, Cuthbertson, P And Stoddart, B., 2000. Situated Learning In The Practice Placement, *Journal Of Advanced Nursing,* 31,(4), 850-856.

Cottrell, S. 2001. *Teaching Study Skills And Supporting Learning.* Basingstoke. Palgrave Publishers Ltd.

Couchman, W. And Dawson, J., 1990. *Nursing And Healthcare Research: A Practical Guide, The Use And Application Of Research For Nurses And Other Healthcare Professionals.* London: Scutari Press.

Creswell, J.W., 1994. *Research Design: Qualitative And Quantitative Approaches.* Thousand Oaks, C.A: Sage.

Creswell, J.W., 2003. *Research Design: Qualitative, Quantitative And Mixed Methods Approaches.* 2nd Ed. London: Thousand Oaks, Sage.

Cutliffe, J R And Ward, M., 2003. *Critiquing Nursing Research.* Wiltshire: Quay Books

Daley, B. J., 2001. Learning And Professional Practice: A Study Of Four Professions. *Adult Education Quarterly,* 52 (1), 39-54.

Daly, W.M., And Carnell, R., 2003. Nursing Roles And Levels Of Practice: A Framework For Differentiating Between Elementary, Specialist And Advancing Practice. *Journal Of Advanced Nursing,* 12, 158-167.

Day, C., Frazer, D. And Mallik, M. 1998. *The Role Of The Teacher/Lecturer In Practice.* London: English National Board.

Dearmun, A.K., 2000. Supporting Newly Qualified Staff Nurses: The Lecturer Practitioner Contribution. *Journal Of Nursing Management* [Online], 8 (3). Available From: Http://Ejournals.Ebsco.Com/Direct.Asp?Articleid=Dnjrey6e4upy91gptq77 [Accessed 10th January 2005].

Denzin, N.K., 1989. *The Research Act: A Theoretical Introduction To Sociological Methods.* 3rd Ed. New York: Mcgraw-Hill.

Denzin N. & Lincoln. 1998. *Handbook Of Qualitative Research.* London: Sage Publications.

Department For Education And Skills (Dfes), 2003. *The Future Of Higher Education.* London: Hmso.

Department Of Health (Doh), 2000. *The Nhs Plan; A Plan For Investment, A Plan For Reform.* London: Hmso

Department Of Health (Doh), 2001a. *Working Together – Learning Together. A Framework For Life-Long Learning.* London: Hmso.

Department Of Health (Doh), 2001b. *Research Governance Framework For Health And Social Care.* London: Hmso.

Department Of Health (Doh), 2002. *Learning For Everyone: A Development Plan For Nhsu* [Online]. London: Hmso. Available From: Http://Www.Nhsu.Nhs.Uk/ Docs/Learning_ For_Everyone.Pdf

Douglas, M.R., Leigh, J.A., And Douglas, C.H. 2001. Uk Registered Nurse Medical Device Education: A Comparison Of Hospital And Bank Nurses. *Nurse Education In Practice,* 1, 85-93.

Elcock, K., 1998. Lecturer Practitioner: A Concept Analysis. *Journal Of Advanced Nursing,* 28 (5), 1092-1098.

Emden, C. And Sandelowski, M., 1998. The Good, The Bad And The Relative, Part One: Conceptions Of Goodness In Qualitative Research. *International Journal Of Nursing Practice* [Online], 4 (4). Available From: Http://Ejournals.Ebsco.Com/Direct.Asp? Articleid=6uqgy2pkvlh94rm33137 [Accessed 20th April 2005].

Emden, C. And Sandelowski, M., 1999. The Good, The Bad And The Relative, Part Two: Goodness And The Criterion Problem In Qualitative Research. *International Journal Of Nursing Practice* [Online], 5 (1). Available From: Http://Ejournals.Ebsco.Com/Direct. Asp?Articleid=Ndu7vfw060he9tlv01ey [Accessed 20th April 2005].

Enb And Doh., 2001a. *Placements In Focus* [Online]. Available From: Http://Www.Dh.Gov.Uk/Publicationsandstatistics/Publications/Publicationspolicyandgui dance/Publicationspolicyandguidancearticle/Fs/En?Content_Id=4009511&Chk=Zlryyo [Accessed 10th January 2005].

Enb And Doh., 2001b. *Preparation Of Mentors And Teachers* [Online]. Available From: Http://Www.Dh.Gov.Uk/Publicationsandstatistics/Publications/Publications Policyandguidance/Publicationspolicyandguidancearticle/Fs/En?Content_Id=4007606&C hk=Cwbwzg [Accessed 10th January 2005].

Fairbrother, P And Ford, S., 1998. Lecturer Practitioners: A Literature Review. *Journal Of Advanced Nursing,* 24 (2), 274-279.

Fairbrother, P And Mathers, N.J., 2004. Lecturer Practitioners In Six Professions; Combining Cultures. *Journal Of Clinical Nursing,* 13 (5), 539-546.

Flanagan, M., 1997. A Profile Of The Nurse Specialist In Tissue Viability In The Uk. *Journal Of Wound Care,* 6 (2), 85-87.

Flanagan, J, Baldwin,S And Clarke, D., 2000. Work-Based Learning As A Means Of Developing And Assessing Nursing Competence, *Journal Of Clinical Nursing,* 9, 360-368.

Field, D.E., 2004. Moving From Novice To Expert – The Value Of Learning In Clinical Practice: A Literature Review. *Nurse Education Today,* 24 (7), 560-565.

Fink, A. 2003. *How To Sample In Surveys.* 2nd Ed. London : Sage.

Fulbrook, P, Rolfe, G, Albarran, J., And Boxall, F., 2000. Fit For Practice: Project 2000 Student Nurses' Views On How Well The Curriculum Prepares Them For Clinical Practice. *Nurse Education Today,* 20 (5), 350-357.

Garcarz, W. And Chambers, R., 2003. Creating And Sustaining A Learning Organization In The Nhs. *Quality In Primary Care, 11, 255-256.*

Gendall, P., 1998. A Framework For Questionnaire Design: Labaw Revisited. *Marketing Bulletin* [Online], 9. Available From: Http://Marketing-Bulletin.Massey.Ac.Nz/Keyword. Asp?Keywordid=47 [Accessed 20th June 2005].

Gibbs, G. And Habeshaw, T., 1989. *Preparing To Teach.* Bristol: Technical And Educational Services Ltd.

Gibson, F., 2001. Focus Group Interviews To Examine The Role And Development Of The Clinical Nurse Specialist. *Journal Of Nursing Management,* 9, 331-342.

Gopee, N., 2001. Lifelong Learning In Nursing: Perceptions And Realities. *Nurse Education Today,* 21 (8), 607-615.

Graham, A.J., 2005. The Development Of A Competency Assessment For Vacuum Assisted Closure Therapy. *Nurse Education In Practice*, 5 (3), 144-151.

Graneheim, U.H. And Lundman, B., 2004. Qualitative Content Analysis In Nursing Research; Concepts, Procedures And Measures To Achieve Trustworthiness. *Nurse Education Today,* 24 (2), 105-112.

Hammond, G. And Pearson, P., 2004. *Centre For Excellence In Healthcare Professional Education: Cetl4healthne* [Online]. Available From: Http://Www.Cetl4healthne.Ac.Uk/ [Accessed 17th September 2005]

Hamric, A.B. And Spross, J., 1983. *The Clinical Nurse Specialist In Theory And Practice.* London: Grune And Stratton, Inc.

Hamric, A.B., Spross, A, And Hanson, C.M., 1996. *Advanced Nursing Practice; An Integrative Approach.* Philadelphia: Wb Saunders Company.

Hanson, W.E. Creswell, J.W. Creswell,J.D Plano Clarke, V.L. And Petska, K.S., 2005. Mixed Methods Research Design In Counseling Psychology. *Journal Of Counseling Psychology* [Online], 52 (2). Available From: Http://Content.Apa.Org/Journals/Cou/52/2/224.Html [Accessed 3rd April 2005].

Hewison, A.. And Wildman, S., 1996. The Theory-Practice Gap In Nursing: A New Dimension. *Journal Of Advanced Nursing.* 24, 754-761.

Hill-Bailey, P. And Tilley, S., 2002. Storytelling And The Interpretation Of Meaning In Qualitative Research. *Journal Of Advanced Nursing,* 38 (6), 574-583.

Honey, P. And Mumford, A., 1992. *The Manual Of Learning Styles.* Maidenhead: Peter Honey.

Hope, A., 2003. Clinical Governance And The Role Of The Lecturer Practitioner In Education In One British Nhs Trust. *Journal Of Nursing Management,* 11 (3), 164-167.

Hudson, R., 2000. *Practice Educators Preparing For New Roles In The New Nhs.* London: Cphva Education And Research Committee.

Humphris, D. 1994. *The Clinical Nurse Specialist, Issues In Practice.* Basingstoke. Macmillan.

Hunt, J.A., 1999. A Specialist Nurse: An Identified Professional Role Or A Personal Agenda. *Journal Of Advanced Nursing,* 30 (3), 704-712.

Hurlimann, B. Hofer, S. And Hirter, K., 2001. The Role Of The Clinical Nurse Specialist. *International Journal Review,* 48, 58-64.

Hutchings, A And Sanders, L., 2001. Developing A Learning Pathways For Student Nurses, *Nursing Standard,* 15, (40), 38-41.

Ibbotson, K., 1999. The Role Of The Clinical Nurse Specialist: A Study, *Nursing Standard,* 14 (9), 35-38.

Jack, B., 2002. Do Hospital Based Palliative Care Clinical Nurse Specialists De-Skill General Staff? *International Journal Of Palliative Nursing,* 8 (7), 336-342.

Johnston, B.T And Boohan, M,. 2000. Basic Clinical Skills; Don't Leave Teaching To The Teaching Hospitals, *Medical Education,* 34. 692-699.

Jones, A., 1995. Reflective Process In Action: The Uncovering Of The Ritual Of Washing In Clinical Nursing Practice. *Journal Of Clinical Nursing,* 4, 283-288.

Jones, H.M., 1996. Introducing A Lecturer Practitioner: The Management Perspective. *Journal Of Nursing Management,* 4 (6), 337-345.

Jowett, J. And Mcmullan, M., 2003. *Evaluative Study Of The Role Of The Practice Educator.* Somerset, Devon And Cornwall Workforce Development Confederation In Partnership With The Institute Of Health Studies, University Of Plymouth.

Knight, C.M., Moule, P. And Desbottes, Z. 2000. The Grid That Bridges The Gap. *Nurse Education Today,* 20, 116-122.

Kolb, D.A., 1984. *Experiential Learning.* New Jersey: Prentice-Hall,Inc.

Lave, J. And Wenger, E. 1991. *Situated Learning : Legitimate Peripheral Participation.* Cambridge : Cambridge University Press.

Lam, T.P., Irwin, M., Chow, L.W.C. And Chan, P., 2002. Early Introduction Of Clinical Skills Teaching In A Medical Curriculum – Factors Affecting Students' Learning. *Medical Education,* 36 (3), 233-240.

Lathlean, J., 1997. *Lecturer Practitioners In Action.* Oxford: Butterworth Heinemann.

Lincoln Y.S.& Guba E.G. 1985. *Naturalistic Inquiry.* Newbury Park, Ca: Sage.

Lutz, W, Lockerbie, L, Chalmers, J, And Hepburn, W., 1992. *Health And Community Surveys. Vol.2 : Questionnaire Design, Interviewing And Recording, Presenting Survey.* London : Macmillan In Association With The International Epidemiological Ass.

Marshall, Z., And Luffingham, N., 1998. Does The Specialist Nurse Enhance Or Deskill The General Nurse? *British Journal Of Nursing,* 7 (11), 658-662.

Martin, P. J., 1997. An Exploration Of The Services Provided By The Clinical Nurse Specialist Within One Nhs Trust. *Journal Of Nursing Management,* 7, 149-156.

Mccormick, R. 1999. *In:* R, Mccormick And C, Paechter Eds. *Learning And Knowledge.* London : Paul Chapman Ltd In Association With The Open University.

Mccreaddie, M., 2001. The Role Of The Clinical Nurse Specialist. *Nursing Standard,* 21 (16), 33-38.

Mcgee, P. Castledine, G. And Brown, R., 1996. A Survey Of Specialist And Advanced Nursing Practice In England. *British Journal Of Nursing ,* 5 (11), 682-686.

Mcsherry, R., 1997. What Do Registered Nurses And Midwives Feel And Know About Research? *Journal Of Advanced Nursing,* 25, 985-998.

Medical Devices Agency 2000. *Equipped To Care: The Safe Use Of Medical Devices In The 21st Century.* London. Medical Devices Agency.

Melia K., 1982. "Tell It As It Is"- Qualitative Methodology And Nursing Research: Understanding The Student Nurses World. *Journal Of Advanced Nursing.* 7 (4), 327-355.

Miller, R.L., Acton, C., Fullerton, D.A. And Maltby. J., 2002. *Spss For Social Scientists.* Basingstoke: Palgrove Mcmillan.

Morse, J.M., 1991. Approaches To Qualitative-Quantitative Methodological Triangulation, *Nursing Research,* 40 (1), 120-123.

Morris, D And Turnbull, P., 2004. Using Student Nurses As Teachers In Inquiry-Based Learning. *Journal Of Advanced Nursing,* 45 (2), 136-144.

Mulholland, J., 2005. *Making Practice-Based Learning Work: Practicebasedlearning.Org* [Online]. Available From: Http://Www.Practicebasedlearning [Accessed 7th November 2005]

Mumford, A., 1995a. Putting Learning Styles To Work: An Integrated Approach, *Industrial And Commercial Training,* 27 (8), 28-35.

Mumford, A., 1995b. Learning Styles And Mentoring. *Industrial And Commercial Training,* 27 (8), 4-7.

Mytton, E.J., And Adams, A., 2003. Do Clinical Nurse Specialists In Palliative Care De-Skill Or Empower General Ward Nurses. *International Journal Of Palliative Nursing,* 9 (2), 64-71.

Nhsu Abolition Order. 2005. Statutory Instrument No 1781. Isbn 0110730453 [Online]. Available From: Http://Www.Opsi.Gov.Uk/Si/Si2005/20051781.Htm [Accessed 17th September 2005].

Nmc., 2002. *Standards For The Preparation Of Teachers Of Nurses, Midwives And Health Visitors.* London: Nmc Available From Http://Www.Nmc-Uk.Org/ (Ymvbgi45i3vjwm 2iknnuebzw)/Aframedisplay.Aspx?Documentid=616 [Accessed 10th January 2005]

Nmc., 2004. *The Nmc Code Of Professional Conduct: Standards For Performance And Ethics.* London: Nmc.

Nmc., 2005. *Review Of The Current Standards For The Preparation Of Teachers Of Nursing And Midwifery: Issues For Change* [Online]. Available From: Http://Www.Nmc-Uk.Org/(Pjenkzqd5qhijdmwsdod5deb)/Aframedisplay.Aspx?Documentid=836 [Accessed 10th January 2005].

Norman, I.J., Watson, R., Murrells, T., Claman, L. And Redfern, S., 2002. The Validity And Reliability Of Methods To Assess Competence To Practise Of Pre-Registration Nursing And Midwifery Students. *International Journal Of Nursing Studies.* 39, 133-145.

Oppenheim, A.N., 1992. *Questionnaire Design, Interviewing And Attitude Measurement.* London: Continuum.

Ormond-Walsh, S.E., 2001. Comparing And Contrasting The Clinical Nurse Specialist And The Advanced Nurse Practitioner Roles. *Journal Of Nursing Management,* 9, 205-207.

Paniagua, H., 2002. Planning Research: Methods And Ethics, *Practice Nursing,* 13 (1), 22-27.

Parahoo, K., 1997. *Nursing Research:, Principles, Process And Issues.* Basingstoke: Palgrove Mcmillan.

Petty, G. 1998. Teaching Today. 2nd Edition. Cheltenham: Stanley Thornes Ltd.

Polit, D.F. And Hungler, B.P., 1989. *Essentials Of Nursing Research: Methods, Appraisal And Utilization.* 2nd Ed. Philadelphis: Lippincott

Punch, K.F., 1998. *Introduction To Social Research: Quantitative And Qualitative Approaches.* London: Sage.

Punch, K.F., 2003. *Survey Research The Basics.* London: Sage.

Quinn, F. M., 2000. *Principles And Practice Of Nurse Education.* 4th Ed. Cheltenham: Stanley Thornes Ltd.

Ramritu, P.L. And Barnard, A. 2001. New Nurse Graduates' Understanding Of Competence. *International Nursing Review,* 48, 47-57.

Ratcliffe, P., 1998. Using The 'New' Statistics In Nursing Research. *Journal Of Advanced Nursing*, 27: 1329.

Reid, B., 1991. *Developing And Documenting A Qualitative Methodology.* Journal Of Advanced Nursing. [16] 544 – 551.

Richardson, A. And Turnock. C., 2003. An Evaluation Of Critical Care Lecturer Practitioners. *Nursing In Critical Care* [Online], 8 (6). Available From: Http://Ejournals.Ebsco.Com/Direct.Asp?Articleid=Rbweygg29lt8m4cghv1e [Accessed 10th January 2005].

Roe, B.H. And Webb, C., 1998. *Research And Development In Clinical Nursing Practice.* London: Whurr.

Rolfe, G, And Fulbrook, P., 1998. *Advanced Nursing Practice.* Woburn: Butterworth-Heinemann.

Ryan-Merrit, M.V, Mitchell, C.A, And Pagel, I., 1988. Clinical Nurse Specialist Role Definition And Operationalization. *Clinical Nurse Specialist,* 2 (3), 132-137.

Sadler-Smith, E., 1996. Learning Styles: A Holistic Approach. *Journal Of European Industrial Training,* 20 (7), 29-36.

Salkind, N.J., 2000. *Statistics For People Who Think They Hate Statistics.* London: Sage

Schon, D.A., 1987 *Educating The Reflective Practitioner.* California: Jossey-Bass Inc.

Silverman, D. 2001. *Interpreting Qualitative Data: Methods For Analysing Talk, Text And Interaction.* 2nd Ed. London. Sage Publications.

Sloan, G. 1999. Good Characteristics Of A Clinical Supervisor: A Community Health Perspective. *Journal Of Advanced Nursing*, 30 (3): 713-722.

Spouse, J. 2001. Bridging Theory And Practice In The Supervisory Relationship: A Sociocultural Perspective, *Journal Of Advanced Nursing,* 33,(4),512-522.

Strauss A. And Corbin J. [1990] *Basics Of Qualitative Research: Grounded Theory Procedures And Techniques.* Newbury Park: C.A. Sage

Strohschein, J, Hagler, P And May, L., 2002. Assessing The Need For Change In Clinical Education Practices. *Physical Therapy,* 82 (2), 160-172.

Tarling, M And Crofts, L., 2002. *The Essential Researcher's Handbook For Nurses And Health Care Professions.* London: Bailliere Tindall.

Thornton, T., 1997. Attitudes Towards The Relevance Of Biological, Behavioural And Social Sciences In Nursing Education. *Journal Of Advanced Nursing,* 26 (1), 180-186.

Tobin, G.A. And Begley, C.M., 2004. Methodological Rigour Within A Qualitative Framework. *Journal Of Advanced Nursing,* 48 (4), 388-396.

Ukcc, 1999. *Fitness For Practice* [Online]. London. United Kingdom Central Council For Nursing And Midwifery. Available From Http://Www.Nmc-Uk.Org/(Ymvbgi45i3 vjwm2iknnuebzw)/Aframedisplay.Aspx?Documentid=627[Accessed 10th January 2005]

Ukcc, 2001. *Standards For Specialist Education And Practice* [Online]. London. Available From Http://Www.Nmc-Uk.Org/ (Pjenkzqd5qhijdmwsdod5deb) / Aframedisplay.Aspx? Documentid=661 [Accessed 10th January 2005]

Ukcc, 2002. *Report Of The Higher Level Of Nursing Practice Pilot And Project.* London: United Kingdom Central Council For Nursing And Midwifery. Available From Http://Www.Nmc-Uk.Org/(Ymvbgi45i3vjwm2iknnuebzw) /Aframedisplay. Aspx?Docu mentid=686 [Accessed 10th January 2005]

Vaughan, B., 1990. Knowing That And Knowing How: The Role Of The Lecturer Practitioner. In Kershaw, B And Salvage, J (Eds) *Models Fro Nursing 2.* London: Scutari Press.

Walkin.L,. 1990. *Teaching And Learning In Further And Adult Education:* Cheltenham: Stanley Thornes Ltd.

Wallace, L.S. Blake, G.H. Parham, J.S. And Baldridge, R.E., 2003. Development And Content Validation Of Family Practice Residency Recruitment Questionnaires. *Family Medicine*, 35 (7), 496-498.

Walliman, N., 2001. *Your Research Project.* London: Sage.

Ward, C And Mccormack, B., 2000. Creating An Adult Learning Culture Through Practice Development, *Nurse Education Today,* 20, 259-266.

Williams, A, Mcgee, P And Bates, L., 2001. An Examination Of Senior Nursing Roles: Challenges For The Nhs. *Journal Of Clinical Nursing,* 10, 195-203.

Williams, B., 2001. Developing Critical Reflection For Professional Practice Throeugh Problem Based Learning. *Journal Of Advanced Nursing*, 34 (1), 27-34.

Williamson, G.R. Webb, C. And Ableson-Mitchell, N., 2004. Developing Lecturer Practitioner Roles Using Action Research. *Journal Of Advanced Nursing,* 47 (2), 153-164.

Williamson, G.R. And Webb, C., 2001. Supporting Students In Practice. *Journal Of Clinical Nursing*, 10 (2), 284-292.

Wilson, H. C., 2000. Emergency Response Preparedness: Small Group Training. Part 2-Training Methods Compared With Learning Styles, *Disasterprevention And Management,* 9 (3), 180-199.

Wilson-Barnett, J., 1997. Contrasts In Professional Progress In The United Kingdom: Education And Services, *Journal Of Advanced Nursing,* 25, 211-212.

APPENDICES-A1 QUESTIONNAIRE

Section 1 - Participation in

Are you involved in providing education or training? Yes ❑ No ❑
If answered No please go to Section 4

For which organisation(s) do you provide education/training? *Please tick as many boxes as apply*

Poole Hospital NHS Trust ❑	South and East Primary Care Trust	❑
Bournemouth Hospital NHS Trust ❑	Bournemouth Primary Care Trust	❑
Poole Primary Care Trust ❑	North Dorset Primary Care Trust	❑
Bournemouth University ❑	Dorset Healthcare NHS Trust	❑
South West Primary Care Trust ❑	Others (please specify)............	❑

In the last three months have you provided? *Please tick one box per item*

	Daily	Weekly	Monthly	Less often	Not at all
Formal lectures	❑	❑	❑	❑	❑
Workshops and/or seminars	❑	❑	❑	❑	❑
One to One training	❑	❑	❑	❑	❑
Mentorship/Preceptorship (a formal relationship with a student to provide support and to act as a learning resource)	❑	❑	❑	❑	❑
Facilitation of staff/student reflection	❑	❑	❑	❑	❑
Clinical supervision (A formal process of providing peer support, may be on a one to one basis or as a group)	❑	❑	❑	❑	❑
Training through a workbook/manual	❑	❑	❑	❑	❑
Computer based training package	❑	❑	❑	❑	❑
Used facilitated group discussion as a teaching method	❑	❑	❑	❑	❑
Critical incident analysis/reflection (may be a case study)	❑	❑	❑	❑	❑
Role modelling	❑	❑	❑	❑	❑
Demonstration of a practical skill	❑	❑	❑	❑	❑
Training through simulation	❑	❑	❑	❑	❑

Coaching (continued support and instruction on how to improve clinical/professional performance)	❏	❏	❏	❏	❏
The opportunity of a student or staff member to shadow you for a morning or day	❏	❏	❏	❏	❏
Other (please specify)........................	❏	❏	❏	❏	❏

Section 2 - About your Students

Who do you provide education/training for? *Please tick as many boxes as apply*

Qualified nurses	❏	Patient	❏
Student nurses	❏	Patient's carer	❏
Auxiliary Nurses	❏	Ancillary Staff	❏
Professions allied to medicine	❏	Others please specify............	❏
Doctors	❏		

Do you assess the learning styles of your potential students?

Yes ❏   No ❏

If you answered No please specify why

_____
_____
_____

Do you provide formal teaching sessions or lectures for any post-registration university courses?

Yes ❏   No ❏

If you answered Yes please specify which course/ unit you contribute to

_____

If you answered No would you like to?   Yes* ❏   No ❏

*Would this be for students on a course/unit related to your speciality?

Yes ❏   No Preference ❏

Do you provide mentorship for any post-registration students undertaking a university course?

Yes ❏   No ❏

If you answered Yes please specify which course/unit you contribute to _____
_____
_____

If you answered No would you like to?

Yes* ❏   No ❏

*Would this be for students on a course/unit related to your speciality?

                              Yes   ☐   No Preference   ☐

Do you provide formal teaching sessions or lectures for any pre-registration university courses?

                              Yes   ☐   No   ☐

If you answered Yes please specify which course/unit you contribute to _____
_____
_____

If you answered No would you like to?
                              Yes*   ☐   No   ☐

*Would this be for students on a course/unit related to your speciality?

                              Yes   ☐   No Preference   ☐

Do you provide mentorship for any pre-registration students undertaking a university course?

                              Yes   ☐   No   ☐

If you answered Yes please specify which course/unit you contribute to _____
_____

If you answered No would you like to?
                              Yes*   ☐   No   ☐

*Would this be for students on a course/unit related to your speciality?

                              Yes   ☐   No Preference   ☐

Section 3 - Development of education

Within the hospital do you develop study days or courses on your specialist subject?

                              Yes   ☐   No   ☐

Are you expected to do so by the hospital?
               Yes   ☐   No   ☐   Don't know   ☐

The following two questions relate to a course as a whole not just the content of an individual lecture or session.

Are you involved in developing/shaping the curriculum or course content for any university pre-registration course?

                              Yes   ☐   No   ☐

If you answered No would you like the opportunity to contribute?

                                                  Yes   ❑   No   ❑

Are you involved in developing the curriculum or course content for any university post-registration course?

                                                  Yes   ❑   No   ❑

If you answered No would you like the opportunity to contribute?

                                                  Yes   ❑   No   ❑

In relation to staff/student assessments have you? *Please tick as many boxes as apply*

(Formal in this context refers to the completion of a written recordable assessment; informal refers to the offering of advice and opinion).	Yes for Post Registration staff	Yes for Pre Registration staff
Constructed an academic assignment which is used within a university for assessment	❑	❑
Formally marked an academic assignment for a university (this could be as first or second marker)	❑	❑
In-formally provided feedback on an academic assignment	❑	❑
Constructed an OSCE *(Objective Structured Clinical Examination)* which is used within a university for assessment	❑	❑
Formally marked an OSCE performance	❑	❑
Informally provided feedback on an OSCE performance	❑	❑
Constructed a competency-based assessment which is used within clinical practice	❑	❑
In practice, formally assessed the competence of a clinical skill	❑	❑
In practice, provided informal feedback on the performance/ completion of a clinical skill	❑	❑

Section 4 - Your Experiences And Opinion

Do you believe that providing education within the practice setting is important for ensuring staff/students are "Fit for Practice"?

                    Yes, a lot   ❑   Yes, a little   ❑   Not at all   ❑

Please state why you feel this way,

_____
_____
_____

_____
_____
_____
_____

Do you consider the role of the nurse specialist 'de-skills' other staff in practice?

Yes, a lot   ❑   Yes, a little   ❑   Not at all   ❑

Please state why you feel this way,

_____
_____
_____
_____
_____
_____
_____

Do you think there are difficulties and/or barriers to providing education in practice?

Yes, a lot   ❑   Yes, a little   ❑   Not at all   ❑

Please state why you feel this way,

_____
_____
_____
_____
_____
_____
_____

Do you feel you have strong educational links with the local university?

Yes, a lot   ❑   Yes, a little   ❑   Not at all   ❑

Please state why you feel this way,

_____
_____
_____
_____
_____
_____

Do you think the provision of education in practice benefits from having strong links with the local university?

Yes, a lot   ❑   Yes, a little   ❑   Not at all   ❑

Please state why you feel this way,

_____
_____
_____
_____
_____
_____
_____
_____

Section 5 - About yourself

My role is a...........

Clinical Nurse Specialist ☐   Practice Educator ☐

Lecturer Practitioner ☐   Other ☐
Please specify..

I am the only person employed within this role for my clinical area/specialty.......

Yes ☐   No ☐

I am employed.....

Full-time ☐   Part-time ☐
(37.5 hours or more)   (less than 37.5 hours)

Do you manage a patient caseload?

Yes ☐   No ☐

How long have you been in your current post?

0 - 2 years ☐   6-10 years ☐

3 – 5 years ☐   11 years and over ☐

What qualifications do you have? *Tick as many boxes as apply*

Professional registration ☐   Degree ☐   Other ☐
Please specify

ENB 998 ☐   Masters Degree ☐

City and Guilds 7307 ☐   Doctorate ☐

Certificate in Education ☐   Diploma ☐

How long have you been qualified as a registered professional?

0 - 2 years ☐   6 -10 years ☐

3 – 5 years ☐   11 years and over ☐

Thank-you for taking the time to complete this questionnaire, your assistance is greatly appreciated.

In: Nursing Education Challenges in the 21st Century
Editor: Leana E. Callara, pp. 115-152
ISBN 1-60021-661-7
© 2008 Nova Science Publishers, Inc.

Chapter 4

NEGOTIATING DIFFERENT EXPERIENCES: HOW RELATIONSHIP FROM THE PERSPECTIVE OF THE STUDENT NURSE

Peter Gallagher

College of Learning , Palmerton North, New Zealand

ABSTRACT

With direct reference to how student nurses acquire, apply and evaluate theory for practical purposes this chapter highlights a number of key lessons for nursing education. The first of which is that educators must acknowledge the personal knowledge and personal experience of each student. Preconceptions must be highly valued and incorporated into the programme of study. This means that as far as is practicable the student must be involved in the design of an individualised programme which must maximise personal experiences and preconceptions. A second implication is that educators must acknowledge that there are three forms of theory to which a student nurse will be exposed and educators must explain those forms of theory to the student. In addition it must be emphasised that all of these forms of theory may be considered as equally valid and that any apparent variance between them should be regarded as an energising force that aids rather than inhibits learning. Third, students should be prepared to expect dissonance and to manage the associated psychological discomfort. As the process of learning to apply theory in practical contexts is an experience that involved emotions, educators must clearly appreciate the importance of emotions in learning and provide opportunities for intra-practicum and post practicum debriefing. Emotional responses should not be viewed as a barrier to learning, but rather as a catalyst to the enhancement of learning. The final lesson for nursing education is that formal, practical and private theories have different roots and any understanding of those different forms of theory cannot be evaluated by the same criteria. Therefore, when educators determine the method that will be used to assess students during a practicum they must involve the student as an active partner. The student should be able to select a means of assessment that most closely corresponds with criteria that relate to related to each of the different forms of theory.

INTRODUCTION

In nursing education there is an orthodox position in respect to the relationship between the theory and the practice of nursing. More commonly this relationship is known by the shorthand expression 'the theory-practice gap'. The notion of a gap is probably the most widely accepted conceptualisation of this relationship and it has assisted educationalists to understand how they might best help student nurses apply theory in practical contexts. However, as an explanation of a complex relationship the orthodox position I consider it to be only a partial explanation because:

- It is over reliant upon the objectivist perspective of learning in which the world of theory is viewed as distinct from the world of practice;
- It fails to regard learning as a unified experience in which the student is influenced by the context in which they learn and at the same time influences that context;
- It fails to recognise that knowledge may be more deeply understood as an integral component, an affiliate, rather than a precursor or a successor to practical activity;
- It is highly dependent upon the mechanistic qualities inherent in the metaphor of the computational mind and thus ignores the more organic notion of embodiment;
- The metaphor of a gap is laden with physical images which contrast with the abstract processes that comprise learning;
- The primary evidence to support the existence of a gap is taken from the ability of one person to articulate or demonstrate to another person their ability to align theory and practice;
- The belief amongst nurses in the existence of a gap is axiomatic and subsequent analyses and attempts to resolve problems presented by the gap are therefore based upon a series of self-supporting concepts.

For a more inclusive understanding of the relationship between theory and practice in nursing, I considered it necessary to regard the relationship as a definitively private and individual experience which must be viewed from the perspective of the student nurse (Gallagher, 2003).

In pursuit of such an understanding I undertook a Grounded Theory (GT) approach to the collection and analysis of data from participants who contributed to two discrete sets of data collection. The first set of data collection employed group interviews and the second set individual interviews. Not surprisingly, given the ubiquitous nature of the orthodox position, the raw data from both sets of data are liberally peppered with metaphorical language and illustrations that appeared to strengthen rather than weaken the orthodox position.

However, when I used the constant comparative method (Glaser & Straus, 1967) to analyse the data, further evidence emerged to confirm that prevalence alone is insufficient to counter an alternative explanation of the relationship between theory and practice. For example, the presence of the orthodox position, in which theory and practice are separate entities from separate domains of experience, is certainly widespread in the data. However, the analysis of the data revealed that when registered nurses and student nurses recalled their experiences of the relationship between theory and practice, they reported those experiences as occasions when thoughts, actions and feelings are simultaneously engaged. This strongly suggested that the experience associated with a perceived dissonance is a holistic experience and not a fragmented experience. Further, the definitions of theory offered by the participants are those that exclusively associate theory with the conventional notion of formal or propositional theory. In spite of these definitions, when it came to illustrations of the application of theory in practical contexts, the participants offer examples that draw upon theory from three different sources and not just one source. Those sources are private (personal), practical (situational), as well as formal (propositional) theory. Finally, the participants believed that an understanding of formal theory is an important precursor to effective nursing practice. However, in their interviews the student nurses described patient care for which the successful outcome was based upon interventions for which they or the more experienced registered nurses had no formal knowledge.

NEGOTIATING DIFFERENT EXPERIENCES: A SYNOPSIS

From my data analysis an alternative and complementary explanation of how student nurses identify, experience and manage any differences they perceive between theory and practice in nursing emerged. That explanation grounded in the experience of student nurses and based around the concept of negotiation is called 'Negotiating Different Experiences', and can be represented by the following diagram (Figure.1).

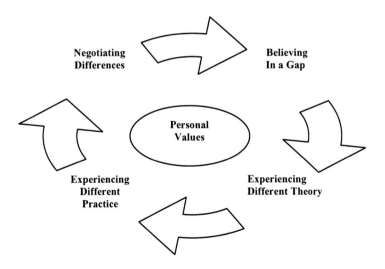

Figure 1. Negotiating Different Experiences.

'Negotiating Different Experiences' is the name I gave to the grounded theory that arose from my exploratory study of the thoughts, emotions and actions a group of New Zealand student nurses associated with their recollections of critical experiences in the delivery of nursing care. These are experiences when the application of one or more of three different forms of theory conflicted with one or all of the key personal values held by each student. The conflict distressed the student and produces a range of strong emotions, mistrust in other nurses and ideas of self doubt. The emotions are not an adjunct to the experience of dissonance; they are central to the holistic nature of that experience. In an effort to reduce the negative feelings that accompany the dissonance between theory and practice, the students sought an explanation for the apparent differences. Some of those explanations contained a direct challenge to their key personal values. The most readily available and the least emotionally charged explanation, and one that also preserves the integrity of personal values, is that a gap exists between the theory and the practice of nursing.

Even before student nurses are exposed to any practicum it is evident that they hold personal values with regard to the skills, attitudes and knowledge that each considers are required for professional nursing. Those values are strongly held and based upon preconceptions which arise from the personal contact that each student had with nurses and common sense notions about nurses in the public domain. Once a student embarks upon an undergraduate nursing degree, two course related experiences are very influential and compel the student to evaluate the validity of their preconceptions. Specifically, those experiences are the exposure that students have to different sources of theory and their exposure to the application of different theories in the context of nursing practice. The tension between these two experiences and their personal values produces a form of intrapersonal conflict which is manifest as emotional discomfort. That discomfort may be private or may be observed by others. As a result of those experiences some of the preconceptions held by students are modified. However, the core personal values that students held about nursing, embedded in their preconceptions, are more resilient and persist throughout the three years of a nursing degree. Those values impact on all learning opportunities and shape the explanation students express of the difference between theory and practice in nursing.

From the range of possible explanations, the notion of a gap is the explanation that offers the least threat to the integrity of personal values and at the same time produces the least emotional discomfort.

BELIEVING IN A GAP

The language that students use to describe the relationship between theory and practice in nursing contains many of the core images of the orthodox position. Furthermore, in a manner similar to other more experienced participants the metaphors of the conduit and the container, which Lakoff and Johnson (1980) considered central to the process of learning, are also evident:

> I didn't really know that there is theory behind anything. We are just put here by God to do the job. So there is a big difference and a big gap between theory and practice. (Alison a first year student nurse)

> I do need to take all the theory into the practice. (Bernadette, a first year student)

I think that there is a big gap… you're talking about what I know about nursing now from the studies I am doing and what actually happening out there? Yes, I think there is a big gap. (Bernadette, a first year student)

Applying Knowledge and Things Learned Into Practical Situations. (Second Year Student Nurse Focus Group)

Personally for me as a student I like as much theory as I can get before I go out on a placement...and even if I'm not going to be using it all on placement at least I've got a good base knowledge. (Pauline, a third year student)

It is clear from these extracts that the relationship between theory and practice in nursing can only be expressed by using the language that is associated with the notions of the orthodox position. In both sets of data collection two key notions surfaced effortlessly and without encouragement. Those notions are that theory is an object found in one location and taken to another location to be stored and processed for later use. Those locations are held to be very different and separated by a physical space.

The widespread presence of the orthodox position came as no surprise and added significant weight to the observation that the orthodox position is both widespread and axiomatic within the nursing profession. However, with particular reference to the contributions of students from the first year three important additional comments are made.

One, in the absence of any practicum experience, this category of student readily uses images derived from the orthodox position. This confirms that linguistic, objectivist, Cartesian and experientialist influences are forces that shape the thinking of student nurses in advance of any practicum experience. Two, the firm belief in the principles of the orthodox position influences the confidence that the first year students express in the relevance of theory in practical contexts even before they are exposed to practicum. Three, in addition to the conventional notions contained in the orthodox position, student nurses also hold very strong personal beliefs about the nature of both nurses and nursing care before they experience a practicum. When the data from first year students and the second and third year student is incorporated into the study, it confirms that the subsequent experiences that students have during an undergraduate programme reinforces rather than weakens their belief in a gap between theory and practice.

PRECONCEPTIONS AND PERSONAL VALUES

In the absence of any formal study of nursing, two categories of informal experience from public rather than professional ideas of nursing combine to provide student nurses with insights into the work of nurses and the qualities that nurses possess. The first category of experience is the personal contact that each student has with nurses or nursing care. The second category is the exposure that students have to the popular representations of nurses in the mass media.

Personal Experience

In respect of the personal contact that students have with registered nurses the students from the second and third years of the programme had undertaken practicum experiences as part of their undergraduate degree. Thus they had come into contact with registered nurses and nursing lecturers. However, of particular interest are the responses of first year students as they recalled occasions of their own experiences of nurses or those of a family member or friend:

My husband has been in hospital recently (Bernadette, a first year student)

Even this morning, I had this blood test (Diane, a first year student)

Probably the practice side would be from what I've seen you know growing up in a family with my mother being a nurse …the way that she probably practices is, I've been into a hospital and seen her working with clients (Fiona, a first year student)

The Popular Representation of Nurses

In addition to personal contact with nurses all of the students said that they watched television programmes or movies which featured nurses. Whilst the impact that the media image of nurses has upon the nursing profession does not form part of this discussion, it is important to point out that nurses; along with police officers, teachers and fire-fighters are members of occupations that are in the public domain. Not only are nurses in the public domain, but nurses and nursing are regularly featured in either documentary or fictional programmes on television and other forms of mass communication. As a consequence representations of the work of nurses are well known to students. The nursing literature has consistently reported that the most common images of nurses in the mass media are those of the handmaiden, the angel of mercy, the battle-axe and the sex-symbol (Gallagher, 1987; Kalisch & Kalisch, 1983; Karpf, 1988; Salvage, 1984). These images of nursing, which have a historical and contemporary reality, persist and are found in the data:

I just thought it is purely practice, practical. That you got taught how to stitch something up and you got taught how to wipe something down. (Margot, a second year student)

She's very kind and open and very relaxed with her clients, and they seem to be very relaxed with her, which is nice. (Fiona, a first year student)

I had a clinical nurse leader lecture me in front of the client. (Third year student nurse focus group)

I just thought it is just women walking around in white coats and looking pretty and assisting people who are ill. (Fiona, a first year student)

The nursing profession usually rejects these popular images of nurses and declares them as inaccurate representations of nurses and nursing (e.g. Fealey, 2004; Meier, 1999; Salvage,

1984). However, it would be difficult to deny that these images are persistent, pervasive and powerful, and that they have provided a source of information about nursing for the general population; the very population from which prospective student nurses are drawn.

When the personal experience of students is combined with commonsense notions of nursing it produces a set of key values that each student associates with professional nurses. Those key values, expressed both implicitly and explicitly in the data, are that nurses are principled people; that nursing is a worthy human activity; and that patients deserve the best care that nurses can provide. These key values are very important to the student and are values that modify learning during the nursing degree and inform personal decisions about the relevance of theory to practice. Personal values also serve another important purpose in that they are the standards against which the students evaluate the formal theory presented to them in their nursing degree, the care that registered nurses offer to patients, the quality of their own nursing care, and the foundations upon which each student extends their knowledge of nursing.

The Influence of Preconceptions in Professional Education

Student nurses hold preconceived ideas about the values of nursing and nursing care, and whether or not those ideas are accurate or converge with professional notions of nursing, is not important. What is important is that student nurses, perhaps even before they begin their nursing degree, develop a personal or private theory of the skills, knowledge and attributes relevant to nursing care. The students accept that at times the formal study of nursing will contradict aspects of their personal experiences. However, as the basis for the values that they associate with nursing work, formal study does not entirely cancel out the impact and influence of personal experience. Personal values emerged frequently in the data and are an enduring feature of the way that student nurses speak about and evaluate the delivery of nursing care.

Personal values, which are central to the process by which student nurses negotiate the relationship between theory and practice, are found to be an important influence in the education of student teachers, and an influence that must not be underestimated (Haney, Czerniak & Lumpe, 2003).

The influence of preconceptions, are one of three important "presage factors" (Biggs, 2003, p. 18) each drawn from personal experience and is demonstrated to be a significant factor in shaping the views and behaviours of students and teachers in respect of how they learned and taught. It is also observed that newly qualified school teachers and student teachers are most likely to select a teaching method or an approach to learning that is proven to be successful during their personal experiences of learning (e.g. Cole & Knowles, 1993; Haney, Czerniak & Lumpe, 2003; Harris, Guthrie, Hobart & Lundberg, 1995; Korthagen & Kessels, 1999; Trigwell & Prosser, 1997). Furthermore, based on their own experiences, teachers often adopted a teaching style that reflected their personal experiences of teaching and learning, and therefore believed that similar approaches to learning would also work the best for the students they taught (Silverman & Casazza, 1996). It is also stated that the performance of experienced teachers is influenced by preconceived notions of teaching and learning and that many teachers functioned without overt reference to educational theories of learning (Eraut, 1994).

The extent to which preconceptions about nurses and nursing has influenced the behaviour of student nurses has received some attention in the nursing literature. In 1993, Andersson was specifically interested in the nature of the preconceptions held by students prior to entering a Swedish nursing programme, and whether those preconceptions altered during the programme. In that study two observations were made which added weight to the importance of preconceptions. One observation was that the preconceptions held by students remained stable throughout the programme. The second was that: "New information offered by the education programme has to 'filter' through perceptions of nursing. Information, knowledge or values, which are not in line with the ideal image of nursing, are rejected or induce perspective transformation" (Andersson, 1993, p. 814). In another study, this time conducted in England, the focus of interest was the interaction between individual preconceptions of nursing, referred to as personal knowledge, and course determined propositional knowledge. The author acknowledged that little is known: "…about how it [personal knowledge] is used to interpret propositional knowledge acquired during students' professional courses" (Spouse, 2000, p. 731). The study reported that some students retained their personal values with more doggedness than others. Further, with an allusion to the relationship between theory and practice in nursing Spouse reported that: "Inevitably interpretative frameworks that students bring to any situation influence their goal achievement. Consequently, beliefs about what nurses do, inform not only their career choice but also the way in which they will engage in it" (Spouse, 2000, p. 737). These references to the significance and persistence of preconceptions supported the observations made in the context of teacher education. Of such preconceptions it was remarked that once established they are very difficult to counter in that: "Preconceptions show a remarkable resistance to traditional attempts to change them" (Korthagen & Kessels, 1999, p. 5).

Preconceptions and Constructivism

Historically, the normative professional curriculum, which usually forms the framework for professional education including that of nurses, had scant regard for the private or personal knowledge held by aspirant professionals (Peters, 2000). If any form of prior knowledge is valued it is usually knowledge of a propositional nature such as those academic subjects deemed relevant to the demands of the traditional academic curriculum (Eraut, 1994). As a consequence the personal knowledge held by student nurses in respect of nurses and nursing is most likely to be viewed as unimportant or at best evidence that the general public is misinformed of the true nature of nursing work (Meier, 1999). For educationalists to disregard the personal theories that students held about the nature of nursing runs counter to a central tenet of constructivist approaches to learning, for which it is considered that the past experiences of the learner are important in the construction of prospective learning experiences (Colliver, 2000; Lesh, Doerr, Carmona & Hjalmarson, 2003; Peters 2000). Constructivism, which is closely associated with the ideas of Dewey, Piaget, Vygotsky, and more recently von Glaserfield (e.g. Begg, 2000; Fox, 2001; Henson, 2003; Peters, 2000). Peters, a nurse educationalist, suggested for the education of nurses the constructivist approach to learning presented a range of possibilities in that:

...prior knowledge influences what new or modified knowledge they will construct from new learning experiences. The learning process is an active one. Learners challenge their comprehension as a result of new learning encounters. If what learners encounter is inconsistent with their current comprehension, their comprehension can be changed (Peters, 2000, p. 167).

EXPERIENCING DIFFERENT THEORY

The core personal values of each student is the axis around which their acceptance or rejection of the validity of different forms of theory to which they are exposed in the undergraduate programme is negotiated. Over the three years of a nursing degree students have a number of learning experiences during which they are introduced to the possibility that there are different forms of theory relevant to nursing care. Those learning experiences are classroom-based formal learning experiences, clinically-based learning experiences in patient care contexts, and learning that is derived from informal personal experiences. The first form of theory to which students are exposed is formal theory, the influence and importance of which is underlined by the definitions of theory found in the data from my study. These are definitions that overwhelmingly associate theory with formal or propositional knowledge:

> The 'book' based part of the learning with no practical hands on of the subject, just reading and assignments to gain learning. (Third year student nurse focus group)

Negotiating Formal Theory

In common with other forms of education that prepare students to enter a profession, nursing education is structured in accordance with the principles of a normative professional curriculum. The normative professional curriculum is usually organised so that the first form of theory to which students are exposed is formal theory (Agryis & Schön, 1989; Benner, 1984; Carr, 1995; Eraut, 1994). Thus from the day that the student nurse starts a nursing programme, formal or propositional theory, associated with textbooks, classrooms and lecturers, forms the basis of their programme. Given the status, power and tradition of formal theory in all forms of higher education, it is not surprising that the students value and trust formal theory. Furthermore, those students who had no practicum experiences express a higher level of trust in both formal theory and the teaching and learning resources associated with formal theory.

In my study all of the students initially learn practical skills under the supervision of nursing lecturers in a classroom designated as the *Skills Laboratory*. The purpose-built *Skills Laboratory* is a simulated nursing environment which uses equipment such as beds, wash basins and a selection of other technical apparatus similar to those found in a hospital ward. In many ways the *Skills Laboratory* looks and feels like a hospital ward except that key human features such as clinical nurses, other health professionals and of course patients, are missing. The students learn how to perform nursing skills by practising on each other or on commercially produced mannequins. Simulation supported by propositional knowledge is, in the absence of learning drawn from practicum experiences, regarded by the students as an important and reliable source of learning:

> It's quite interesting... I suppose we all need to start at the very beginning and be taught properly I suppose. (Fiona, a first year student)

> You have got to have the theory first. I feel ...to a certain extent obviously you've got to have basic knowledge before you can go out and do your practice otherwise you're not going to be safe ... it gives you a background to what you need to do it's quite important. (Catherine, a first year student)

However, it should not be construed that the knowledge associated with textbooks, classrooms and other artefacts of formal education is fixed in that:

> It is an illusion that there is knowledge in books or documents. They contain language, which is a string of words, deposited in them by authors. The words have meaning for the author and the readers and interpreters, each one of whom has built up her subjective meanings according to her individual experiences (Von Glaserfield, 1993, p. 30).

The view held by Von Glaserfield is important as it regards formal knowledge, in particular formal knowledge that may underpin practical nursing skills, as subject to interpretation. However, it is not a perspective that is shared by all of the nursing lecturers. The nursing lecturers are more likely to conclude that there is one correct way to perform nursing care, and that is the way that the student is taught in the classroom:

> Students may be taught a skill [in the classroom] and it will be the right way, they go to clinical and see it performed completely different and sometimes completely wrong. They will come back to class and repeat what they have learned because the 'clinician did it that way, it must be right'. Which shows me, that what I teach is not as important to what they see. (Nurse Lecturer focus group)

With respect to the validity of types of theory other than formal theory, the above response from a nursing lecturer suggests that the actions of educationalists contribute to the power and primacy of formal theory in an undergraduate nursing degree. The structure of the undergraduate degree means that for students in their first year of study, formal theory is the only theory to which they are exposed, and the only theory which is made explicit. Therefore, from the outset only formal theory is afforded authority and legitimacy, thus by default nursing lecturers reinforce the hierarchy of knowledge present in the conventional curricula of professional education (Schön, 1987), namely a hierarchy of knowledge in which propositional knowledge is generally regarded by nurse academics as the most important form of knowledge for nurses in the care of patients.

As a precursor to the execution of practical skills, the primacy of formal knowledge is also reinforced by the way in which students learn and practice hands-on nursing in the simulated environment of the *Skills Laboratory*. One of the important qualities of the *Skills Laboratory* is that it provides an emotionally and physically safe environment for the students to learn and practice skills under the guidance of a lecturer. If a student makes mistakes whilst learning, no actual or potential harm is caused to patients. However, despite the 'role-play' nature of learning in the *Skills Laboratory* the students consider it is important to perform practical skills correctly:

> It [simulation] is all quite entertaining. But it does make it, almost makes it, feel that it's not until we get go out do out and actually do some practicum out on the ward. Something like that it's actually going to put it together properly it's not going to completely fall into place I don't think, until then. (Fiona, a first year student)

The students know that they want more than simulated practical nursing skills from a nursing course. And whilst simulation is considered a very important form of learning, it is valued only as forerunner to learning and applying those skills in the clinical environment. The opportunity that an upcoming practicum presents to learn nursing in the actual clinical area is a prospect mixed with a sense of excitement and anticipation:

> I'm looking forward to that [an upcoming practicum] I know its just observation and I am quite happy about that …I'd be quite happy to take a blood pressure or a temperature. But yes I am quite happy just to watch and sort of, I mean I've got expectations of this course but until I really get in to the community and really see the *real stuff* [strong emphasis] you know the how you do it. (Fiona, a first year student)

The desire on the part of students to get out in to a real world, do 'it' and engage in the real work of nursing, or at least the hands-on aspects nursing work is also identified in a discussion amongst the lecturers in the first round of focus groups:

> For some [referring to the students] nursing is a huge mystery in the first year they expect to emulate those on 'Shortland Street' [A New Zealand television soap opera situated in a hospital] and be "doing" they cannot seem to relate many of the first year subjects to nursing at all. We [lecturers] sometimes suffer delusions of grandeur that we teach them [students] nursing assuming they will undertake practice that is appropriate and thoughtful, but what do they want, "the action" cause baby that's where it's at as far as they are concerned. (Nurse Lecturer focus group)

The 'doing', the 'it', and the 'action' are just a few of the shorthand terms that the participants use to refer to what they consider to be the real work of nurses. For students and lecturers the real work of nurses is something that can only be experienced during a practicum outside of the physical boundaries of the college. In a very simple way the notion of separation between theory and practice is reinforced. 'Doing', 'it' and 'action' cannot be simulated and therefore they are notions most usually associated with the hospital and the everyday work of nurses. The 'doing' and the 'action' are also key components not only of learning nursing but also of becoming a person who is a nurse:

> Learning to think like a professional now requires learning to build one's own theory of practice, which in turn requires engaging in situations of practice. Practice must play a central role in the process by which students learn to think like practitioners (Agryis & Schön, 1989, p. 186).

Learning to 'think like a professional' requires that the practitioner draws upon another form of theory; that theory is situational or practical theory, which can only be learned by engaging in patient-centred experiences.

Negotiating Practical Theory

As the programme advances student nurses are increasingly exposed to the actual work of nurses and thus the students learn more and more nursing in the company of experienced registered nurses. Often students observe registered nurses draw upon a form of theory which is determined by factors in the context in which that nursing care is undertaken (Manias, Aitken & Dunning, 2004). This form of theory has been named situational knowledge or practical theory and it is a form of theory that can only be acquired through experience:

"Therefore knowledge development in applied discipline consists of extending practical knowledge [know how] through theory-based scientific investigations and through charting of the existent 'know how' developed through clinical experience in the practice of that discipline (Benner, 1984, p. 2-3).

One student described how a registered nurse employed an injection technique that varied from the technique which she had been taught:

Even this morning I had this blood test and they, the nurse said "You'll be told never to do this, but this is how I do it"...and she and she, then the needle is on an angle as opposed to instead of straight on to the...I'm not sure what it's called...and she said "You'll be told never to do this but this is how we do, I do it because I find it comfortable and I've never had any problems with it". So I thought okay so it really is, it really is the case of how you do it... (Diane, a first year student)

At the time she also noticed that the nurse found it difficult to articulate the reasoning behind her practical theory. This made Diane unsure if practical theory has the same validity as formal theory:

... so I'd say she is taught you know how you do it this way you do it you don't ever do it differently and then she shifted off and did it her own way anyway. So I think that people just do it how they want to [Laughs]... I think a lot of nurses develop how it suits their own way of doing things. (Diane)

Students also refer to specific examples of patient care when they draw upon personal or private theories. The sources of which are the life experiences of each student, which must also include the experiences each had as a student nurse.

Negotiating Private Theory

In the course of their undergraduate degree, student nurses apply their private theories in the delivery of patient care. Such theories are closely related to the key personal values held by each student and private theories are most evident when the students refer to the professional demeanour that they think nurses should exhibit; the interpersonal skills that nurses should employ in patient contexts; and the ethical standards that they expect of nurses:

> They [the nurses] are friendly enough and polite and kind (Bernadette a first year student)

> So people come up to me and tell me you have a nurse's voice when you start doing the blood pressure you start talking like a nurse. (Diane, a first year student)

> You know that you have to do you know what's expected of you, and you know that at the end of the day you have got to make sure everything is in the rightful place, done at the right time, and you can't be laid back and you've got to be really alert and slightly, sort of you don't have a life of your own. [Laughs] (Emma, a first year student)

> You rely on your experience and your knowledge of human patterns and human behaviours and how people will react...and okay sometimes you get it wrong ...but if you've got something that you honestly believe is right then you go with it. (Grace, a first year student)

> So with regards to how you treat someone I think ...you know, if you don't know how to treat another human being like you would be treated you probably shouldn't be a nurse. You might not; you might not last long in the profession. (Fiona, a first year student)

These five illustrations, each selected to support an assertion that student nurses become aware of the existence of different forms of theory are purposely taken from the contributions of the first year students. They demonstrate that even in the very early stages of the programme students are exposed to the possibility that there may be more than one form of theory that guides nursing practice.

For the first year student nurses the origin of their personal theory clearly lies in their life experiences:

> I actually over the years I have picked up quite a few life skills ... being a supervisor of a conference centre and dealing with people I know that a lot of staff liked working with me because I is very empathetic towards their needs. (Emma, a first year student)

> I is in the bank [referring to a previous job] and... I is a teller and you could only spend so much time with a person and if they are asking you questions that you couldn't answer then you passed them on because you had to keep that queue going and it sort of kind of the same in nursing, ... It's just the way you treat people [Laughing]. (Fiona, a first year student)

However for the second and third year students, it is unclear if the origin of personal theory each employs in patient contexts is from their social or recent educational experiences. However, what is clear is that as the students progress in their nursing programme, their interpersonal interactions with patients are influenced by personal theories:

> Just chatting with the patients, spending a little more time than the least possible. Just a few more moments when talking with them changes them and their attitude towards you. (Second year student nurse focus group)

Spending time with an elderly man who did not want to leave hospital and having him open up to me that his wife bullied him and he is scared to go home. Not sure why he chose me. (Third year student nurse focus group)

In the process of learning to become a professional nurse the combination of the private theory acquired from life's experiences, the practical theory acquired as a student nurse and the key values held by each student produces a very influential force. It is a force that is a major determinant of the way the student perceives the relevance and appropriateness of theory in practical situations:

As I've experienced it the relationship between theory and practice sometimes interact with each other but sometimes commonsense comes in first.

… It is commonsense that got me through [rather] than theory. Does that make sense? (Helen, a third year student)

Peter Gallagher. Do you want to tell me more about commonsense?

Helen….[extended pause]… It's like your actions; you do without even reading your book like you know all about safety and all the rest of it so you wouldn't need to go to a book to know what's in safe practice and that. Does that yes, answer your question?

As student nurses engage in longer periods of practicum, they increase their own experience of nursing and also observe registered nurses care for patients in the real world of nursing. As a consequence, the students become more aware that in common with the registered nurses they frequently employ forms of theory other than formal theory. Moreover, as the theories that emerge from practice are of a holistic nature they can not be explained in the same terms as formal theory in that contextualised theory:

… Is seen as an embodied, reflexive process of responsive action. As such theorizing involves tuning in to and critically considering bodily sensing, intuitive and emotional responses, existing theories and research, contextual forces, and so forth. These responses are seen as forms of knowing that can in-form and re-form our in-the moment actions, that is to say, theoretical practice (Hartrick Doane & Varcoe, 2005, p. 83).

EXPERIENCING DIFFERENT PRACTICE

Once the students are exposed to their first practicum they encounter a number of experiences that gradually erode their confidence in the primacy of formal theory. Those experiences relate to occasions when they observe or carry out nursing care for which it appears there is no single correct way of performing nursing care. The first of these experiences is the realisation that formal theory is only one of a number of different standards to which the student is expected to perform; and it is a realisation that is present even before the student engages in practicum:

I realised that theory is not identical to how you will be practising out there in the real world. The theory is sort of idealistic. Whereas what you're doing in practice ..., means, you have to work differently with different people in different situations. (Diane, a first year student)

The second and third year student nurses know in advance of each practicum that they will have to perform differently to meet different expectations. They also know that having to meet different expectations rather than a single prescribed standard of nursing care is important in that it contributes to success during a practicum. The following expectations frequently surfaced in the data:

1. The clinical team
2. The nurse lecturer
3. The patient or client
4. The mandatory course requirements
5. The personal and private expectations of each student

Negotiating Expectations

The students soon discover that during a practicum if they want to be regarded as part of the clinical nursing team, they must conform to the unspoken expectations and values of that particular nursing team (Cahill, 1996; Melia, 1984; Swain, Pufahl & Williamson, 2003):

We are put in a position where we're nursing, young, beginning practitioners and we're out of [name of college] for two, three weeks at a time. You run the risk, I feel, of either alienating yourself from the staff or being a know-it-all that no-one wants to help... (Norah, a second year student)

The students also find out that success during a practicum is ensured if they meet the individual expectations of the nursing lecturer who works alongside, and perhaps more importantly assesses the student during a practicum:

Different lecturers have different styles, do it one way: WRONG. [The participant used upper case to add emphasis to this word]. Change it [The way I do things] for new lecturer; WRONG. (Second year student nurse focus group)

Another expectation of practicum, one that is that valued highly by students is the feedback that they receive from patients:

It is nice to hear from a patient leaving, that they wish you well for the future and tell you that you will make a good nurse. It is sad that only patients say this usually, but it can be argued that they are the ones we deal with so perhaps their opinion is the most important. (Third year student nurse focus group)

In addition to these three sets of informal expectations in order to pass a practicum the student also has to meet the compulsory requirements of educational assessment:

... I suppose it's just getting signed off really is the very final result. (Catherine, a first year student)

Practice is going out into the hospital, community or where ever and trying to learn things as well as doing assignments, learning objectives and attempting to pass the placement. (Third year student nurse focus group)

The final and no less important set of expectations are the individual expectations that each student has of their own performance in the care of patients. This is a set of expectations that very closely relates to the personal values that each student nurse holds about the nature of nursing:

I'd let myself down...because I didn't act professionally. I mean, I didn't do the best in my practice. (Irene, a third year student)

The students are fully aware that it is in their best interests to meet different expectations. They also knew that inconsistent performance to different and at times fickle standards is a necessary and frustrating part of the practicum:

As students, in one placement we are told by a lecturer we had to do them [complete patient assessment documentation]. However, the ward staff told us the opposite - in fact demanded that they not be done in that format. (Third year student nurse focus group)

I felt that [the name of college] and clinical [the name of the practicum placement] each wanted different things from us and we are puppets. You are constantly changing the way you do things from what you know they should be done like, to how you know the person assessing you or precepting [A neologism that alludes to the preceptor] you wants it done, so that you can pass. (Third year student nurse focus group)

For student nurses the attempt to meet different expectations produces unsettling and dissonant feelings which are associated with the application of theory in practical contexts. Furthermore, those feelings are compounded by circumstances when the student notices obvious differences between the theory and the practice of nursing.

Noticing Differences

There are circumstances when students become acutely aware of differences between the theories they are taught and the practice that they perform or observe. Those circumstances can be grouped as four categories of experience. The first category is those occasions when the student deems that theory is correct and that some registered nurses choose to ignore that theory:

Their [the registered nurses] practice is not matching what I am learning and experiencing ... and the respect that you give to people and the way that we're told you know...do no harm and they are not treating him as a human being. They we're treating him as "Oh he's slightly demented and he's incontinent. So therefore we are not going to pay that much attention to his care". (Margot, a second year student)

The second category is those circumstances when formal theory appears correct but does not provide an explanation for aspects of nursing care for which contextual features are a significant factor:

They [the registered nurses] explained, that they [the patient] gets the surgery and all that. But they could not explain one situation and what happened afterwards didn't quite match up as such...When it came to the care and everything else it didn't quite - the person, the signs, and the [pause] symptoms. The signs and the symptoms and everything else isn't quite what they had said. It is quite contradictory, what... the way we had to deal with the patient. (Kevin, a second year student)

The third category relates to situations when the students consider that the formal theory presented to them in the classroom is idealistic or unrealistic:

But in actual fact when something is done differently in reality. We kind of, well I is left wondering whether we are perhaps being taught , of course are being taught the ideal here [in the college], but I do sometimes step back and wonder if the ideal can actually be practiced or is it a bit airy fairy. (Leah, a second year student)

What is taught in theory is usually from a fantasy world where everything is done a particular way. Once out in the REAL world, things are done differently. Nurses do daily tasks completely different from the way taught in theory, so it requires more learning, and the student is left wondering what is the use in attending theory anyway? (Third year student nurse focus group)

And a final category is the circumstances when the student realises that the process by which formal theory is applied to a practical situation is not always a methodical or premeditated process. Instead, both the student and experienced practitioners perform nursing care which at the time is thought to be correct and appropriate. It is usually only afterwards, when they reflect upon the performance, that the student reviews the suitability or otherwise of an intervention:

I didn't ask the right questions yet I knew later on that I should have done this and done that. (Irene a third year student)

So I still have those memories of what I should have done what I perhaps should have said or how I should have approached the nurse, but I didn't. (Leah a second year student)

Or do you do whatever you feel is right. (Norah a second year student)

We sometimes suffer delusions of grandeur that we teach them nursing assuming they will undertake practice that is appropriate and thoughtful. (Nurse Lecturer focus group)

In each of the above categories the awareness that there is a difference between theory and practice in nursing is always accompanied by an emotional response:

I found that there is so much going on that I was thinking of the first 50 things that I should do instead of the very first thing! It took another colleague walking into the room and saying

"How many joules are you charging the defibrillator for?" For me to FOCUS and do what I is supposed to DO!!!!!! yikes!!!!!! (Registered Nurse focus group

The emotions conveyed by this illustration from an experienced registered nurse are of a quite different quality than those emotions expressed by student nurses. The difference is highlighted in the range of responses from a discussion amongst students who were asked to recall how they felt when theory and practice did not align:

Crap.
Pissed off.
What the hell are they teaching us?
Incompetent and doubting myself.
Inadequate.
Incompetent, useless and a failure.
Out of my depth and out of control, isolated with no where to turn.
What's the point of this am I ever going to be good enough.
(Third year student nurse focus group)

When they perceive a difference between theory and practice, the discomfort students feel results from the tension between the experience that brings about that perception, and the key personal values that each student holds about the nature of nursing. The tension generates intrapersonal conflict which is produced when an individual is faced with a clash between two sets of values (Huber, 1996; Marquis & Huston, 1998). Privately the students compare the experience with their key personal values. If there is close alignment between the two, then no disruptive emotions are produced and the student has no reason to question the quality of the nursing care they witness. However, if the experience appears to present an overt or covert challenge to the substance of their personal values, the dissonance is experienced as intrapersonal conflict: an uncomfortable experience that it had to be addressed. For the students learning from practical contexts is an experience in which actions, thoughts and emotions are inseparable in that: "Knowledge depends upon being in a world that is inseparable from our bodies, our language and our social history - in short embodiment" (Varela, Thompson, & Rosch, 1997, p. 149).

For the students, the emotional responses that accompany practical experiences form an integral and inseparable component of their learning. However, the more unsettling feelings also contribute to the total experience of dissonance and are therefore a very powerful experiential reinforcement that there is a real difference between the theory and the practice of nursing. In the moment that the students experience dissonance they not only think that there is a difference between theory and practice in nursing: they also sense that difference.

NEGOTIATING DIFFERENCES

For students of nursing the practicum is a very powerful class of experiential learning which engages their whole person (Beard & Wilson, 2002; Kolb, 1984). In experiential learning, emotions form a central part of learning and the disruptive emotions that accompany the experience of a gap between theory and practice are a sentient reinforcement for each student of the instability that exists between theory and practice in nursing. In order to deal with the conflict the student has to choose between a number of courses of action; each of which will challenge their efforts to maintain one or all of their personal values, and will either increase or decrease their emotional discomfort.

The first course of action, or rather inaction, is for the student to do nothing and say nothing. The student is highly conscious that they have to complete their nursing degree, and to reduce the possibility that they may be penalised for challenging the practice of a registered nurse they choose not to point out to those concerned the differences between the theory and the practice that they observe:

> I felt that my ideals will wait until I am registered. I will go with the flow to get through.
> (Second year student nurse focus group)

If they select this particular course of action the student knows that they have silently colluded with poor practice or inadequate theory. By not speaking out the student behaves in a manner that is in dispute with their own personal values. And when the student reflects upon the incident, they regret their inaction. Furthermore, the student knows that to remain silent may contribute to success, but silence also increases the intensity and extends beyond the practicum, the timescale of the emotional discomfort felt by the student. Another course of action is for the student to blame others for the experience and thereby transfer negative feelings to their lecturers, the registered nurses, other student nurses or classroom based-learning experiences. The student then dislikes or mistrusts those who are considered responsible for the negative feelings. The transfer of blame is an act that also preserves personal values. If a student nurse realises that the difference between theory and practice is of their own making, and that they have personally failed to live up to their own set of values they doubt their ability as a future professional, which in turn has an impact on their self-esteem. A less common course of action is for the student to approach those associated with the uncomfortable feelings; to confront those people, and seek the rationale behind the behaviour that they observed. This is a course of action that poses a direct challenge to the authority of others and thus increases the immediate emotional discomfort for the student. However, it is also a course of action that preserves the integrity of the student's personal values. In one interview Margot recalls how upset she felt when she saw nurses care for a patient in a manner that fell far short of her personal values. I asked Margot to tell me about her experience:

P.G: What is the end result for you?

Margot: For me? I don't know. A bit of jadedness crept in. I became a bit hardened. I went in there a little fluffy bunny. A brand new bouncy student and came out thinking great [pronounced ironically] the real world sucks [laughs] and [pause]... It made me think about what I would do differently.

In all of the learning experiences that produce intrapersonal conflict it is evident that the personal values of each student are the standards against which nursing care is evaluated. The attempt to resolve intrapersonal conflict, retain personal values and at the same time alleviate uncomfortable feelings is a complex balancing act during which the student searches for a satisfactory explanation of the differences between theory and practice. In that search, the personal values are the focal point around which each student negotiates a satisfactory explanation.

To recap, those values are: that nursing is a worthy occupation; that nurses always behave morally, and that patients always receive the best possible care. So just how do student nurses rationalise the differences they perceive between the theory and the practice of nursing?

Explaining Differences

In an effort to explain the difference between theory and practice, a number of explanations are available to the student. However, all but one of those explanations erodes one or all of the key values held by the student nurse.

The first explanation is that the knowledge base of either the registered nurse or the student nurse is of an unacceptable or unsatisfactory standard and for the student it follows that the person concerned is unfit to be a nurse. A second explanation is that the registered nurses who perform so poorly do so because they had a lower standard of professional education than the student. A third explanation is that the registered nurses are jaded or disillusioned after many years of nursing work. A fourth explanation is that historically the working environment for nursing has been under resourced. A fifth explanation is that some registered nurses, in full knowledge that they are carrying out inappropriate care, choose to cynically disregard formal theory. A sixth explanation is that the theory taught or present in textbooks is either outdated or unrealistic in the context of the real world of the clinical setting. Each of the above explanations presents a challenge to the integrity of key values held about nurses and nursing.

However, one possible explanation for the difference that students experience is contained in the orthodox position. That explanation is that there are two nursing worlds, one a world of theory and the other a world of practice, separated by a conceptual gap. This is an explanation that contains a notion of inevitability and thus it offers the least threat to personal values, it is emotionally neutral, and it is an explanation that is widely understood by the rest of the nursing profession.

THE IMPLICATIONS AND SOME LESSONS FOR NURSING EDUCATION

The theory that emerged from this study complements the orthodox position, in that it is a theory which acknowledges that there are a variety of features in the educational environment that contribute to the emotional discomfort experienced by students, and that those features require attention. Contextual features, important for effective learning, are conceptualised by Hall and Kidman as: "A relational map of teaching and learning", of which the: "The central core of the map is the interface between the students, the content of the course (paper or module), and the teacher. These are the cornerstones of any formal teaching-learning context (Hall & Kidman, 2004, p. 332). A simple way to understand how 'Negotiating Different Experiences' complements other educational initiatives in nursing education designed to improve the relationship between theory and practice, is to think of 'Negotiating Different

Experiences' in terms of the container and conduit metaphors (Lakoff & Johnson, 1980), for which there are two containers and multiple conduits. The first container holds the knowledge required for practice, and the second container is the student nurse. The conduits are the various educational strategies, such as those that enhance the roles of lecturers and clinicians, the design and sequencing of formal subject matter, each of which is devised to improve the ability of student nurses to apply that knowledge in a practical context. It is important to emphasise that 'Negotiating Different Experiences' does not propose educators should ignore contextual features that contribute to learning. Rather, it is a theory that advises nurse educators to afford the same degree of attention to the ways that students learn nursing as is afforded to the conditions in which that learning takes place.

In addition, and perhaps more importantly, 'Negotiating Different Experiences' also identifies that the experience of bringing together theory and practice in nursing is a holistic experience for which the individual characteristics of each student are a very significant component. The idiosyncratic nature of the experience of dissonance holds some important lessons for improving the way in which students learn how to apply theory in practical contexts. Those lessons are that nurse educators should make a number of changes to undergraduate nursing programmes. The modifications required will not need wholesale revision of curricula and will not compromise the ability of students to meet the prescribed competencies set by the professional bodies that award registration. The specific changes that can be made concern individual rather than collective approaches to learning, the forms of theory relevant to nursing care, the nature of practical assessment, and the role of emotions in learning. It is those adjustments to nursing programmes that will be discussed in this concluding section.

INDIVIDUAL RATHER THAN COLLECTIVE APPROACHES TO LEARNING

Students may be taught a skill and it will be the right way, they go to clinical and see it performed completely different and sometimes completely wrong, they will come back to class and repeat what they have learnt because the 'clinician did it that way, it must be right' Which shows me that what I teach is not as important to what they see. (Nurse Lecturer focus group)

A nursing degree in New Zealand, in common with nursing programmes in other countries, must ensure that at the end of the programme student nurses meet predetermined professional competencies. How those competencies are interpreted and the detail of each programme is a matter for each educational institution. Most usually the prescribed professional competencies are subsumed in the overall aim of a programme, before being broken down into a number of learning outcomes which are often expressed in behavioural terms. The learning outcomes are then used as the building blocks of a nursing programme for which the orthodox notions of input, process and output generally shape programme design and delivery. In this form of curriculum delivery the students, the teacher, and the subject matter are usually timetabled to a set location for predetermined periods of time. For the practical purposes of teaching each student nurse is a member of a cohort that comprises other students who enrolled at the same time. The maximum size of each cohort is usually determined by the physical and human resources of the tertiary institution at which the nursing programme is offered.

This approach mirrors other forms of professional education for which the focus of teaching and learning is the perceived need of a group, rather than the individuals who make up that group. Thus each student is expected to learn subjects that educators determine relevant, in a manner that educators consider to be the most effective, and in a sequence that educators also hold to be the most suitable. These principles are common objectivist principles that pervade many forms of conventional education. The following observation made about the role of educators in the design of curricula for the formal schooling of children over thirty years ago are as valid when applied to the contemporary context of nursing education:

> They [educators] arrange the material in some order of increasing complexity, an order usually thought of as the "natural" or "normal" way to approach the subject. They decide what minimum amount of knowledge will be acceptable. They decide on a schedule, the time periods in which the student is to learn particular batches of material (Becker, 1972, p. 92).

More specifically, for student nurses the key components of their programme are determined in advance with little, if any, consideration for their previous experience and knowledge of nursing. Furthermore, the overall design of the nursing programme is such that formal or propositional knowledge is presented to students in advance of each of their practicum experiences. This is a pattern of teaching and learning that conforms to the principles of the normative professional curriculum. Within the culture of academia it is considered that there is a hierarchy of knowledge, of which applied knowledge has the lowest status (Agyris & Schön, 1987; Eraut, 1994; Schön, 1987). The normative professional curriculum also contends that the student will best learn in practical contexts if they are guided by knowledge framed in objectivist terms: "The university based schools of the professions... have assumed that academic research yields useful professional knowledge and that the professional knowledge taught in the schools prepares students for the demands of real-world practice" (Schön, 1987, p. 9-10).

At the time that I conducted my study the Nursing Council of New Zealand mandated that fifty percent of an undergraduate nursing programme must take place in practical settings (NCNZ, 2001:2004). Therefore, a significant portion of the learning that occurs for student nurses is by definition experiential in nature. For the nursing students who participated in my study the majority of practicum experience takes place in the second and third years of their programme. Thus the shape and pattern of the nursing programme reinforces to students the importance of formal or propositional knowledge in advance of practical experience whereby groups of students are 'allegedly' prepared for each practicum in advance of that practicum. However, based upon the data from my study the effectiveness of attempts to prepared students for practicum in a collective rather than an individual manner is limited for the following reasons.

First, when the complexity and variety of experiences that each student encounters during a practicum are permutated, it would be very difficult for educators to claim that it is possible to prepare students collectively for what is a definitively individual practicum experience. Second, any preparation for practicum based upon propositional knowledge or simulated practice does not take sufficient account of the holistic nature of the practicum as a form of experiential learning in that: "Knowledge does not exist solely in books, mathematical formulas, or philosophical systems; it requires active learners to interact with, interpret, and elaborate these symbols" (Kolb, 1984, p. 121). It is self-evident that two central components of learning that can not be authentically simulated in the classroom are the emotions that students experience when they learn in the real world of nursing, and the immediate reflections that practicum experiences generate. A third reason why preparing students for practicum collectively is flawed is that the individual knowledge and experience of each student are ignored by collective approaches to the preparation of students for practicum learning. Therefore for nurse educators to continue to design nursing programmes based upon the key principles of the orthodox position, in which collective and standardised approaches to teaching, learning and assessment predominated, is founded on an erroneous premise.

Recommendation

My first recommendation concerns an educational principle that should underpin a programme for nurses, for which I propose the emerging theory of enactivism. Enactivism builds upon and extends constructivism, whilst also explaining non-cognitive knowing, intuition and the role of emotions in learning (Fenwick, 2001). The holistic nature of practical learning, so evident in my data supports the enactivist perspective for which the focus of learning is: "Not on the "learning event" and its components (which other perspectives might describe in fragmented terms: person, experience, tools, community and activity) but on the *relationships* binding them together in complex systems" (Fenwick, 2001, p. 248).

There are a number of reasons why enactivism dovetails with the data generated by my study. The first of which is that enactivism supports the experience of the participants in that the learning that eventuates from practical contexts is a process by which the student is wholly engaged and has an active rather than a passive role:

> But for me I know that if you're left to do it your own way you don't do it exactly as the textbook tells you. You learn to do it how you feel comfortable. (Diane, a first year student)

The second is that for students their knowledge, is formed or enacted by experience and as such that knowledge is invented or devised as consequence of their total experiences rather than discovered from an existing fixed reality:

> Practice is what one does in order to get a desired outcome. We may be aware or unaware of the theoretical base of those practices if we do them out of habit. Practice does not imply thoughtful practice. (Nurse Lecturer focus group)

And finally, in the enactivist perspective of learning, the learner makes sense of the world based upon previous and concurrent experiences of that world and uses those experiences to address new challenges and solve new problems:

> I think it goes on instinct and just knowing and feeling comfortable about yourself and your role is, and how you practice. (Third year student nurse focus group)

By suggesting that nurse educators adopt an overtly enactivist approach to learning I am not proposing that student nurses should be left to their own devices and engage in unstructured practicum learning experiences. On the contrary, student nurses must be enabled to feel confident that what they experience is very important and is valued by nurse educationalists. In order to achieve that goal the following should be introduced to the nursing programme:

- The personal values of the student nurse must be respected, valued and a formal way must be found to incorporate personal values into a nursing programme;
- The sources of private, practical and formal knowledge should be made clear to the students so that they can distinguish more clearly between different forms of knowledge;
- Alternative approaches to the assessment of practice, which are less reliant on third party observation should be devised;
- The important role that emotions play in learning during a practicum should be optimised.

THE IMPORTANCE OF PERSONAL EXPERIENCE

A focus on personal growth and development and a better understanding of who we are in relation to our nursing practice. (Nurse Lecturer focus group)

In the context of nursing education the student must not be regarded as tabula rasa, a blank canvas upon which the essential qualities of professional nursing can be pasted. It is clear from my study that the individual characteristics of each student are important features that modify and mediate all forms of learning. The personal characteristics of each student are as equally important as those contextual features found in the care settings in which practical learning occurs. Nursing Educators must put aside some of the orthodox conventions so prevalent in many forms of professional education and openly acknowledge that all students have extensive and varied life experiences. In addition, nurse educators should ensure that the individual experience and personal characteristics of each student receive significant focus when a nursing programme is planned. The basis of the conventional professional curriculum, established on orthodox principles, should be reviewed and the starting point for learning the personal experiences of the student which must be regarded as valid and incorporated into the programme.

It is evident that before students engage in practical experiences and probably even before they enrol on a nursing programme they are exposed to many aspects of nursing and health care. More importantly, that exposure not only forms the basis of their understanding of nursing but is also confirms that students have clear preconceptions of the skills, knowledge and attitudes required by nurses. These are core values, which along with other values are strongly held, but are by no means fixed, which is illustrated by the following extract taken from an interview with Alison:

Actually to begin with I thought that there is no theory in nursing. To me nursing is more of a practical hands on job, way of life. So the theory is a bit of a slap across the wrist for me. I didn't really know that there is theory behind anything. We are just put here by God to do the job. So there is a big difference and a big gap between theory and practice. (Alison, a first year student)

In this extract Alison offers her personal interpretation of how she will 'learn to become a nurse'. However, she also expresses surprise when very early in the programme she realises that one of her preconceptions—the depth of study required by nurses— is not borne out by her experience as a student nurse. It could be argued that her beliefs contain naive and idealised notions of professional nursing, and that those innocent aspects of her beliefs will ultimately be dispelled by the reality of nursing work. However, for nurse educationalists what is of greater general significance than the detail of Alison's' preconceptions is that such preconceptions are very, very important and the personal values they contain influence many aspects of learning during the time spent as a student of nursing and beyond into professional practice (Korthagen & Kessels, 1999; Spouse, 2000). In other forms of education it is established that the personal knowledge held by students is a strong influence that mediates learning (Belenky, Clinchy, Goldberger & Tarule, 1986). Yet, it appears that in the design and delivery of an undergraduate nursing curriculum it is generally assumed that amongst student nurses, ignorance of the nursing profession and nursing care is the lowest common denominator:

There will be people coming in to us that have had absolutely no…They've got no idea about nursing or maybe they haven't come from a nursing background and I suppose we all need to start at the very beginning and be taught properly I suppose. (Emma, a first year student)

And even if the views held by students are found to be inaccurate perspectives, they are perspectives that must be respected, and should be used as the basis to debunk any false notions students hold. To assume that student nurses know nothing or at best very little about professional nursing is unacceptable to the students. Further, it is an assumption that makes the student believe that they are being patronised:

Tried to generate discussion on topic and seek assistance and is talked over and disregarded - made to feel like an idiot whilst being talked to like a baby!!!!. (Third year student nurse focus group)

The illustrations that students provided of those occasions when interpersonal skills are the focus of nursing interventions there are clear examples of the application of skills and knowledge that is drawn from theory of a personal rather than a formal nature

The interpersonal relationship that nurses develop with others is both explicit and implicit in nursing, and has been considered the single-most feature that distinguishes nurses from other health care professionals (Peplau, 1991). The untutored and unique interpersonal qualities of each student are very important as they form the basis of each student's professional nursing skills, knowledge and attitudes. The importance of prior experience to the clinical practice of nursing students is illustrated by the strong influence that personal experience has on the development of the interpersonal skills student nurses employ in the care of patients.

I've been care giving for about 30 odd years, with time off for bus driving but you know, you rely on your experience and your knowledge of human patterns and human behaviours and how people will react. (Grace, a first year student)

Nursing is a human social activity that arises out of the tendency of humans to nurture and care for each other, and as with any other social action, nursing has to be learned. Professional nursing however, is a social action that has been constructed as an occupation and one important feature of nursing which is shared with other occupations such as teaching and social work is that they all require highly skilled interpersonal relationships with other humans.

Recommendation

In order that student nurses are enabled to gain a greater understanding of the relationship between the theory and practice of nursing, educators should develop nursing programmes which openly acknowledge, respect, and value personal experience. This means that each student must be involved in the design of their own individualised programme, which must also be constructed so that the personal experiences and personal values of each student can be optimised. One way that personal experiences and values can be optimised is to ensure that from the outset of an educational programme each student is obliged to maintain a personal journal which is used to trace their personal understanding of nursing from naïve preconceptions to professional awareness. In conjunction with the entries made in that journal, significant time should be allocated for regular, open and supported discussions so that students may share their preconceptions and personal values with other students. In addition to these initiatives, and within the constraints of a programme driven by professional competencies, significant time should be allocated on the timetable for students to determine their own learning needs. And to facilitate individualised learning some of the subject driven content of nursing programmes should be replaced by learning experiences that enable students to engage in personal development. I suggest that established models of clinical supervision (Butterworth, Faugier & Burnard, 1998; Hawkins & Shohet, 2000; Morton-Cooper & Palmer, 1994; Van Ooijen, 2003), prevalent in many of the helping professions including nursing, should become a core component of an undergraduate nursing degree.

THE NEED TO DIFFERENTIATE BETWEEN DIFFERENT FORMS OF THEORY

There is usually some theory why we do things even if it is 'because we've always done it this way'. Every time someone thinks about their practice, reflects upon it, asks why they do it they are theorising.

'Wisdom' is not always relevant to theory -- the exploration of others' wisdom can increase awareness of theory -- critical evaluation and interpretation of theory. (Nurse Lecturer focus group)

The second lesson for nursing education arises from the perception that the dissimilarity between different forms of theory, which is wrongly interpreted by students as a conflict between the sources of theory, not as a possibility that there may be other alternative and complementary sources of theory.

However, in the educational culture of nursing education the desire to meet the requirements of the awarding body with respect to curriculum content means that the content of nursing programmes takes precedence over the processes by which nursing is learned in that: "Truth or reality is restricted to the context applicable to the event under consideration, recognising that no theory or knowledge of nature should be understood as final" (Good, Wandersee & St Julien, 1993, p. 80).

The nursing lecturers, who participated in my study, whilst aware of the existence of knowledge sources other than formal or propositional knowledge, did not generally share their awareness with student nurses in any formalised way. In fact, the inability of student nurses to discriminate between the personal, practical or formal theory that registered nurses draw upon in the conduct of nursing care, is a feature that makes a major contribution to the perception of dissonance. In the absence of a clear explication of the different forms of theory available to registered nurses, students resort to the most readily available explanation provided by the orthodox position. Namely, that there is a gap between the theory and the practice of nursing, and that theory and practice are experiences of a very different kind. The ease with which the students attribute the difference between theory and practice to the existence of a gap in lieu of other explanations is illustrated by the following four examples.

Irene, on being asked to recall an illustration of a gap between theory and practice, selects an occasion when she realises that her assessment of a patient's health status is inadequate:

> When I went home that night I actually got into my books and I looked up what septicaemia is what the signs and symptoms … and what I is to look for and how it is to be treated and so the next time it happens I'm going to know. (Irene, a third year student)

In this example, the theory is correct and the practice would have been correct if Irene had known the relevant theory at the time. In short, there is no gap between theory and practice; contextual factors prevented Irene from applying the relevant theory. Irene concedes that it is her formal knowledge base that is deficient; it is formal theory to which Irene turns in an effort to resolve her discomfort.

In another example Bernadette perceives a gap between theory and practice when she notices that the nurse who cares for her husband does not adhere to some basic theoretical principles associated with hygiene:

> She hasn't washed her hands and yet she came straight in from heavens knows where and is handling equipment and him [her husband] and that is one of the first things we we're taught. When you go into a clinical setting environment wash your hands between patients. (Bernadette, a first year student)

In this illustration, the nurse in question deliberately chose to disregard formal theory and behaves inappropriately. For this situation there is ample theory available to draw upon that is both accurate and relevant. The omission on the part of the nurses is intentional, and it cannot be construed that because the nurse ignores formal theory that there is a gap between the theory and her practice. Experienced practitioners are often faced with situations in which they draw upon theory which develops as a result of their experience (Benner, 1984). In a focus group one registered nurse provides an illustration of how the care of a dying patient is influenced by private theory:

> I watched a man meet eternity, and all I did is let him be with his family. This is never in a book or research project, and I have no idea why what we did worked. It might not for another client, or at another time... It is luck...grace. (Registered nurse focus group)

In a fourth example, an experienced nurse uses practical theory which has emerged from personal clinical experience as the rationale for an nursing intervention:

> There is a theory that some clients in the mental health setting need to be nursed in a "de-stimulated setting" because it is thought that their internal thought processes being chaotic combined with a highly stimulated setting makes things worse. My experience is that often it makes things worse, imagine being alone with your confused, disorganised thoughts. In my practice, careful management of the environment the person is in and helping them manage the impact is the thing to do. (Registered nurse focus group)

The basis of the practical or situational theory is often difficult to articulate, as it is a form of theory that may have derived from experiences that are either personal or professional in origin. Although they did not use the terms practical theory and private theory, Chenitz and Swanson (1984) allude to those notions when they argue that: "the detailed descriptions and explanations of nursing process are...submerged in practice" (p. 206). To surface those explanations they considered that a change to theory generation is required whereby: "...attention to theory development is given to generation of theory through analysis of data systematically collected from observations of nursing as it occurs" (Chenitz & Swanson, 1984, p. 208).

Recommendation

Students will only be able to make the distinction between the different forms of theory that experienced practitioners use in practical contexts if they understand that there are different forms of theory in the first instance. Furthermore, students will only consider different forms of theory as valid, if the validity of those forms of theory is made explicit to them, and if each different form of theory is equally weighted in terms of importance. The ability to differentiate forms of theory will be only heightened if from the outset of their pre-registration programme the epistemology and validity of those theories is made clear. If students understand that there are other explanations for the apparent differences in nursing interventions they will be better equipped to explore the reasoning behind those nursing interventions. If the targets outlined above are to be achieved; then from the outset a nursing programme must include a discrete component of learning that makes the epistemology of the different forms of theory explicit. That component should be threaded throughout the programme as the student encounters more and more contexts in which different forms of theory are surfaced. Furthermore, when students raise concerns about the differences that they perceive between theory and practice, those concerns should be addressed in an atmosphere which is free from any apportion of blame.

THE ROLE OF ASSESSMENT IN PRACTICUM

I agree it takes time to integrate theory into practice and for some subjects this integration may be a few years down the track. (Nurse Lecturer focus group)

At the time that my study was conducted the awarding body in New Zealand had an expectation that most student nurses would complete their nursing degree within three years of their first enrolment. In addition there was a prescribed a minimum time scale of 1500 hours, during which it was expected that student nurses would gain practical experience in seven discrete clinical contexts. The timescale in which a programme must be completed and the variety of placements directly influence the structure of an undergraduate nursing programme. These are two factors that contribute to a powerful illusion that it is possible to learn the knowledge, attitudes and skills central to nursing practice in a manner that is somehow controlled, tallied and assessed in a linear and logical manner for which: "Learning is presumed cumulative and knowledge incremental" (Brew, 1993, p. 87). Evidence to support the presence of these essentially objectivist principles; which are central to the orthodox position are found in many aspects of undergraduate nursing programmes. What is of a particular interest in the context of my study is the influence of being formally assessed has on the ability of student nurses to apply theory in practical contexts.

Over the course of the three years of their degree, the population of student nurses pursue a programme in which they are allocated to separate practicum placements and in which the competence of each student is summatively assessed. In order to assess competence, nursing interventions, including those of a holistic nature are dissected into observable external behaviours considered amenable to description and measurement. To be judged successful in a practical assessment the student is expected to either demonstrate a range of practical skills to a third-party, or alternatively offer an oral or written explanation. The regular and frequent summative assessment of students during a programme raises concerns as to the educational purpose and educational relevance of assessment during a practicum (Rowntree, 1987). Whilst I acknowledge that the practicum has many purposes I believe that the primary educational purpose of the practicum is to provide students with the opportunity to learn nursing in the clinical setting. For many students the multiple challenge presented by having to conform to the work place culture, learn new topics, consolidate previous learning and appreciate the application of theoretical principles in practice, is an unreasonable target to achieve in a relatively short period of time:

Practice is going out into the hospital, community or where ever and trying to learn things as well as doing assignments, learning objectives and attempting to pass the placement. (Third year student nurse focus group)

The frequency and intensity of assessment means that in order to pass a placement some students compromise other aspects of clinically-based learning. Such compromises mean that the opportunity to gain a more complete understanding of the relationship between theory and practice is missed. It is noted that the learning that eventuates from merely wanting to be successful is more likely to be of a superficial nature than of a deep nature (Marton & Saljö, 1997). For nursing education, the ability to understand the relationship between theory and practice in nursing requires that the student makes links between different notions and concepts. This form of understanding is one that requires learning at a deep rather than superficial level (Hillier, 2002). Furthermore, it is noted that assessment invariably detracts from deep learning as the student only learns that which they need to know in order to pass (Biggs, 2003; Hillier, 2002).

Traditional forms of practice–based assessment place a high level of confidence in the close relationship between explanation and understanding. For example, if a student is required to demonstrate that they can effectively counsel a patient, that student might be asked to explain the psychological principles associated with the concept of counselling. However, this would only provide insight into the ability of a student to recall theory and would not provide adequate evidence of the student's ability to relate theory to a practical situation. A student nurse who is studying counselling theory might be able to recall the theory associated with being an active listener, understand how to phrase questions, how to encourage the speaker to continue, and how to bring about timely closure. However, that student whilst achieving high academic grades in counselling theory might not be able to demonstrate the application of counselling theory in a practical situation. The ability to demonstrate or explain should not be construed as confirmation of synergy between thought and action or the ability of the individual to be able to link theory with practice:

> A third difference between knowing by apprehension and by comprehension is most critical for our understanding of the nature of knowledge and its relationship to learning from experience. Apprehension of experience is a personal subjective process that cannot be known by others except by the communications to them of the comprehensions that we use to describe our immediate experience (Kolb, 1984, p. 105).

In addition, the ability to perform competently does not always mean that a person can articulate the relevant theoretical explanations (Sandelands, 1991; Wittgenstein, 1953). In practical forms of assessment the student will only perform to the level that they need to perform in order to pass the particular assessment. What happens before and after the assessment might or might not be differ but it will almost certainly be a different type of performance (Biggs, 2003). Finally, the assessment of practice is a subjective act, and it is an act of observation in which the observer is as much part of the activity as the observer and that which is observed (Maturana, 1987).

The traditional ways in which student nurses are assessed are based upon the principles of the orthodox position. These are principles that pervade many aspects of the design of the conventional professional curriculum, and they contrast with more constructivist notions of learning in which the student is regarded as an active participant in their own learning. When student nurses learn in a workplace they make their own choice of what will be learned in that: "He need not, when he wants learn a certain procedure wait until its time in a prearranged schedule; nor need he learn something he is not ready for, thinks uninteresting, frightening or unnecessary. The learner makes his own curriculum" (Becker, 1972, p. 99). It is evident in the data that in practical settings, student nurse intentionally select that which they learn. By the same token it follows that students should be equally as able to select that which will be assessed, the frequency by which they will be assessed, and the means by which they should be assessed.

Recommendation

In relation to the purpose and process of assessment, the role of assessment during the practicum should be re-examined and the following important considerations incorporated in to the specific methods by which practical nursing is assessed.

First, the practicum must be viewed primarily as a learning experience and because regular and frequent summative assessment serves to increase anxiety, and the fear associated with failure appears to distract from any learning. Therefore, summative assessment conducted whilst the student is still in the process of learning, should be kept to a minimum or even discarded altogether. Anxiety and fear are negative emotions that impact upon deep learning, which in turn contribute to the experience of dissonance between theory and practice. Therefore, unilaterally lecturer determined success criteria should not form the basis of assessment. Instead when nurse educators devise methods to assess the practice of student nurses they must involve the student as an active partner. This means that, not withstanding the mandatory requirements of formal assessment, the individual student should be more involved in the selection of a range of assessment of methods and determine the timing of an assessment.

THE IMPORTANCE OF EMOTIONS IN LEARNING

> We often confront students at a vulnerable time and place and make them feel silly--we need to establish a safe space for learning and acknowledging gaps in knowledge (Nurse Lecturer focus group)

The practicum does not take place in a simulated environment, it occurs in locations in which nurse's work and thus like other aspirant health professionals the student:

> ... Learns on the job, in a place where people do in a routine way whatever members of his trade do. He finds himself (sic) surrounded from the outset by the characteristic sights, sounds, situations, activities and problems he will face if he remains in the trade (Becker, 1972, p. 98).

For student nurses, the practicum is an authentic form of experiential learning, a form of learning in which: "…individuals have, or are given in the teaching and learning process, a direct or simulated encounter with the external world" (Jarvis, Holford, & Griffin, 2003, p. 55). As experiential learning is a holistic experience, student nurses not only learn the knowledge and skills essential to nursing; they also learn how to become a nurse:

> …as everybody starting work soon realizes, there is a world of difference between abstract knowledge in books and the practical knowledge required for, and acquired in everyday

experience-between reading what to do, seeing others do it, and doing it for yourself (Dey,1999, p. 101).

For the contemporary student nurse in New Zealand the practicum is in many ways a more well-ordered learning experience than was the case in an era when student nurses were apprentice employees. However, there continue to be many similarities between these two periods of our nursing history. The most noticeable of which are that both sets of students learn from their exposure to the real work of nursing, are exposed to other health professionals, and most importantly both engage in the care of actual patients.

When combined these three factors constitute a very powerful form of experiential learning, for which emotions are not merely adjuncts to learning. Quite simply, emotions are a central component of the total learning experience (Benner, Tanner & Chesla, 1996; McClelland, Dahlberg, & Plihal, 2002). If students can be assisted to understand how to utilise emotions; those emotions will only serve to benefit rather than detract from their learning. In my view emotional responses should not be viewed as a barrier to learning. Instead they should be utilised in a manner similar to the way a registered nurse moves from advanced beginner to competent practitioner, a process in which:

> Emotional responses are no longer characterized by diffuse or global anxiety. Instead competent nurses' emotional responses to a situation now give them better access to what is happening to the patient. Emotions in practice thus begin to be a screening or alerting process rather than a perceptual impediment or block (Benner, Tanner & Chesla, 1996, p. 88-89).

In the more structured learning environment of an educational institution, when educators, including nursing educators, facilitate experiential learning they should to take significant steps to ensure that any strongly felt emotions evoked during a formal learning experience are used to maximise learning (Brackenreg, 2004). Those who facilitate experiential learning consider that some emotions are so powerful that they could remain long after the intended learning has been facilitated. Should such an occurrence arise the skilled facilitator usually ensures that potentially negative emotions are dissipated by using debriefing exercises before closing the session (Brackenreg, 2004; Morrison & Burnard, 1997; Heron, 1992).

However, for student nurses the experiential learning that eventuates as a direct result of a practicum is not subject to the same degree of control as forms of experiential learning that occur in a classroom or simulated environment. In the clinical setting major incidents such as the sudden and unexpected death of a patient or a violent incident are events that are usually followed by a post-incident debriefing session. However, most of the time, potentially uncomfortable learning experiences, such as those that the students recalled in my study, are unnoticed by the clinical team and the opportunity for students to talk about those experiences is more likely to be in an informal setting:

> There is nowhere to go to vent your feelings while on placement except to each other, if you try to talk to the lecturer you are scared of failing. (Third year student nurse focus group)

> [I] usually discuss with other students at lunch time and [we] have a big bitch session. (Third year student nurse focus group)

Furthermore, in the clinical setting it is unlikely that the relatively mundane event in which a student nurse perceives a gap between theory and practice is of sufficient concern to warrant any extended discussion amongst the clinical team. However, the student nurses encounter a number of experiences during a practicum that contribute to the intensity of emotions that students feel whilst attempting to learn.

The first of those experiences is the possibility that by not performing correctly or by failing to take any action the student may cause physical or emotional harm to patients:

> I had a student who thought she had broken the bounds of safe practice when she responded to the hug of an elderly woman (Nurse Lecturer focus group)

A second important experience that contributes to the emotions felt by the student is the sense that one's performance is constantly being observed or tested, and of particular note are those experiences of being observed associated with formal assessment:

> Each lecturer has a different method and states that their method is the one and only correctly researched based method and that it should only be done that way. Thus students are constantly trying to learn each lecturer's requirements so that they can perform this way for that lecturer. (Third year student nurse focus group)

The third experience that stirs strong emotions during the practicum relate to the desire of the student to be part of the clinical team:

> I challenged an awful lot of people and I rocked that boat. And being in nursing as a student rocking the boat is terrible [Her intonation indicated a high level of discomfort]. (Margot a second year student)

However, in the orthodox position the emotions associated with learning to apply theory in practical contexts are afforded less attention than other aspects of learning. To consider the relationship between theory and practice in solely Cartesian terms, for which mind, body, and feelings are separate, is to render the relationship as an emotionally neutral experience. The Cartesian conceptualisation is one that contrasts sharply with the data from my study, in which the relationship between thoughts and actions is a holistic experience. And as a consequence it is an experience in which the perception of dissonance between theory and practice is highly emotionally charged.

Recommendation

As the process of learning to apply theory in practical contexts is an experience that always involves emotions, educators must clearly acknowledge the importance of emotions in learning and provide the student with ample opportunity for intra - practicum and post - practicum debriefing. In most circumstances emotions should be used as a catalyst that enhances learning, as opposed to the notion that students should disguise or repress emotions. For that to be successful, the process of learning from experience requires an opportunity for the student to engage in structured reflection (Beard & Wilson, 2002; Kolb, 1984). With specific reference to the assessment of practice, the role the educator during a practicum should be one that focuses less on assessment and more on guidance and support (Severinsson, 1998; Spouse, 2001).

The theory, 'Negotiating Different Experiences', contends that the emotions associated with the perception of a gap between theory and practice are more than a product of that perception. Instead the emotions are part of the dissonance. Therefore if the unpleasant emotional content of dissonance is reduced, then the perception of a gap between theory and practice would correspondingly be reduced. The student nurse should be enabled to facilitate reflection for which a number of strategies including: learning circles (Hiebert, 1996); reliving practicum experiences in the form of educationally focused drama (Ekebergh, Lepp & Dahlberg, 2004) or clinical supervision (Severinsson, 1998; Spouse, 2001) are recommended strategies. As a consequence of reflection, the student will be in a better position to appreciate the rationale behind nursing interventions that previously they perceived as based upon inappropriate theory or interventions that had no theoretical basis at all. Therefore, as nursing educators strive to enhance the relationship between theory and practice, they should seek to lessen the frequency and intensity of those events which produce the negative emotions that students associate with the experience of dissonance and maximise the positive emotions that accompany learning.

CONCLUSION

The data for this study was gathered from the students, lecturers and clinicians who formed part of the population of one specific educational site, and over a specific period of time in the history of nursing education in New Zealand. As such the data and the subsequent analysis of that data are a reflection of the perceptions of those, and only those, who chose to participate in this study. However, with the above caveat firmly in mind, the undergraduate nursing degree and the experiences of student nurses in this study bear many similarities to other nursing programmes in New Zealand and other countries in the western world.

The degree of relevance of the lessons and recommendations that arise from my study should be conceived as a series of concentric circles, at the core of which is the lessons that emerged from this study. In the outer circles are the populations for whom the theory has relevance. The closer the population is to the core; the more direct is the relevance of 'Negotiating Different Experiences'.

The circle nearest the core contains those who participated in this study, and the next circle the students and educational staff at the site at which the study was conducted. As the circles move further away from the core, the next two circles are the system of nursing education in New Zealand and the systems of nursing education systems in other western countries respectively. In the most outer circle are other forms of vocational education for which it is acknowledged that students experience similar problems in attempting to understand the relationship between theory and practice in their respective disciplines.

In the orthodox position it is argued that in general, nurses believe that the gap between theory and practice is an inevitable and undesirable by-product of the process of learning to assimilate concepts from two separate domains of experience. However, this study has demonstrated that any failure to align theory and practice did not lie exclusively in factors that are external to the student. In this study a complementary analysis of that experience has shown that the personal biography of each student is also an intimate part of the process of learning to apply theory in practical contexts. Therefore, the recommendations from the lessons contained in this chapter advise that the primary focus for educators should be the individual student and not the external environment in which the student learns. As these recommendations concern the ways in which nursing is learned, they are recommendations that can be introduced to nursing education without the need for an extensive reorganisation of a curriculum. Instead educators can continue to develop and introduce educational innovations focused on external factors whilst at the same time attending to the process by which individual students learn to apply theory in practical contexts.

REFERENCES

Agryis, C., & Schön, D, A. (1989). *Theory in practice: Increasing professional effectiveness.* San Francisco: Jossey Bass Ltd

Andersson, E. P. (1993). The perspective of student nurses and their perceptions of professional nursing during their nurse training programme. *Journal of Advanced Nursing, 18*(5), 808-815.

Beard, C., & Wilson, J. P. (2002). *The power of experiential learning: A handbook for trainers and educators.* London: Kogan Page.

Becker, H., S. (1972). School is a lousy place to learn. In B.Geer (Ed.), *Learning to work* (pp. 89-109). Beverly Hills: Sage.

Begg, A. (2001). Enactivism: A personal interpretation. Retrieved October 12, 2001, from http//ioe.stir.ac.uk/docs/Begg%20Enactivism%20.DOC

Belenky, M. F., Clinchy, B. M., Goldberger, N. F., & Tarule, J. M. (1986).*Women's ways of knowing: The development of self, voice and mind.* New York: BasicBooks, Incorporated.

Benner, P. (1984). *From novice to expert: Excellence and power in clinical nursing practice.* Menlo Park, CA: Addison-Wesley.

Benner, P., Tanner, C. A., & Chesla, C. A. (1996). *Expertise in nursing practice: Caring, clinical judgment, and ethics.* New York: Springer Publishing Company.

Biggs, J. B. (2003). *Teaching for quality learning at university: What the student does.* (2nd ed.). Philadelphia, P.A.: Society for Research into Higher Education and Open University Press.

Brackenreg, J. (2004). Issues in reflection and debriefing: How nurse educators structure experiential activities. *Nurse Education in Practice, 4*(4), 264-270.

Brew, A. (1993). Unlearning experiences. In D. Boud., C. Cohen., & D. Walker. (Eds.), *Using experience for learning* (pp. 87-98). Buckingham, United Kingdom: The Open University Press.

Butterworth, T., Faugier, J., & Burnard, P. (1998). *Clinical supervision and mentorship in nursing.* Cheltenham, U.K.: Stanley Thornes.

Cahill, H. A. (1996). A qualitative analysis of student nurses' experiences of mentorship. *Journal of Advanced Nursing, 24*(4), 791-799.

Carper, B. A. (1978). Fundamental patterns of knowing in nursing. *Advances in Nursing Science, 1*(1), 13-23.

Carr, W. (1995). *For education: Towards critical educational inquiry*. Buckingham, England: Open University Press.

Chenitz, W. D., & Swanson, J. M. (1984). Surfacing nursing process: A method for generating nursing theory from practice. *Journal of Advanced Nursing, 9*(7), 205-215.

Cole, A.L., & Knowles, J.G. (1993). Shattered images: Understanding expectations and realities of field experiences. *Teaching & Teacher Education 9*(5/6), 457-471.

Colliver, J, A. (2002). Constructivism: The view of knowledge that ended philosophy or a theory of learning and instruction? *Teaching and Learning in Medicine, 14*(1), 49-51.

Dey, I. (1999). Grounding grounded theory: Guidelines for qualitative enquiry. San Diego: Academic Press.

Ekebergh, M., Lepp. M. , & Dahlberg, K. (2004). Reflective learning with drama in nursing education a Swedish attempt to overcome the theory praxis gap. *Nurse Education Today, 24*(4), 622-628.

Eraut, M. (1994). *Developing professional knowledge and competence*. London: The Falmer Press.

Fealey, G., M. (2004). 'The good nurse': Visions and values in images of the nurse. *Journal of Advanced Nursing, 46*(6), 649-757.

Fenwick, T. J. (2001). Work knowing "on the fly": Enterprise cultures and co-emergent epistemology. *Studies in Continuing Education, 23*(2), 243-258.

Fox, R. (2001). Constructivism examined. *Oxford Review of Education, 27*(1), 23-35.

Gallagher, P. (1987). Media image of nursing, *Nursing, 3*(18), 674-676.

Gallagher, P. (2003). Re-thinking the theory practice relationship in nursing: An alternative perspective, *Contemporary Nurse, 14*(2), 205-210.

Glaser, B. G., & Strauss, A, L. (1967). *The discovery of grounded theory: Strategies for qualitative research*. Chicago: Aldine Publishing Company.

Good, R. J., Wandersee, J. H., & St Julien, J. (1993). Cautionary notes on the appeal of the new "Ism" constructivism in science education. In K. Tobin (Ed.), *The practice of constructivism in science education* (pp. 71-87).Hillsdale, New Jersey: Erlbaum Associates.

Hall, C., & Kidman, J. (2002). Teaching and learning: Mapping the contextual influences. *International Education Journal, 5(3)*, 331-343.

Haney, J.J, Lumpe, A.T., & Czerniak, C.M. (2003). Constructivist beliefs about the science classroom learning environment: Perspectives form teachers, administrators, community members, and students. *School Science and Mathematics 103*(8) 366-376.

Harris, R., Guthrie, H., Hobart, B., & Lundberg, D. (1995). *Competency-based education and training: Between a rock and a whirlpool*. Melbourne: Macmillan Education.

Hartrick Doane, G., & Varcoe, C. (2005). Towards compassionate action: pragmatism and the inseparability of theory/practice. *Advances in Nursing Science, 28*(1), 81-90.

Hawkins, P., & Shohet, R. (2000). *Supervision in the helping professions: An individual, group and organizational approach*. Buckingham, (England): Open University Press.

Henson, K. (2003). Foundations for learner-centred education: A knowledge base. *Education, 124*(1), 5-16.

Heron, J. (1999). *The complete facilitator's handbook*. London: Kogan Page.

Hiebert, J. L. (1996). Learning circles: A strategy for clinical practicum. *Nurse Educator, 21*(3), 37–42.

Hillier, Y. (2002). *Reflective teaching in further and adult education*. London: Continuum.

Huber, D. (1996). *Leadership and nursing care management*. Philadelphia: WB Saunders.

Jarvis, P., Holford, J., & Griffin, C. (2003). *The theory and practice of learning.* (2nd Edition). London: Routledge Falmer.

Kalisch, P. A., & Kalisch, B. E. (1983). *The media image of the nurse.* New York: Springer Press.

Karpf, A. (1988). *Doctoring the media: The reporting of health and medicine.* London: Routledge.

Kolb, D. A. (1984). *Experiential learning: Experience as the source of learning and development.* New Jersey: Prentice–Hall.

Korthagen, F.A. & J., Kessels, J.P.A. (1999). Linking theory and Practice: Changing the pedagogy of teacher education *Educational Researcher 28*(4), 4-17.

Lakoff, G., & Johnson, M. (1980). *Metaphors we live by.* Chicago: The University of Chicago Press.

Lesh, R., Doerr, H. M., Carmona, G., Hjalmarson, M. (2003). Beyond constructivism. *Mathematical Thinking and Learning, 5*(2 & 3), 211-233.

Marquis, B. l., & Huston, C. J. (1998). *Management and decision making for nurses: 124 case studies.* Philadelphia: Lippincott.

Manias, E., Aitken, R., & Dunning, T. (2004). Decision-making models used by 'graduate nurses' managing patients' medications. *Journal of Advanced Nursing, 47*(3), 270-278.

Marton, F., & Saljo, R. (1997). Approaches to learning. In F, Marton, D. Hounsell, & N.J. Entwhistle (Eds.), *The experience of learning* (pp. 39-58). Edinburgh :Scottish Academic Press.

McClelland, J., Dalhlberg, K., & Plihal, J. (2002). Learning in the ivory tower. *College Teaching, 50*(1), 4-8.

McCutheon, H. H. I., & Pincombe, J. (2001). Intuition: An important tool in the practice of nursing. *Journal of Advanced Nursing, 35*(3), 342-348.

Maturana, H. R. (1987). Everything said is said by an observer. In W. Thompson (Ed.), *Gaia: a way of knowing* (pp. 37-47). New York: Lindisfarne Press.

Meier, E. (1999). The image of a nurse—myth vs. reality. *Nursing Economic$, 17*(5), 273-276.

Melia, K. (1987). *Learning and working: the occupational socialisation of nurses.* London: Tavistock Press.

Moccia, P. (1992). Reconceptualising the environment. In P. Moccia (Ed.), *New approaches to theory development* (pp. 23-37), New York: National League for Nursing.

Morrison, P., & Burnard, P. (1997). *Caring and communication: Facilitators' manual.* (2nd Ed.). London: Macmillan Press Ltd.

Morton-Cooper, A., & Palmer, A. (1994). *Mentoring preceptorship and clinical supervision: A guide to professional roles in clinical practice.* Oxford: Blackwell Science.

Nursing Council of New Zealand. (2001/2004). *Nursing schools/departments handbook for pre-registration nursing programmes.* Wellington: Author.

Peplau, H. (1991). *Interpersonal relations in nursing: A conceptual frame of reference for psychodynamic nursing.* New York: Springer.

Perry, M. A. (2000). Reflections on intuition and expertise. *Journal of Clinical Nursing, 9*(1), 137-145.

Peters, M. (2000). Does constructivist epistemology have a place in nurse education? *Journal of Nursing Education, 39*(4), 166-171.

Rowntree, D. (1987). *Assessing students: How shall we know them?* New Jersey: Kogan Page.

Salvage, J. (1985). *The politics of nursing*. London: Heinemann Nursing.

Sandelands, L. (1991). What is so practical about theory? *Journal of Social Behaviour, 20*(3), 235-262.

Schön, D. (1987). *Educating the reflective practitioner.* San Francisco: Josey-Bass.

Severinsson, E. I. (1998). Bridging the gap between theory and practice: A supervision programme for nursing students. *Journal of Advanced Nursing, 27*(6), 1269-1277.

Silverman, S. L., & Casazza, M. E. (1996). *Learning and Development: Making connections to enhance teaching.* San Francisco: Jossey-Bass.

Spouse, J. (2000). An impossible dream? Images of nursing held by pre-registration students and their effect on sustaining motivation to become nurses. *Journal of Advanced Nursing, 32*(3), 730-739.

Spouse, J. (2001). Bridging theory and practice in the supervisory relationship: A socio-cultural perspective. *Journal of Advanced Nursing, 33*(4), 512-522.

Swain, J., Pufhal, E., & Williamson, G. R. (2003). Do they practise what we teach? A survey of manual handling practice amongst student nurses. *Journal of Clinical Nursing, 12*(2), 297-306.

Trigwell, K., & Prosser, M. (1997). Towards an understanding of individual acts of teaching and learning. *Higher Education Research & development 16*(2), 241-252.

Van Ooijen, E. (2003). *Clinical supervision* made easy*: The three step method.* Edinburgh: Churchill Livingston.

Varela, F. J., Thompson, E., & Rosch, E. (1997). *The embodied mind: Cognitive science and human experience.* Cambridge Massachusetts: The MIT Press

Von Glaserfield, E. (1993).Questions and answers about radical constructivism. In K. Tobin. (Ed), *The practice of constructivism in science education* (pp. 23-38). Hillsdale, New Jersey: Lawrence Erlbaum Associates.

In: Nursing Education Challenges in the 21st Century
Editor: Leana E. Callara, pp. 153-170
ISBN 1-60021-661-7
© 2008 Nova Science Publishers, Inc.

Chapter 5

TEACHING AND ASSESSING INTERPERSONAL SKILLS IN MENTAL HEALTH NURSING: WHY AND HOW DO WE NEED TO INVOLVE SERVICE USERS?

Jon Perry and Sue Linsley

Faculty of Health and Social Work,
University of Plymouth,
Earl Richards Road North, Exeter,
Devon EX2 6AS, United Kingdom

ABSTRACT

This chapter focuses on the idea that the development of mental health nursing as a profession in the United Kingdom depends on the strength of our ability to train our students interpersonally to a high level. The chapter gives the historical context of the development of a therapeutically active role for mental health nurses since the 1940s and the end of the asylum system. It goes on to argue that the development of interpersonal skills and the values and attitudes that are required for their effective use is essential if mental health nursing is to meet the challenges of this new role. Further background is given covering the social and political forces that have led to the development of mental health service user movement since the 1970s hospital scandals. We go on to discuss why these factors have impacted on the unique nature and development of mental health nursing as a profession, and user involvement as a political and social force.

The chapter puts forward a definition of interpersonal skills as the point of delivery for nursing care, reviews the literature on service user involvement in interpersonal skills training and assessment across medical and nursing professions and provide a commentary on and direction for nursing research and curriculum development in this area as developed by the authors.

"The words we choose matter, and will serve either to perpetuate the problem or resolve it" (Hulme 1999 p176).

INTRODUCTION

This chapter sets out to chart both the historical development and contemporary influences shaping the teaching of interpersonal skills in mental health nursing. It puts forward the view that three key influences have shaped the need for nurses with effective interpersonal skills, and the style of interpersonal skills teaching required to satisfy this need. Firstly, social and political changes since the 1800's in the United Kingdom (U.K.) saw the growth of humane treatment for mental illness, the rise and fall of the asylum system, the birth of the NHS and the growth of community based care for mental health problems. This has created the need for a large flexible, responsive and economically viable nursing workforce. Similar processes were experienced in the United States (U.S.) where an asylum system expanded in response to a call for humane treatment and was eventually dismantled in response to the post war deinstitutionalisation movement. This movement highlighted inhumane treatment and conditions and pressure for cuts in expensive social welfare programmes in the 1980s. The consequent development of U.S. mental health nursing has followed a simlar course, though U.S. nursing theory is more developed than in the U.K., particularly regarding theraputic interpersonal interactions (Silverstein 2006) and U.S. authors have been influential in developing U.K. nursing theory (Tilley 1999). This chapter will chart these developments in the U.K. and will draw on a wide body of literature in making an argument for a user involved approach to teaching interpersonal skills. A second theme is the growth of public empowerment and consumerism in the health arena, most specifically the growth of the service user movement in mental health which has added pressure for this workforce to offer both human qualities and specific clinical skills (Department of Health 2006b). Lastly debates within mental health nursing as to its proper purpose have developed in the post war period as nursing evolved and continues to evolve as a profession. This debate appears to find common ground in the need for skilful interactions with clients, varying mostly in debating the emphasis it places on the different determinants of mental illness. The chapter will also set out a direction for the teaching of interpersonal skills designed around the involvement of service users. We view this type of involvement as the single most important contemporary development in mental health nursing education. We have developed and will set out an approach to such involvement which seeks to synthesise and implement existing best practice in both interpersonal skills teaching and service user involvement.

WHAT ARE INTERPERSONAL SKILLS?

Within the literature definitions of the terms communication and interpersonal skills have considerable overlap and are frequently used interchangeably (Brereton 1995). Some authors make a distinction between interpersonal and communication skills (Duffy et al. 2004). They define communication skills as the performing of specific tasks and behaviours and interpersonal skills as focusing on the process of forming and maintaining relationships and monitoring and responding to the effect of communication on others. This definition views interpersonal skills as being of a higher order than communication skills. These higher order skills were described at the Kalamazoo II conference on assessment of medical communication and interpersonal skills as "humanistic qualities" required to form and maintain therapeutic relationships (Mangione 2002; Duffy et al. 2004). A useful working definition of interpersonal skills is that these skills are used to reach a goal in collaboration with another person within the context of a helping relationship (Cormack 1985). This would require the helper to deploy the main components of such skill which have been described as "appropriate   knowledge…behavioural   skills…positive   attitude…availability   of opportunity"(Brereton 1995). Hargie and Dickson emphasis both the macro skills involved in social encounters such as mutual respect for rights and the elements of a skilled performance involving the formulation of goals and implementation of actions to achieve them, linked to an iterative process of monitoring goals and actions and adjusting them in response to outcomes (Hargie et al. 2004). A comprehensive and detailed definition of interpersonal skills can be achieved by combining the definitions discussed above using the definition set out at the Kalamazoo conference as a framework (Duffy et al. 2004) (see table 1 below).

Table 1. Elements defining interpersonal skills
(Cormack 1985; Hargie *et al.* 1996; Duffy *et al.* 2004)

- Respect for the rights of the client[1] and yourself
- Mindfulness - being personally present and responsive in the moment without pre-judgment
- Purpose – Having a therapeutic goal in mind and working toward this in a respectful and mindful manner
- Paying attention to the client using open verbal, nonverbal, and intuitive communication
- A focus on the importance of the relationship
- Having a caring intent, not only to relieve suffering but also to be curious and interested in the client's ideas, values, and concerns
- Flexibility or the ability to monitor the relationship in real time and adjust actions as necessary.

THE EMERGENCE OF MENTAL HEALTH NURSING

The central feature of this definition is that it combines learnt skills with values and attitudes which can only be obtained by exposure to expertise derived from experience of having been a client. In the United Kingdom recent policy and advice has made it clear that it is the combination of the application of learnt skills and values that provides the foundation of an effective approach to gaining competent interpersonal skills (Nursing and Midwifery Council 2004 ; Department of Health 2006a; Department of Health 2006b). Within mental health nursing education we now have the opportunity to offer a style of service user[2] involvement that can genuinely meet the challenge set by these documents and by the needs

---

[1]:the term client is used to indicate an individual in a helping interaction who is receiving help.
[2] the term service user is used to indicate an individual who has experienced mental illness and has expertise in service use which can be used in training and education.

of our clients. This has become possible because of a process of social and political change over a period of some two hundred and fifty years of mental health care. How then did we get to this point, what were these influences and how did they impact on the development of mental health nursing?

From William Tuke, Quaker philanthropist to Hildegard Peplau the mother of modern mental health nursing, interpersonal skills have been placed at the heart of the nurse's role. Tuke introduced 'moral therapy' as a response to the inhuman conditions he witnessed at the York Asylum in the late 1700's. He highlighted the role of what were then known as attendants to the insane, viewing their interactions with their charges as being a powerful influence in returning the insane to a 'moral path'. As we will see later in this chapter Peplau has been one of the most influential thinkers in mental health nursing in the post war period, and placed interpersonal skills at the heart of her model for nursing.

The history of mental health nursing in the UK is one of evolution away from a role as "doctors' helper" and "patient's keeper" that existed within the asylum based system of psychiatric care which prospered between the world wars. Asylums have been described as a requirement of a developing industrial society in which it was economically convenient to remove those who were unproductive. Nurses (still called attendants at this time) within the asylum system were largely involved in the smooth running and maintenance of status quo within these institutions, which in many cases were self sustaining communities that offered little effective treatment or therapy. Pressures on mental health services brought about by the Second World War led to shortages of medical staff and a growth in mental illness. This growth was due in no small part to returning service personnel with post traumatic disorders. Ironically this had the effect, to an extent, of allowing nurses to become more involved as practitioners in their own right, rather than the purveyors of medical clinical decision making.

Mental health nursing as we now recognise it began to emerge in the UK in the post war period. As nurses were given increasing responsibility for therapeutic involvement with their patients, beyond the traditional roles of the attendant in an asylum, some began the work of creating and defining a mental health nursing profession based upon interpersonal skill. Two such nurses were Annie Altschul (Nolan 1999) and Hildegard Peplau (Barker 1999) who worked with returning soldiers at Army mental hospitals in London.

Annie Altschul was an Austrian refugee in England during the Second World War who had become disenchanted with the rigidity of general nurse training and practice and consequently, chose to train as a psychiatric nurse at Mill Hill, part of the Maudsley Hospital specialising in the treatment of mental illness in the armed forces. Altschul was greatly influenced by the collaborative approach adopted at Mill Hill. She went on to have a very influential career becoming principal tutor at the Maudsley and promoting the skills of understanding and promoting human relationships as an essential component of psychiatric nursing (Nolan 1999). In so doing Altschul did a great deal to raise the profile of Hildegard Peplau and the significance of her seminal work, "Interpersonal relations in nursing" (1952). Peplau emphasised the importance of talking as therapy based on psychodynamic principles. Peplau and Altschul were amongst the earliest nurses engaging in the post war debate as to the proper scope and direction for psychiatric nursing. Altschul was able to be particularly influential in the training of nurses, she introduced the idea of training in the skills of creating and maintaining therapeutic relationships, seeing these as central and substantial parts of nurse training (Tilley 1999). Altschuls and Peplau were the foremost mental health nurses of the post war period. Their legacy is a research and development focus on interpersonal skills within nursing.

The post war period was a time of great social and political change which saw the birth of the National health service (NHS) in the UK. Immediately post war and in the years following the setting up of the NHS health professionals existed within a paternalistic comfort zone (Klien 1995). The public were happy to ascribe decision making power to professionals, and to influence institutions such as the NHS solely through the politics of representation. This comfort zone however has been short lived.

The current pace of change and disruption to nursing roles is greater than ever experienced in the past, and this has steadily intensified over the last 50-60 years. This has, in no small part, been due to the closure of the asylums and also the shift in power dynamics between professionals and their clients in the wake of growing consumerism in health and the radicalism of campaigning mental health service user organisations (Hopton 1997a; Barker *et al.* 1999; Repper 2000). The catalysts for this shift in the public relationship with health services were both political and social.

FAILURE AND CHANGE IN SOCIAL POLICY AND THE IMPACT OF CONSUMERISM AND PRESSURE GROUPS ON THE DEVELOPMENT OF MENTAL HEALTH NURSING

Hospital scandals involving the abuse and depravation of patients in psychiatric hospitals across the UK during the late 1960s and early 70s raised human rights issues in the popular press and sparked off early incarnations of the service users' movement. The "People Not Psychiatry" group was set up in London in 1969 and aimed to provide support through informal networks. Its principles emphasised acceptance, uniqueness and an individuals right to a self determined life-style. In December 1972 the Mental Patients Union was formed again in London. They produced a pamphlet claiming that psychiatry was an instrument of capitalist repression (Roberts 1981).

Also in 1972 the National Association for Mental Health changed its name to MIND and appointed a new director with a civil rights campaigning background. This organisation had been viewed as part of the establishment but now shifted its emphasis to lobbying for patients rights (Darton 1999).

Expedient reaction to public opinion and budgetary considerations were a major influence on the then minister for health Enoch Powell when he made the famous 1961 "water tower speech" which predicted a 50% fall in mental hospital beds over the next 15 years (Freeman 1998). The subsequent "Hospital Plan" began the process of closing the Victorian asylums. By 1990 the National Health And Community Care Act (Johnson *et al.* 2000) went still further in this direction. The creation of community nursing, gathered momentum to meet the needs of a developing community based mental health service. However, community nursing predated the end of the asylum system. Community nurse roles had been developed at Warlingham park Hospital in the in the post war period and most notably at Moorhaven hospital in Devon where John Greene developed the role and began to describe its elements, in particular its person centred and interpersonal nature (Nolan 2003). Community nurses had less time for a medical model based on a positivistic scientific tradition and became increasingly interested in a role which placed the unique interpersonal nature of the nurse client relationship at its heart (Brooker *et al.* 1986; Nolan 2003).

A ROLE AND PURPOSE FOR MENTAL HEALTH NURSING?

The net effect then of these political changes has been to further increase the pressure for mental health nursing to examine its role and purpose (Barker *et al.* 1999). Nurses were no longer able merely be the facilitators of institutional care but also had to look beyond subservience to the medical establishment largely wedded to a system of "scientific" physical treatment. The shift of focus to community care has served to steer mental health nursing still further along the path set by Altchul and Peplau toward a role defined by the interpersonal and client centred nature of our relationships with our clients. This shift was encouraged during the move toward community care because nursing activity was viewed by politicians seeking to reform the mental health system as more flexible and pragmatically based and above all cheaper than a system dominated by medicine.

It would be misleading however to claim that mental health nursing is not divided between scientific and humanistic traditions along similar lines to psychology and to an extent psychiatry (Repper 2000; Forchuk 2001). The debate within mental health nursing, has on one side those who stress the need for development of specific interventions aimed at diagnosed conditions and see the determinants of mental illness as biologically and genetically determined (Gournay 1995). The other side of this debate stresses the importance of nurse client relationships and an holistic view of those clients and their difficulties (Barker *et al.* 1999). However the need for skilful interpersonal delivery of therapeutic interventions can provide a common ground for both these traditions built upon the " priorities of service users in the current social context" (Repper 2000 p579) (Brooker 2001).

Peplau and Altschul sought to encompass both sides of this debate in their approach to mental health nursing. They both emphasised the importance of individualised care whilst recognising the nurses role in implementing treatment proscribed in response to specific diagnosis. Indeed the existing sides of this debate vary more in the emphasis they place on the causes of mental illness than in the need for an interpersonal approach in nursing as it is defined in this chapter. Champions of behaviourally based psychosocial interventions (Gournay *et al.* 1998)can no more deny the need for the ability to work in collaboration with clients and evidence the knowledge skills and attitudes required for effective communication (Chadwick *et al.* 1996) than would the developers of what are often termed holistic approaches, such as the Tidal Model, who stress them as key components of their approach (Barker 2001).

Authors from both sides of the debate are attempting to provide new and appropriate frames of reference for mental health nursing. In this endeavour no one working in the field can advocate the purely mechanistic application of therapeutic technique no matter how wedded they may be to an evidence base that indicates that a technique has demonstrated efficacy. Neither the positivist scientific or humanistic tradition can therefore minimise the need for nursing interpersonal skill developed within a context of service user involvement and collaboration (Perkins *et al.* 1996; Barker 1998; Barker 2001). Mental health nursing has come along way since Tuke strove to reform an inhumane system of care and treatment. The need for interpersonal skills is established by external policy makers and within nursing itself. What is the current state of interpersonal skill in nursing and how should it change to involve service users?

COMMUNICATION, INTERPERSONAL SKILLS AND SERVICE USER INVOLVEMENT WITHIN MENTAL HEALTH NURSING

The importance of and difficulty in attaining good and effective interpersonal skills amongst nurses is well recognised within nursing literature (Cormack 1985; Telford 1985; MacLeod-Clark 1988; Dickenson *et al.* 1989) . As long ago as the 1950s seminal research carried out by Isabel Menzies Lyth (1988) reported on the effect of high levels of stress and anxiety in nursing as being to minimise inter-personal communication between nurse and patient and to foster professional distancing as a way of managing that anxiety. Resistance by nursing staff to the humanistic and interpersonal style required for a form of mental health nursing which is built upon the needs and priorities of its users has been a theme that has been examined through the concept known as "emotional labour" (McQueen 2004 p 1.). The idea that nurses feel threatened by the perceived personal cost involved in the humanistic delivery of care is well documented (Phillips 1996; McQueen 2004). The concept of emotional labour was originally developed by Arlie Hochschild (1983), and refers to paid work requiring the maintenance of an outward appearance which could conflict with internal emotional states. This work is carried out to create particular emotional feelings in clients and is in effect a form of acting. Hochschild believed that this way of managing difficult situations can have an ultimately negative effect in that the surface acting required to emotionally manage a difficult situation can become incorporated into a more general style of emotional management. Hochschild called this deep acting, in which the individual distances themselves from emotions caused by work situations as a way of coping. More recently, within nursing, the concept of emotional intelligence first developed by John Mayer and Peter Salovey (1990) has been seen as a vital attribute that should be valued and developed amongst nurses attempting to deliver humanistic care as a way of avoiding the damaging effects of emotional distancing. Ultimately emotional distancing exists because of a power imbalance that allows those in positions of power to objectify the individuals in their care, effectively dehumanising them in order to protect themselves from the possibility of emotional pain. This is in the long term a self defeating strategy as it tends to escalate expressed emotion as those in distress attempt to be heard and gain a response to their pain from those entrusted with their care.

The impact of emotional distancing is evidenced in the literature. A report by the standing nursing and midwifery advisory committee which researched the perceived care deficit in inpatient mental health, identified a "lack of a basic humane response in some of our hospitals" (Standing Nursing and Midwifery Advisory Committee 1999). Similar concerns have been highlighted by the chief nursing officer who has called for a "values based" approach and included interpersonal skills as a "best practice competency" for modern mental health nurses (Department of Health 2006b). This type of policy and research has served to generate increasing awareness and concern among nurse educators striving to effectively teach interpersonal skills (Ashmore *et al.* 1997; Burnard 1999; Ashmore *et al.* 2004).

This type of pressure to improve interpersonal skill in the nursing workforce is timely. There is an increasing body of evidence to support the view that mental health services and particularly services provided for clients with what is termed severe mental illness are failing those who they seek to help. Frequent re-admission, overly restrictive observation based care, poor quality of life, social exclusion and a high suicide rate are all commonly cited indicators of this failure (Sainsbury Centre for Mental Health 1998; Standing Nursing and Midwifery Advisory Committee 1999; Barker 2000; Department of Health 2001), as are the mental health related tragedies documented in (amongst others) the Clunis, falling shadow and Cummings reports (Ritchie 1994; Blom-Cooper *et al.* 1995; Laming Lord 2000). There is increasing recognition that in order to improve, our mental health services must work collaboratively with service users and service user ownership of and power within services must increase (Barker *et al.* 1999; Appleby 2000; Bowles 2000; Department of Health 2001; Bowles *et al.* 2002). In order to begin the job of creating a collaborative and empowering mental health service mental health workers must be trained in a way that gives them the necessary interpersonal skills values and attitudes required to form mutually respectful relationships with service users (Heron 1990; Speedy 1999 .; Watkins 2001)

Whilst it is true to say that a growing consumer 'voice' has had a considerable impact on policy making in mental health (Rycroft-Malone *et al.* 2001; Fox 2003) the impact it has made on the clinical practice of mental health practitioners is far less certain. Indeed there is evidence to suggest that the multiple emerging concepts influenced by this trend, such as user involvement, negotiated care, collaborative care, patient participation, and person centred care, which feature in nursing literature are frequently reduced to procedural implementation which pays lip service to these concepts without adopting their common ethos of humanistic delivery of care.

Given then that the potentially threatening nature of interpersonal communication with users of health care is well established (Menzies Lyth 1988; Booth *et al.* 1996; Martin 1998; Bray 1999) and problems in this area have been recognised in clinical practice (Ricketts 1996) and the education of nurses (Chant *et al.* 2002). It comes as no surprise then that the teaching of interpersonal skills in nurse education has become a cause of concern to nurse educators (Ashmore *et al.* 1997; Burnard 1999; Ashmore *et al.* 2004). Such concerns have led the authors as part of a mental health nurse's teaching team to review and change their curriculum. We have sought to use the best available evidence to support and design this involvement. The following sections review the evidence base for user involvement and provide indications for the best style for that involvement.

USER INVOLVEMENT IN HEALTH EDUCATION
AND CURRICULUM DEVELOPMENT

Even though there is a large body of literature covering user involvement in mental health services (McIntyre et al. 1989; Perkins et al. 1996; Hopton 1997b; Newnes et al. 1999; National Institute for Mental Health 2003) much of this focuses on the empowerment of service users in planning and controlling their care and on the skills and attributes required of professionals in practice (Brandon 1996; Heller 1996; Egan 2002; Simpson et al. 2002). There is far less written about the involvement of users in the education of mental health professionals and less still about their involvement in student assessment. Within this literature however it has been reported that the involvement of service users in professional education has been shown to have a variety of positive effects which can only be realised if opportunities are taken and if barriers once identified are overcome (Department of Health 2001). A set of guidelines have been produced for user involved education and a Cochrane review of its efficacy is underway (Tew et al. 2004; Simpson et al. 2005).

Much of the existing educational literature has focused on involvement in curriculum design. In a qualitative study of user views of pre-registration nursing curriculum Rudman (1996) reports that an eclectic knowledge base that valued difference, recognised the importance of social context, the need for an emphasis on inter-personal skills training and the reduction of professional distancing were the main emerging themes. Forrest and Risk et al.(2000) also used a qualitative approach to examine user's views of what should be the focus of nursing education and reports that users valued professionals' interpersonal and human qualities above the implementation of specific techniques. These findings are consistent with the existing evidence on user preferences regarding nursing approaches (Barker et al. 1997, Barker et al. 1999, Repper 2000) and provide invaluable indicators of the deficits in educational practice and the challenges and barriers that need to be overcome in order to meaningfully involve service users in the educational process. An evaluation of the process of developing partnerships with service users in mental health curriculum planning identified as a key themes the need to address the practicalities of breaking down boundaries to involvement which included; issues of representation, training for users involved in research to prevent service user drop out and lack of skill and training on the part of academic staff in user involvement (Masters et al. 2002). This paper mostly examined the difficulties of collaborative curriculum design. In conclusion it stated that the breaking down of traditional boundaries had led to the development of an effective curriculum planning process.

MEASURING THE IMPACT OF INVOLVEMENT

In addition to the literature focusing on curriculum design some authors have attempted to describe and directly measure the impact of user involvement in the teaching process. An inquiry into the effect of service user feedback during practice placement found that a majority of students were receptive to user feedback but had reservations about its reliability. Students did not find feedback given to a group as a whole useful in changing their practice and indicated a preference for individual feedback (Morgan et al. 1997).

A 1999 study used a videoed role played assessment of a client to promote discussion(Wood et al. 1999). In a comparative design two groups discussed the video, one was facilitated by service users and lecturers and the other by lecturers only. Both qualitative and quantitative methods were used to measure user centeredness and make comparisons between the user involved and lecturer only groups. Results indicated that user involvement led to a more user centred approach and a reduction in professional distancing; they also showed an increased use of the "human qualities" most valued by service users.

A qualitative study of mental health nurse lecturers perceptions of user involvement in their programmes identified; the current level of and barriers to involvement, role identification and power imbalances as key themes (Felton et al. 2004). This paper also highlighted the need for changes in infrastructure to enable the involvement of service users in education and for more research on the efficacy of such involvement. Barnes evaluated the impact of service user involvement in post graduate interprofessional mental health training and reported a beneficial effect from user involvement (Barnes et al. 2000). These evaluations of the impact of user involvement in the classroom have shown some efficacy in bringing about change in nursing students. They also begin to highlight some of the inherent difficulties in increasing user involvement in the traditional structure of higher education. Consistency of marking by service users has been identified as an important component of reliability in assessment (Wilkinson et al. 2002). Felton (2004) and Morgan (1997) identified student and lecturer anxiety regarding the "capability" of service users to provide feedback to students and the "validity" of their feedback. This lack of confidence in service user capability is potentially a barrier to meaningful involvement, particularly in areas where service users are involved in student assessment. Unless evidence is gathered regarding the reliability and validity of service user feedback and summative marking of student assessment, concerns about their involvement could prevent full integration of service users into mental health nursing curricula that is both fit for purpose and effective. Research needs to be carried out in this area in order to demonstrate the true impact of service user involvement.

USER INVOLVED INTERPERSONAL SKILLS TEACHING

In collaboration with our service user colleagues we have sought to directly address emotional distancing and poor levels of interpersonal skill. The principles of collaborative conversation and client centred relationship formation are central to our curriculum. These are based upon foundations for practice set out by authors such as Repper and Perkins (1998) Hulme (1999) and Egan(2002) . They emphasise the importance of; understanding experiences from the client's frame of reference, a flexible person centred approach, the exploration of client's preferred futures and empowerment through client choice and informed decision making. We believe that lecturer led theoretical and experiential teaching based on these principles only obtains meaning in the classroom when it is combined with the involvement of service users, and service user ownership of and power within our curriculm (Barker et al. 1999; Appleby 2000; Bowles 2000; Department of Health 2001; Bowles et al. 2002). This move toward increasing involvement has developed from a belief that in order to begin the job of creating a collaborative and empowering mental health service, mental health workers must be trained in interpersonal skills in a way that instils the values and attitudes required to form mutually respectful relationships with service users (Heron 1990; Speedy 1999 .; Watkins 2001). Furthermore that service users should be viewed by students not only as people that they come into contact with during practice placement, but as powerful and influential actors within the process of education and qualification. In order to disrupt the normal nurse client power dynamic in this way we have sought to develop client involvement and "live" or "virtually live" skills based teaching and assessment methods and to carry out research to evaluate the impact of these innovations (Perry *et al.* 2006). These methods combined didactic teaching of theoretical techniques with skills based practice in clinical role play using video playback for group supervision and assessment.

This type of approach has already been adopted to varying degrees within nurse education to meet the needs of service users and professionals who are now stressing the importance of "acceptance, respect, and a non-judgemental attitude" (Faulkner *et al.* 2000) as integral in the formation of helpful relationships between users and practitioners (Sainsbury Centre for Mental Health 1998). Performance based assessments provide an opportunity for students to demonstrate that they can deliver these qualities, however in order to measure their level of ability it has been our experience that a different form of assessment is required which directly incorporates service user experience. There is little research that considers service user involvement in interpersonal skills assessment of health professionals (Biehn *et al.* 1979; Merkel 1984; Thomson 1994; Greco *et al.* 2002), this maybe because such research is problematic in that the relative quality of different assessment methods is hard to measure.

Table 2. Aims for interpersonal / communication skills session

Two aims

1. The first aim is to help students develop a style of conversation to include:

- Warmth
- Comfort
- Genuineness – "Be yourself" "Don't say things unless you mean them"
- Clarity – How easily understood is the student?
- Empathy / support – How easily does the student "tune in" and react to the clients emotions / needs

2. The second aim is to help them ask questions which might be helpful in a skilful manner, this includes being able to show the ability to:

- Ask "why" and "how" type questions – "Why did that happen?" "How could that have been different?"
- See things from different angles – No one absolute truth
- Unfazed - by anger, upset or other strong emotions but able to acknowledge and talk about them
- Enquire – Open ended questions not requiring specific answers
- Take Interest in the detail – Asking questions which open with- how much, how often, how easy, how difficult, and how long – How to phrase such questions
- Get the story – Time and encouragement for people to tell their story - "Could you tell me a little bit more about that?"
- Focus – Homing in on something which is clearly significant or helpful
- Checking understanding - summarising

The key features of this development have been service user involvement in teaching and marking for an interpersonal skill's module taught to second year mental health students. Involvement in teaching has included an awareness raising session in which service users spend a day with students looking at the experience of hearing voices. A variety of experiential techniques and narrative accounts are used in these sessions, to address student attitudes to their clients and their experiences. A recovery model of mental health difficulty and the use of survivor narratives of psychotic experiences underpins these sessions (Deegan 1988; Anthony 1993; Romme *et al.* 1993). A second session again involving a full day with the students has more recently been incorporated into the module. This involves service users in directly running experiential learning of interpersonal skills. This day has been developed using a set of aims developed collaboratively by service users and the academic team. The aims are as above in table 2.

The assessment developed for this module also involves service users. The assessment takes the form of a videoed role play in which students interview a client. Role players are professional actors employed from a local agency. A scenario used for the role play has been developed by the team to provide sufficient background for the actor to respond to a reasonable line of questioning during interview; however one reason for using trained professional actors is that a degree of improvisation is required in order to deal with the wide variety of types of interview. The actors are prepared in advance by the team. Preparation includes practice interviews and discussions regarding the presentation of the client. The scenario is unseen by the students before the assessment. The assessment itself is run over the course of two days; students are scheduled to attend for specific time slots to do their interviews. These are observed by video link by members of the team to ensure smooth running and recorded for later marking.

A panel of experts consisting of practitioners and service users is convened to assess student's interpersonal skills. Practitioners are qualified nurses in practice with local services and have a range of clinical experience. The service users involved have all experienced severe mental health problems. Service users and practitioners are trained in using the assessment tool and specific support and debriefing is made available for the service users involved if required. Marking criteria were that the students demonstrated basic interpersonal skills and the use of techniques which had been taught during the module (these were termed interventions for the purposes of this assessment). The marking tool developed in partnership with service users, is a global rather than itemised scale asking for an overall impression of student performance rather than an itemised rating of the elements of an interview. There is evidence to suggest that global scales are more valid and reliable as a tool for assessing aspects of competency that require a set of expertise and experience rather than a more functional task that can be broken down into a set of discrete actions which can be assessed on a checklist style inventory. A study of the use of global rating by expert examiners in assessing medical student's clinical competence found such an approach effective. This included the extent of compassion and courtesy shown (Cohen et al. 1991).Wilkinson (2002) in a study of standardised patient (role players) global rating of medical student competence used correlation of aggregated service user global rating from eleven observed structured clinical examination (OSCE) stations with overall OSCE marks as an indicator of the validity of standardised patient rating. Wilkinson found that the use of global rating by service users provided a valid measure of student competence. This study used both actors and real patients as role players and service user raters, but did not include mental health clients. However both Wilkinson and Cohen identified the use of global rating as being appropriate for assessing interpersonal rather than technical or procedural skills. The marking is carried out by convening a panel consisting of one lecturer, one practitioner and two service users. Videoed student interviews are watched by the panel initial marks are given without discussion, a moderating discussion then takes place and a final mark is awarded.

A qualitative evaluation of these developments (reported in full elsewhere) (Perry *et al.* 2006) identified significant features for students including that role play is of central importance as a learning experience. Within the assessment process the use of neutral actors and their consistency was viewed as equally important. The impact of and steps to reduce student anxiety also featured, such as mock exams and experiential practice. This evaluation also indicated that our teaching of interpersonal skills should include fewer mechanistic interventions and more emphasis on engagement and collaboration. Finally that feedback from users is valued and can contribute to addressing professional socialisation and the use of emotional distancing which can impact on students as well as more experienced staff.

CONCLUSION

To conclude, in this chapter the gradual shift from a medical perspective to a more psychosocial approach to care within mental health nursing has been explored, highlighting the influence of Altschul and Peplau. This exploration argues that whether one subscribes to the science of mental health practice (Newell *et al.* 2000) or the artistry of mental health care, (Barker 2001; Watkins 2001) that to engage with our clients it is fundamental that we embark upon a radical collaboration with service users (Chadwick 2006) so that essential interpersonal skills can be mastered in an eloquent and sophisticated fashion. For students of mental health nursing to be fit for purpose and to meet the requirements highlighted in the Chief Nursing Officers Review (Department of Health 2006b) it is vital that they have the opportunity to meet with users of the service to learn from their rich life experience and are assessed to meet *their* standards. The high order skills of gleaning accurate narratives and containing people's distress through what can be termed collaborative conversations (Smail 1995; Hulme 1999) need to be practised and performed with the safety net provided by role played patients and where feedback from experienced individuals can provide increased self awareness. From this vantage point a real knowledge about the effectiveness of one's own interpersonal skills can be learned and developed. We are advocating therefore a resurrection of the values based, humanistic interpersonal process, (Peplau 1952) whilst accepting Clarke's (1999) view that it is what we do with client's that is integral as opposed to a particular paradigm. The elements of this approach to teaching interpersonal skills are not new in themselves. The combination of theoretical input consolidated by skills rehearsal and developed through supervision by teachers and peers has long been a favoured approach to the training of counsellors (Gallagher *et al.* 1992) and elements of this approach have been incorporated into many nurse education programmes. It is the combination of this approach with a radical collaboration (Chadwick 2006) with service users in education that makes this approach innovative and we feel provides a new direction for interpersonal skills teaching. Users of mental health services have the key to the therapeutic experience and this needs to be harnessed to develop and assess the interpersonal skills of engagement thus ensuring mental health nurses are competent, capable, and fully honed in Barker's (2003), 'craft of caring'.

REFERENCES

Anthony, W. A. 1993. Recovery from mental illness: The guiding vision of the mental health service system in the 1990s. *Psychosocial Rehabilitation Journal*, 16, (4) 11-23.

Appleby, L. 2000. Safer services: Conclusions from the report of the national confidential inquiry. *Advances in Psychiatric Treatment*, 6, 5-15.

Ashmore, R. and Banks, D. 1997. Student nurses perceptions of their interpersonal skills: A re- examination of burnard and morrison's findings. *International Journal of Nursing Studies*, 34, (5) 335-345.

Ashmore, R. and Banks, D. 2004. Student nurses' use of their interpersonal skills within clinical role-plays. *Nurse Education Today*, 24, (1) 20-29.

Barker, P. 1998. The future of the theory of interpersonal relations? A personal reflection on peplau's legacy. *Journal of Psychiatric and Mental Health Nursing*, 5, 173–180.

Barker, P. 1999. Hildegard e peplau: The mother of psychatric nursing. *J Psychiatr Ment Health Nurs*, 6, (3) 175-176.

Barker, P. 2000. The tidal model: Theory and practice.

Barker, P. 2001. The tidal model: Developing an empowering person-centered approach to recovery within psychiatric and mental health nursing. *Journal of Psychiatric & Mental Health Nursing*, 8, 233-240.

Barker, P., Jackson, S. and Stevenson, C. 1999. What are psychiatric nurses needed for? Developing a theory of essential nursing practice. *The Journal of Psychiatric and Mental Health Nursing*, 6, (4) 273-82.

Barker, P. J. 2003. *Psychiatric and mental health nursing: The craft of caring.* Arnold; Distributed in the USA by Oxford University Press.

Barker, P. J., Reynolds, W. and Stevenson, C. 1997. The human science basis of psychiatric nursing: Theory and practice. *Journal of Advanced Nursing*, 25, (4) 660-667.

Barnes, D., Carpenter, J. and Bailey, D. 2000. Partnerships with service users in interprofessional education for community mental health: A case study. *Journal of interprofessional care*, 14, (2) 189-200.

Biehn, J. and Molineux, J. 1979. Patient evaluation of physician performance. *Journal of Family Practice*, 565-569.

Blom-Cooper, L., Hally, H. and Murphy, E. 1995. *"The falling shadow: One patient's mental health care 1978-1993".* Duckworth, London.

Booth, K., Maguire, P. M., Butterworth, T. and Hillier, V. F. 1996. Perceived professional support and the use of blocking behaviours by hospice nurses. *Journal of Advanced Nursing*, 24, (3) 522-527.

Bowles, A. 2000. Therapeutic nursing in acute psychiatric wards engagement over control. *Journal of Psychiatric and Mental Health Nursing*, 7, (2) 179-184.

Bowles, N., Dodds, P., Hackney, D., Sunderland, C. and Thomas, P. 2002. Formal observations and engagement: A discussion paper. *Journal of Mental Health and Psychiatric Nursing*, 9, (3) 255-261.

Brandon, D. 1996. Normalising professional skills. In: Heller T., R.J., Gomm R., Muston R. & Pattison S. (Ed) *Mental health matters.* McMillan/Open University Press,, Basingstoke.

Bray 1999. *Journal of Psychiatric and Mental Health Nursing*, 6, (4) 297-305.

Brereton, M. 1995. Communication in nursing: The theory-practice relationship. *J Advanced Nursing*, 21, (2) 314-24.

Brooker, C. 2001. A decade of evidence-based training for work with people with serious mental health problems: Progress in the development of psychosocial interventions. *J Mental Health*, 10, (1) 17-31.

Brooker, C. and Simmons, S. 1986. *Community psychiatric nursing.* Heinemann, London.

Burnard, P. 1999. *Counselling skills for health professionals.* Stanley Thornes, Cheltenham.

Chadwick, P. 2006. *Person centered congnitive therapy for distressing psychosis.* Wiley & Sons, Chichester.

Chadwick, P., Birchwood, M. and Trower, P. 1996. Cognitive therapy for hallucinations, delusions, and paranoia. Chichester: Wiley.

Chant, S., Jenkinson, T., Randle, J., Russell, G. and Webb, C. 2002. Communication skills training in healthcare: A review of the literature. *Nurse Education Today*, 22, (3) 189-202.

Clarke, L. 1999. *Challenging ideas in psychiatric nursing.* Routledge, London

Cohen, R., Rothman, A. I., Poldre, P. and Ross, J. 1991. Validity and generalizability of global ratings in an objective structured clinical examination. *Academic Medicine*, 66, (9) 545-548.

Cormack, D. 1985. The myth and relaity of interpersonal skills use in nursing. In: Kagan, C. (Ed) *Interpersonal skills in nursing : Research and applications.* Croom Helm, London. pp 107-115.

Darton, K. 1999. History of mind - the national association for mental health. http://www.mind.org.uk/Mind/Templates/Content%20(RelatedTopics).aspx?NRMODE= Published&NRORIGINALURL=%2fInformation%2fFactsheets%2fHistory%2bof%2bm ental%2bhealth%2fHistory%2bof%2bMind%2b%2bThe%2bNational%2bAssociation%2 bfor%2bMental%2bHealth%2ehtm&NRNODEGUID=%7b382DAF0C-38F8-4497- 92CD-8025D4FB70B7%7d&NRCACHEHINT=NoModifyGuest#The_National_ Association_for_Mental_Health__NAMH_.

Deegan, P. E. 1988. Recovery: The lived experience of rehabilitation. *Psychosocial Rehabilitation Journal*, 11, (4) 11-19.

Department of Health 2001. *The mental health policy implementation guide department of health.* Department of Health, London. pp.

Department of Health 2006a. *Best practice competencies and capabilities for pre-registration mental health nurses in england: The chief nursing officer's review of mental health nursing.* Department of Health, London. pp.

Department of Health 2006b. *From values to action: The chief nursing officer's review of mental health nursing.* Department of Health, London. pp.

Dickenson, D., Hargie, O. and Morrow, N. 1989. *Communication skills training for health personnel: An instructors handbook.* Chapman and Hall, London.

Duffy, F. D., Gordon, G. H., Whelan, G., Cole-Kelly, K. and Frankel, R. 2004. Assessing competence in communication and interpersonal skills: The kalamazoo ii report. *Acad Med*, 79, (6) 495-507.

Egan, G. 2002. *The skilled helper: A problem management and oportunity development approach to helping.* Brooks/Cole Publishing Company, Albany, NY.

Faulkner, A. and Layzell, S. 2000. *Strategies for living: A report of user-led research into people's strategies for living with mental distress.* Mental Health Foundation, London. pp.

Felton, A. and Stickley, T. 2004. Pedagogy, power and service user involvement. *Journal of Psychiatric & Mental Health Nursing,* 11, 89-98.

Forchuk, C. 2001. Evidence-based psychiatric/mental health nursing. *Evid Based Ment Health,* 4, (2) 39-40.

Forrest, S., Risk, I., Masters, H. and Brown, N. 2000. Mental health service user involvement in nurse education: Exploring the issues. *Journal of Psychiatric and Mental Health Nursing,* 7, (1) 51-57.

Fox, J. 2003. Consumerism, part 1: The different perspectives within health care. *Br J Nursing,* 12, (5) 321-6.

Freeman, H. 1998. Mental health policy and practice. *journal of mental Health,* 7, (3) 225-239.

Gallagher, M. S. and Hargie, O. D. W. 1992. The relationship between counsellor interpersonal skills and the core conditions of client centred counseling. *Counselling Psychology Quarterly,* 5, (1) 3-14.

Gournay, K. 1995. What to do with nursing models. *J Psychiatr Ment Health Nurs,* 2, (5) 325-7.

Gournay, K. and Birley, J. 1998. Thorn: A new approach to mental health training. *Nurs Times,* 94, (49) 54-5.

Greco, M., Spike, N., Powell, R. and Brownlea, A. 2002. Assessing communication skills of gp registrars: A comparison of patient and gp examiner ratings. *Medical Education,* 36, (4) 366-376.

Hargie, O. and Dickenson, D. 2004. *Skilled interpersonal communication.* Routledge, Hove.

Hargie, O., Hargie, O. and Hargie, O. D. W. 1996. *A handbook of communication skills.* Routledge.

Heller, T. 1996. Doing being human. In: Heller T., R.J., Gomm R., Muston R. & Pattison S. (Ed) *Mental health matters.* McMillan/Open University Press, Basingstoke.

Heron, J. 1990. *Helping the client.* SAGE, London.

Hochschild, A. R. 1983. *The managed heart: Commercialization of human feeling.* University of California Press, Berkeley.

Hopton, J. 1997a. Towards a critical theory of mental health nursing. *J Adv Nurs,* 25, (3) 492-500.

Hopton, J. 1997b. Who are we listening to? *Nursing Times,* 93, (41) 44-5.

Hulme, P. 1999. Collaborative conversation. In: Newnes, C., Holmes, G. and Dunn, C. (Eds) *This is madness* PCCS Books, Ross-on-Wye.

Johnson, M. and Cullen, L. 2000. Solidarity put to the test. Health and social care in the uk. *International Journal of Social Welfare,* Volume 9, (Issue 4) Page 228.

Klien, R. 1995. *The new politics of the nhs.* Longman, Harlow.

Laming Lord, H. 2000. *"The report of the independent enquiry into the care and treatment of ms justine cummings".* Somerset Health Authority and Somerset Social Services, Taunton. pp.

MacLeod-Clark, J. 1988. The continuing challenge. (communication skills are vital if individualised patient care is to be practised). *Nursing Times and Nursing Mirror,* 84, (24) 26-27.

Mangione, S. 2002. Assessment of empathy in different years of internal medicine training. *Medical Teacher*, 24, (4) 370-373.

Martin, G. W. 1998. Ritual action and its effect on the role of the nurse as advocate. *Journal of Advanced Nursing*, 27, (1) 189-194.

Masters, H., Forrest, S. and Harley, A. 2002. Involving mental health service users and carers in curriculum development: Moving beyond 'classroom' involvement. *J Psychiatric & Mental Health Nursing*, 9, (3) 309-16.

McIntyre, K., Farrell, M. and David, A. 1989. Inpatient psychiatric-care - the patients view. *British Journal of Medical Psychology*, 62, 249-255.

McQueen, A. 2004. Emotional intelligence in nursing work. *Journal of Advanced Nursing*, 47, (1) 101-108.

Menzies Lyth, I. 1988. *The functioning of social systems as a defence against anxiety.* The Tavistock Insitute of Human Relations, London.

Merkel, W. T. 1984. Physician perception of patient satisfaction - do doctors know which patients are satisfied. *Medical Care*, 22, (5) 453-459.

Morgan, S. and Sanggaran, R. 1997. Client centered approach to student nurse education in mental health practicum: An inquiry. *Journal of Psychiatric & Mental Health Nursing*, 4, 423-434.

National Institute for Mental Health 2003. *Attitudes to mental illness 2003 report nimhe.* National Institute for Mental Health in England, London. pp.

Newell, R. and Gournay, K. 2000. *Mental health nursing: An evidence-based approach.* Churchill Livingstone, London.

Newnes, C., Holmes, G. and Dunn, C. 1999. *This is madness: A critical look at psychiatry and the future of mental health services.* Llangarron, UK: PCCS.

Nolan, P. 1999. Annie altschul's legacy to 20th century british mental health nursing. *Journal of Psychiatric & Mental Health Nursing*, 6, (no. 4) 267-272.

Nolan, P. 2003. The history of community mental health nursing. In: Hannigan, B. and Coffey, M. (Eds) *The handbook of community mental health nursing.* Routledge, London.

Nursing and Midwifery Council 2004 *Standards of proficiency for pre-registration nurseeducation.* NMC, London. pp.

Peplau, H. E. 1952. *Interpersonal relations in nursing: A conceptual frame of reference for psychodynamic nursing.* Putnam, New York.

Perkins, R. and Repper, J. 1996. *Working alongside people with long term mental health problems.* Chapman & Hall, London.

Perry, J. and Linsley, S. 2006. The use of the nominal group technique as an evaluative tool in the teaching and summative assessment of the inter-personal skills of student mental health nurses. *Nurse Education Today*, 26, 346-353.

Phillips, S. 1996. Labouring the emotions: Expanding the remit of nursing work? *Journal of Advanced Nursing*, 24, (1) 139–143.

Repper, J. 2000. Adjusting the focus of mental health nursing: Incorporating service users' experiences of recovery. *J Mental Health*, 9, (6) 575-87.

Repper, J. and Perkins, R. 1998. Principles of working with people who experience serious mental health problems. In: Brooker, C. and Repper, J. (Eds) *Serious mental health problemsin the community: Policy, practice and research.* Bailliere Tindall, London.

Ricketts, T. 1996. General satisfaction and satisfaction with nursing communication on an adult psychiatric ward. *J Advanced Nursing*, 24, (3) 479-87.

Ritchie, J. 1994. *"The report of the inquiry into the care and treatment of christopher clunis"*. London. pp.

Roberts, A. 1981. Mental health history timeline. http://www.mdx.ac.uk/www/study/sshtim.htm.

Romme, M. and Escher, S. 1993. *Accepting voices.* Mind Publications.

Rudman, M. 1996. User involvement in the nursing curriculum: Seeking users' views. *J Psychiatric & Mental Health Nursing*, 3, (3) 195-200.

Rycroft-Malone, J., Latter, S. and Yerrell, P. 2001. Consumerism in health care: The case of medication education. *J Nursing Management*, 9, (4) 221-30.

Sainsbury Centre for Mental Health 1998. *Acute problems: A survey of the quality of care in acute psychiatric wards.* Sainsbury Centre for Mental Health, London. pp.

Salovey, P. and Mayer, J. D. 1990. Emotional intelligence. *Imagination, Cognition, and Personality*, 9, 185-211.

Silverstein, C. M. 2006. Therapeutic interpersonal interactions: The sacrificial lamb? *Perspectives In Psychiatric Care*, 42, (1) 33-41.

Simpson, E. L., Barkham, M., Gilbody, S. and House, A. O. 2005. Involving service users as trainers for professionals working in adult statutory mental health services (protocol). *The Cochrane Library*, (3) 1-4.

Simpson, E. L. and House, A. O. 2002. Involving users in the delivery and evaluation of mental health services: Systematic review. *British Medical Journal*, 325, (7375) 1265-1268.

Smail, D. 1995. *How to survive without psychotherapy.* Constable, London.

Speedy, S. 1999 . The therapeutic alliance. In: Clinton, M. and Nelson, S. (Eds) *Advanced practice in mental health nursing.* Blackwell Science, Oxford.

Standing Nursing and Midwifery Advisory Committee 1999. *Mental health nursing: "addressing acute concerns".* Standing Nursing and Midwifery Advisory Committee, London. pp.

Telford, A. 1985. Interpersonal skills training: Therapeutic tool and professional necessity: Part 1. *Community Psychiatric Nursing Journal*, 5, (2) 17-21.

Tew, J., Gell, C. and Foster, S. 2004. *Learning from experience: Involving service users and carers in mental health education and training.* Mental Health in Higher Education, Nottingham. 1-62 pp.

Thomson, A. N. 1994. Reliability of consumer assessment of communication-skills in a postgraduate family-practice examination. *Medical Education*, 28, (2) 146-150.

Tilley, S. 1999. Altschul's legacy in mediating british and american psychiatric nursing discourses: Common sense and the 'absence' of the accountable practitioner. *Journal of Psychiatric & Mental Health Nursing*, 6, (4) 283-295.

Watkins, P. 2001. *Mental health nursing: The art of compassionate care.* Butterworth-Heinemann, London.

Wilkinson, T. J. and Fontaine, S. 2002. Patients' global ratings of student competence. Unreliable contamination or gold standard? *Medical Education*, 36, (12) 1117-1121.

Wood, J. and Wilson-Barnett, J. 1999. The influence of user involvement in the learning of mental health nursing students. *NT Research*, 4, (4) 257-70.

In: Nursing Education Challenges in the 21st Century   ISBN 1-60021-661-7
Editor: Leana E. Callara, pp. 171-194   © 2008 Nova Science Publishers, Inc.

Chapter 6

EMOTION BECOMES VOICE, VOICE BECOMES A POEM: USING POETRY IN NURSING CURRICULA TO ENCOURAGE A HOLISTIC APPROACH TO CARE PLANNING

David Sharp[1] and Ryan Futrell[2]
[1] Department of Nursing, Cedarville University
[2] Department of English, Cedarville University

ABSTRACT

This chapter draws upon on a study carried out with B.S.N. students during psychiatric clinical experience in which the concentration on interpersonal relationships and therapeutic conversation encouraged students to look beyond the diagnostic label (Olson, 2002).

Coudriet describes how the nurse enters an instant with his or her own life spinning and full of stresses and doubts, "constelling themselves with the suffering of her patients." (2004; p100). It is this "constelling" by nursing students that this study sought to tap into. For each week of a seven or eight week clinical rotation in psychiatric settings, students were asked to reflect upon their experiences and to write these experiences in the form of a poem. Coudriet suggests that when the nurse and patient meet they bear witness to each other regarding not only the story of their lives, but also to the moment of meeting itself. "It is this very act, this fundamental act of witness, of compassion, that becomes emotion, becomes memory, becomes sound, becomes voice, and becomes a poem." (2004; p100).

The content of the 179 poems generated in this study was subjected to thematic analysis. A number of themes were identified from the poems including initial uncertainty and fear of the students ; ways in which the students come to terms with caring for the clients; feelings of confusion and helplessness experienced by the students during the clinical rotation; and issues relating to moving beyond that particular clinical experience

At the conclusion of the clinical rotation the students were asked to provide an anonymous evaluation on the use of poetry. Most students reported that the experience made them "think deeper" and get in touch with their own feelings, even although they might never have written poetry before. They did not report any disadvantages in using poetry as a reflective tool compared to other methods they had been exposed to, and most preferred it as a means of assessment. They reported enjoying the creative aspects of the poetry and enjoyed "a new way of thinking" that enabled them to view the "clinical experience as a whole."

INTRODUCTION

Nursing students are encouraged to provide holistic care for patients, yet they are taught and evaluated primarily form a scientific, empirical perspective (Kidd and Tusaie, 2004). Within nursing education there is a growing awareness of the need to uncover the meaning of caring (Priest 2000) and ascertain how a deeper understanding of the components of caring can be applied in practice. One method of helping student nurses achieve a deeper understanding of the holistic nature of patient care is through the use of poetry in the nursing curriculum (Olson, 2002). "Poetry helps nurses find meanings in their everyday life and make note of experiences they might have otherwise ignored." (Raingruber, 2004, p19). In so doing it "allows the thoughts and feelings about everyday human experiences to escape the unconscious workings of the mind" (Hunter 2002, 141). For BSN nursing students experiencing a clinical rotation in psychiatric settings their "everyday human experiences" were the challenges of working in secure environments with clients with mental health problems, many of whom were acutely ill or had committed crimes.

Facing such a new and different clinical experience produces many emotional challenges for the student. The aim of this study was to use poetry as a reflective tool to allow the student nurses to review their practice on a daily basis. The phenomena of such lived human experience commonly finds expression through the medium of poetry (Hunter, 2002). In expressing their experiences in this way it was anticipated that the students would be able to identify some of the emotions they were dealing with in this clinical environment. Linney (2000) stresses the ways in which poetry helps us to reflect, and by so doing, remember what is important in our lives, including our professional lives.

In a short article in *Clinical Nurse Specialist,* Coudriet (2004), from the Department of English at the University of Massachusets, summarizes succinctly the emotional dimension involved in the caring aspects of the nursing role. He notes that as healers nurses are involved in countless intimate moments with patients, continually entering and leaving such personal moments. "In no other world can each moment contain such large stories" (2004, p100). Nurses are privileged to witness the pain and healing, survival and death of strangers. Into this "single instant of contact" the nurse brings her/his own stresses, doubts and suffering. The stresses and doubts of the nurses "constelling themselves with the sufferings of her patients." In this way, Coudriet speculates, the lives of the nurse and the patient become intertwined as each bear witness to the moment of contact.

And it is this very act, this fundamental act of witness, of compassion , that becomes emotion, becomes memory, becomes sound, becomes voice, and becomes a poem. Coudriet (2004, 100)

It is this journey from witnessing to poetry, suggested by Coudriet, that the authors sought to capture for the student nurses. In so doing they should be able to identify feelings of compassion toward the patients. It was anticipated that emotions that were evident when working in this particular clinical environment; deeper memories of the experience; and their voice regarding the experience would be able to be expressed in the form of poetry. Olson (2002, p46) concludes that "nursing and poetry are inextricably linked, with each patient representing a living poem, ready to teach us important lessons about others and ourselves." Student nurses who write poetry should therefore be able to give voice not only to their feelings about the patients, but also to their feelings about themselves working with those patients. Melies (1997, p94) suggests that nursing, as a human science "has at its core an understanding of experiences as lived by its members."

This emphasis on reflection and identifying emotional issues in nursing practice addresses one of the dimension of knowledge identified by Carper (1978) as aesthetics, or art of nursing. A dimension that is seen as being relevant to nursing, but one which is difficult to quantify and measure to ascertain its existence or impact on patient care. In Carper's (1978) well know thesis on nursing knowledge, four patterns of knowledge in nursing are described. The first is empirics, or the science of nursing; the second is ethics, the knowledge underlying judgments; the third is personal knowledge, including knowing one's self; and the fourth is aesthetics, the art of nursing. Within most nursing curricula emphasis is given to the science of nursing in delivering care and the ethical dimensions relating to that care delivery. Science is easy to find, for example in textbooks, and apply through the teaching of theory and practice. Ethics are increasingly becoming a staple in the nursing curriculum (Bastable, 2003) and often form the basis for classroom centered debate in the curriculum. Knowledge of one's self is not usually incorporated into the nursing curriculum and the art of nursing is often mentioned but not acknowledged as being a taught component in a nursing course. Often the 'art' of nursing is viewed as something a student nurse will develop as they move from 'novice' status to that of 'expert' as postulated by Benner (1984) in her well known of thesis outlining the journey a neophyte nurse takes as she moves in status "From Novice to Expert".

This study sought to use provide student nurses with access to the third and fourth dimensions of nursing knowledge as postulated by Carper (1978). Through reflecting on their practice by recording a daily diary that would be used to generate a poem, the students would gain an insight into their own emotional experience. In so doing they would be able to assess their own place in the nurse/patient relationship, reflecting on the 'art of nursing' as they witnessed it and understood it in themselves. It was also anticipated that by bearing witness to the relationship with the patient, the student nurse would also be able to reflect on the care the patient was receiving, that is the scientific, empirical aspects of knowledge, as well as the ethics involved in providing that care. Clinical experiences for students are somewhat transient in that they last only a short period of time. Poetry should enable the students to reflect on this experience in some detail, as Connelly (1999, p420) suggests, "the power of poetry is to insist on immediacy."

Holmes and Gregory (1998) chart the use own use of poetry to explore nursing knowledge in relation to Carper's ways if knowing in nursing. One of the writers, Vicki Holmes, describes how working on several medical units over a period of twelve years had left her with "many experiences, feelings and images," which culminated in an awareness of something that was difficult to articulate (Holmes and Gregory 1998, p1193). Holmes discovered that the process of writing a poem about a significant incident that had occurred twelve years previously allowed her to release, through words and images, the meaning contained in the experience," (Holmes and Gregory 1998, p1193). Holmes goes on to describe feelings related to the incident that included powerlessness, helplessness, shock and anger, sorrow, and pleasure. Writing a poem was a way to discover new knowledge relating to these feelings and memories, in this way meaning could be derived from events and actions that might otherwise have been considered to be insignificant.

THE USE OF POETRY IN NURSING EDUCATION

Watson (1994) suggested that using poetry in nursing provides a way to see and know the core of nursing practice as it makes substantial that which might otherwise remain invisible. Hunter (2002, p141) contends that "poetry is used in nursing education, to enhance nursing theory, to teach students more about themselves, the clients they care for, and, on occasion, in nursing research." Although the use of poetry in nursing education does not appear to be widely used, there is an expectation that student nurses should go through the process of learning how to care for people using narrative approaches such as journaling. Kidd and Tusaie (2004) point out that although undergraduate nursing students might be required to write a weekly journal reflecting on their experiences in a mental health area, the students had difficulty discerning what was meaningful to them, often feeling overwhelmed and frustrated by such an assignment. It was noted that in a process of journal development over a two year period "it became clear students were able to express themselves more freely using poetry," (Kidd and Tusaie 2004, p404).

Freedom of expression through poetry was evidenced by Holmes reflected on a clinical experience that was twelve years old (Holmes and Gregory 1998), yet it is unusual for students to be asked to examine their own emotions in this way. As Friedrich (1999, p19) suggests, poetry has the potential to provide the student with "a time for reflection, a time to hear other's experiences, a time for replenishment, a time for growth." For student nurses each new clinical experience is a time for growth that brings with it a raft of challenges and emotions. Part of the professional approach to nursing is that these emotions should be held in check and dealt with out-with the educational setting. When faced with clinical situations in mental health settings the emotions relate to experiencing situations where there is a great deal of ignorance, uncertainty and even fear. Students in these situations are expected to use therapeutic use of the self (Olson, 2002). In this study it was expected that by examining themselves, in relation to the emotions they were experiencing, they would be better able to understand the mental health clients they were coming into contact, and having to work, with during their clinical experience in psychiatry.

Poetry is used a reflective tool with clients in mental health settings in one-to-one interventions as well as informal and formal groups. McArdle and Byrt (2001, p517) describe the ways in which expressive writing, including poetry, has been used to "enable people with mental health problems to enjoy and express themselves, develop creativity and empowerment, affirm identity and give voice to views and experiences." The benefits of using poetry with the mentally ill has been described in numerous studies such as those carried out by Carty (1988) and Madden (1990), and Chouvardas (1996) used this approach to improve therapeutic communication with schizophrenic patients. Mental heath service users themselves use such writing to describe their experiences in published anthologies such as *Beyond Bedlam: Poems Written Out of Mental Distress,* (Smith and Sweeney, 1998). Similar experiences of mental health clients have also been used to construct resources that are used by course participants, including heath professionals, to gain insight into the experiences of mental heath service users. An example is the poetry included in the mental health text *Speaking Our Minds,* published by The Open University in the UK and used in some of the mental heath courses it offers (Read and Reynolds, 1996).

This form of self realization available to users of mental heath services is usually ignored when working with students facing the challenges of a mental heath placement, yet poignancy and memorability of poetry enables the writer to become familiar with a potentially emotional climate (Ogden, 1999). Such poetry "alerts the health care professional to client problems and opportunities for learning that might otherwise be missed." (Connelly 1999, p422). Looking beyond the diagnostic labels attached to clients, the student nurse is expected to emphasize interpersonal relationship and therapeutic communication. (Olson, 2002). This involves techniques that might be novel and unfamiliar applied to a client group that may be perceived as new and challenging, yet this dimension is often ignored within educational approaches for nurse. McArdle and Byrt (2001, p518) note that "in many texts on mental health nursing, there is little or no mention of nurses' involvement in expressive or therapeutic uses of reading and writing." Exceptions include a chapter on creative and expressive approaches by Simms in the text by Wright and Giddey (1993), and a section on setting educational objectives in the affective domain for nurse teachers by Jeffries and Norton in a guide for faculty teaching by Billings and Halstead (2005).

The use of poetry enables discovery and reflection on other's feelings whilst developing empathy (Akhtar, 2000). Treistman (1986) used poems to teach nurses about nursing care whilst Raingruber (2004) used her own poems with clients and students to create dialogue about events that occurred in mental health settings. Barilan et al (2000) described how poetry could be used with medical students to help to develop patience and questioning, interaction and compassion. As mentioned previously, Holmes wrote a poem to explore her own feelings of dealing with a previous clinical event (Holmes and Gregory, 1998). Thinking about feelings in nursing has also been encouraged through the use of the Japanese poetry known as haiku. A Japanese haiku poem traditionally consists of three lines: the first line having five syllables, the second having seven syllables, and the third having five syllables (Reichold, 1996). Schuster (1994) and Anthony (1998) have both used haiku poetry with nursing students to explore feelings and perceptions and Taylor (1985) used it for providing insight into issues related to the elderly.

Poetry has also been used previously to test knowledge in nursing students (Smith 1996), as well as for monitoring students (Peck 1993). Stowe (1996) and Smith (1996) both used poetry in classroom situations. Stowe using poetry to increase compassion and empathy as well as problem solving and conflict resolution, Smith using poems to examine the students' ability to make assessments and plan care based on the content of poems.

The previous studies that perhaps come the closet to the present study are those by Olsen (2002) using poems by students to reflect on their experiences in psychiatric units and Kidd and Tusaie (2004) asking students to submit poems as part of a journaling assignment during the last week of mental health experience. These studies are similar to each other in that they asked students to reflect on mental health clinical experience as students neared the end of that experience. They differed from the present study where students were asked to write poems each week to provide an on-going reflection of their mental health student experience.

Olsen (2002) found that examples of poetic work by students allowed nursing students to "expand their thinking beyond the often cold and harsh realities of clinical situations." (p50). He found that students embraced this approach, even those who were initially cynical, as they developed more insight into the reality of the patients. Whilst recognizing the lack of expertise the student nurse had in writing poetry, Olsen noted a deeper level of understanding about themselves and the patients that the students were achieving

> Regardless of the literary merits of what was written, the poems touched a deeper and more complete sense of humanity than had been possible in other, more traditional, assignments, such as process recordings or care plans (2002, p50).

Olson noted that this exercise demonstrates what Chinn and Kramer described as the intersection of aesthetic and personal knowing in that "all knowing is personal," (1999, p6). Raingruber suggests that (2004, p20) "reading and writing poetry should be incorporated to a greater extent into clinical and educational practice within mental health nursing." In an area, such as mental health, where the nuances of conversation or relationships might not be immediately apparent to the student nurse, poetry allows for components in the interaction between the student nurse and the client to come to the fore. As Holmes and Gregory (1988, p1194) note: "In its portrait and its permanence, poetry refuses to let experiences, feelings and images remain inconsequential, mundane or insignificant."

Using an expressive approach, Kidd and Tusaie (2004) asked undergraduate nursing students taking part in mental health clinical experience to write a weekly journal reflecting on their experiences. Unfortunately this process was eventually thought to stifle the students' ability to examine personal and client goals, therefore students were encouraged to write a poem about their clinical experience. Using this new approach students began to express themselves more freely and it was noted that "Perhaps it was time for faculty to learn from students," (2004, p404).

Raingruber suggests that (2004, p20) "reading and writing poetry should be incorporated to a greater extent into clinical and educational practice within mental health nursing." In an area, such as mental health, where the nuances of conversation or relationships might not be immediately apparent to the student nurse, poetry allows for components in the interaction between the student nurse and the client come to the fore. As Holmes and Gregory (1988, p1194) note: "In its portrait and its permanence, poetry refuses to let experiences, feelings and images remain inconsequential, mundane or insignificant."

The Present Study

The aim of this poetry project was to produce an interpretive study in which writing poetry on a regular basis was used to explore the lived experience of BSN nursing students during their mental health clinical experience. Hunter (202, p145) suggests that when a student nurse is assigned to write a poem about a clinical day, she may express feelings "about her lived experience concerning fears, feelings and new found knowledge." Although Hunter speculates that these emotions could relate to a clinical situation such as such as "starting her first intravenous line on a patient" (2002, p145), the authors were interested in using this reflective process in mental health settings.

The subjects involved in this study were groups of between six to eight students allocated for mental health clinical experience to a Behavioral Health Organization (BHO) in central Ohio, USA. The BHO is comprised of two acute admission units and two forensic nursing units. Each unit has approximately twenty eight beds. One admission unit and one forensic unit were used for student experiences. The admission unit cares for male and female clients with acute mental health problems, the average length of stay being two weeks. The forensic nursing unit is also a mixed unit caring for clients with enduring mental health problems who have committed crimes. Both units present new and unique challenges for student nurses who have never previously worked in these mental heath environments. During the mandatory five hours induction and orientation sessions to the BHO, the students often appear excited, nervous and unsure of themselves. By the time they completed the clinical experience, several weeks later, the clinical instructor noted that most students now felt at ease in the mental health environment, relaxed with the clients and displaying insightful and empathetic behavior. It was the emotion and insight attached to these changes in behavior, from nervous newcomer to confident student, that the researchers sought to gain insight into using poetry as a tool.

Students spent two days per week in the mental heath units for a period of seven or eight week (depending on the impact of public holidays on the clinical rotation). Students used the BHO as their clinical base during this period, rotating out to community based mental heath sites for a total of two weeks. This gave each student a total of five or six weeks experience in the BHO. The project has been running for two academic years and this study used 39 subjects who have completed this experience.

Students were advised to keep a daily journal in the BHO. It was recommended that they write a brief diary each evening following their clinical day in the BHO. Each week this journal should be used to inspire the student to write a poem about their experiences. Somewhat surprisingly, most students did not seem fazed by this new and potentially challenging approach to academic work. There were no complaints or objections from the students over the two year period the project has been running. (If students had objected to this approach there were arrangements in place to offer them an alternative clinical experience where poetry was not used as a reflective tool).

One of the requirements for mental health clinical component of this BSN course was that students complete a reflective exercise on their mental heath clinical experiences. Students allocated to the two units at this particular BHO were informed that their reflective assessment exercise would consist of submitting a poem at the end of each week relating to their experiences in the BHO. To assist the students in this task they were briefed by the nursing clinical instructor as well as a faculty member who teaches poetry in the English Department of the university. The students met as a group and were given instructions on composing the poems along with a pack of poems (compiled by the English department faculty member) as examples of different types of poetry that might also act as a possible source of inspiration. The students were advised that if they required any further advice on writing the poems they could contact the faculty member from the English Department via e-mail or they could arrange an appointment. Several of the students availed themselves of this opportunity by contacting the faculty member or by seeking him out in person.

Each week the students would submit their poems to the nursing faculty clinical instructor. He would read the poems and attempt to discern any themes or issues that appeared to be emerging from the clinical experiences of the previous week. For example, some of the students might initially mention feeling afraid or nervous, or express feeling of compassion for the clients. This information would be used in the pre-conference session held at the beginning of each clinical day between the nursing instructor and the students. The information gleaned from the poems might also be used for promoting discussion during the post-conference sessions held at the end of each clinical day, under the direction of the clinical instructor, when students were given the opportunity to explored some of the issues they had been dealing with in the units.

The reflective exercise using the poems was worth a total of 10 % of the total assessment for this mental health course. Students were not judged on their literary skills or ability to construct a particular form of poetry. Instead they were given credit for taking part in the exercise each week and for producing a portfolio of their work at the end of the mental health experience.

Following completion of the mental heath course the students who attended the BHO for clinical experience were asked to complete an anonymous evaluation form on the poetry exercise, as well as a consent form seeking permission to use their poetry at a future date.

Handling Qualitative Data

Apart from providing the clinical instructor with on-going, weekly, information concerning the feelings and progress of the student nurses, the poems also provided a rich source of qualitative data relating to the lived experience of nursing students on a mental health clinical rotation. As such, this form of narrative can be described as "Tales from the Field," (Van Maanen, 1988). Qualitative data with their emphasis on "lived experience," are well suited for locating the meaning placed on the events, processes and structures that student nurses experience as part of their working lives (Miles and Huberman 1994, p10). Richardson (1992) even goes as far as to suggest that data obtained in the usual way through interviewing subjects and transcribing the data, can be presented in the form of a poem. As an example Richardson interviewed an unmarried mother and converted the thirty six pages of interview notes into a three page, five stanza poem. Denzin and Lincoln (1998, p356) suggest that "poetry may actually better represent the speaker than the practice of quoting snippets in prose." Poetry may engage the reader in a practical and powerful analysis of the social world in a way that is not possible using prose. Denzin and Lincoln (1998, p357) quote Robert Frost's statement that a poem is "the shortest emotional distance between two points," the speaker and the reader. It was anticipated that in the present study the production of poems by the students would allow them to distill the thoughts and feelings they had during the clinical experience and present them in a way which could be analyzed using traditional methods of qualitative data analysis.

Using standard protocols for analyzing qualitative data, open coding was selected as a method as this is an "analytic process through which concepts are identified and their properties and dimensions are discovered in the data," (Strauss and Corbin, 1998, p101). The content of each poem was coded through recognition of "persistent words, phrases, themes or concepts within the data," (Field and Morse, 1991, p99). Through the abstraction process of conceptualization, the data in the poems were broken down into "discrete incidents, ideas, events, and acts that were given a name," (Strauss and Corbin, 1998, p105). These 'names' are used to classify the data, allowing comparisons to be made between the poems produced by different students and for themes that were common to emerge. In this way matrices can be formed that allowed relationships between data to be discovered and developed (Field and Morse, 1991, p104). This allows the researcher to discover categories of data. These are "concepts, derived from the data, that stand for phenomena," the phenomena being important analytic ideas that emerge from the data.(Strauss and Corbin, 1998, p114). As categories are identified they are developed in terms of properties and dimensions and further differentiated "by breaking it down into its subcategories, that is, by explaining the when, where, why, how, and so on of a category," (Strauss and Corbin, 1998, p114). Conceptualization (via categorization) allows the large amounts of data in the poems to be reduced to smaller, more manageable pieces of data. In this way patterns in the data can be established and theory building can be commenced as themes emerge from the data (Strauss and Corbin, 1998, p121).

The lead researcher in this study had had previous experience in qualitative research techniques and was familiar with the various stages in the process required to produce categories of data for conceptualization. To ensure validity the poems and data produced were given to the other member of the research team to confirm the categories identified (Polit and Hungler, 1997, p533). Agreement was reached between the researchers on the themes emerging from the data.

Themes Emerging from the Study.

Mindful of Olson's contention that over analysis of students' poetry may "obscure the basic truths they reveal," (2002, p51), the content of the 179 poems generated in this study was subjected to basic thematic analysis as outlined above. Through this analysis process four categories of data emerged from the poems:

a) Initial uncertainty and fear: "I expected that I would be nervous."
b) Coming to terms with the clinical environment: "Resolve grows.
c) Confusion and control: "I want to help so badly."
d) Moving on: "Sad because…"

Analysis of Poems

The ways in which students dealt with clinical experiences in Mental Health can be examined in relation to the four themes outlines above. (Excerpts of poems are copied as written by the students.)

a) Initial uncertainty and fear: "I expected that I would be nervous."

Students reported a range of emotions related to their clinical experience in a mental health setting. These feelings were particularly noticeable when they were discussing how they felt about going into this clinical environment for the first time. Students would state that "I expected that I would be nervous." Typically students admitted:

I entered the admissions unit the first day
I was scared,

and,

My first day, and I'm scared out of my socks
I fear so much, the patients, my reactions,
What I will do or say;
So many what-ifs abound
What if I say something wrong?

Students had the expectation that this clinical rotation would be less challenging academically than other courses, but more challenging in other directions:

Some say this course is easy
I had heard you just sit and talk
But I think this was a mind strain
And not a breezy walk.

One challenge was that they were conscious of entering a locked environment, often finding this intimidating

The breath of freedom
Fills my nostrils as I past the guarded entryway.

Another student expressed this as :

Shutting us in.
Sunshine, fresh air, a good run, freedom...

Along with this feeling of being cut off from the outside world (of "reality"), there was the fear of being in strange place.

The heavy doors that read "AWOL Risk"
Swing in so that I may enter.
Shutting with a profound clunk
Shutting out reality.

And this feeling of being shut off would increase the fear level associated with this challenging new experience:

Before I go in I'm scared,
I'm anxious, but not in a good way,

I don't want to do this.

Similarly, students dealt each day with these emotions as they journeyed to the clinical area:

Long ride to the mental hospital,
Nervous of what to expect.
Waiting in the waiting room,
Many nerves firing through my head.

Many of these feelings experienced by the students were anticipated by them before the clinical experience.

I expected that I would be nervous,
I expected I would be uncomfortable,
I expected that you would be confused,
That you wouldn't be able to hold a conversation.

These fears regarding role uncertainty and safety were the major issues in the early weeks of the clinical experience:

The first thing I feel is fear,
I don't know what to say.
How can I talk to these women?

Similarly,

Is it safe, will I be all right?
Maybe I will drop out.
I could just turn back.

And by another student,

I expected that you would be insane.
I expected you to be inappropriate.
I expected I would have to defend myself-
That you would attack me.

b) Coming to terms with the clinical environment: "Resolve grows."

As the students moved through their clinical experience they began to come to terms with their new working environment and their feelings changed. One student summed up the approach to care she was developing as:

Cautious at first
Aware continually

Respectful at present
Empathetic always.

Adjusting to the pace of the clinical environment, where there is much sitting around and communicating with patients, was a challenge for some students, some of whom found:

Boredom
Boredom smells like day-old clothes and stale air.

and mixed with boredom, fear,

Maybe it is because these areas bore me.
Maybe it is because these areas scare me.

Most students, however, did seek to find a way forward in the experience to connect with the clients, expressed by one student as:

Amidst the fear and uncertainly, resolve grows
Resolve to find a way
To connect and make a difference
However small and insignificant.

Relationships with the clients that provided deeper understanding began to develop and were acknowledged by the students:

A few more patients I have come to know
And with the others I deeper grow
Some fight for my attention
While others leave to go back to their own dimension.

Initially there was a lot of self doubt amongst the students concerning their abilities to connect with the clients:

What if I don't interact with them enough?
What if I don't know what to say?

Similarly,

What are we to do?
What am I expected to do with the patients?

Students acknowledged that the task of developing relationships with these clients was challenging given that each client was an individual with unique needs:

It's challenging
Each individual requires being approached differently.

As students began to develop relationships with the clients the nature of the challenge was found to be both physically and emotionally tiring. Examples from a couple of students express feelings such as :

Amazing how much has changed.
I feel completely rearranged, emotionally drained.

and

Depressed and tired I come away
But the learning experience it worth is all.

In fact, some students expressed these challenges in terms of questioning what sort of person would willingly select this daily experience as a career:

It 's tIrIng
Day after day dealing with the same issues
It's easy to want them to simply snap out of it-stop acting or thinking in such a way
I'm tired after 4 weeks…who does this for their career?

These doubts were also sometimes stated somewhat more directly as:

I do not think I could work here,
Too depressing, too many lives to mend.

Eventually the students developed feelings of empathy and caring towards the clients of whom they had initially been afraid of. Often they expressed a real concern for them, promoting their case and fearful of their plight:

My heart goes out to them,
I don't want to leave.
I almost want to cry.

Or when reflecting on a common humanity:

I see hurt by the label "insane" put on them by the world,
I see a person who wants a companion,
I see a person who was created by God.

Sometimes the student would put themselves in the place of the client, attempting to explain the world as they thought they might perceive it:

Stuttering and confused
I feel abused
Five years I was in prison
Months behind the walls of this asylum.

From a similarly subjective viewpoint the students would express insight into the care delivery system they had witnessed. Often they acted as the client's advocate:

A man on a guerney
Tied down with restraints
Put in the seclusion room
Drugged to keep him down.

A similar view of care issues was sometimes expressed in relation to situations where the progress of the client would be reviewed by the multi disciplinary team in the unit:

Four meetings hurried through
In just over an hour or so
Not much has changed in the past week
'Keep doing what you're doing
And you'll be out soon.'
But as soon as the client leaves
Reality of a few more months is disclosed.

Some students had not been looking forward to this particular clinical rotation and did not enjoy the experience, often feeling challenged by the lack of clinical procedures and the emphasis on communicating with clients. One student in particular was very forthright in summarizing these feelings:

Give me a hypoglycemic diabetic.
They start off unconscious. I give them sugar.
They are "fixed."
You can't "fix" people with mental illnesses.
Give me an unconscious patient.
This kind of patient can't hit on me or attack me.
Unconscious patients are harmless.

c) Confusion and control: "I want to help so badly."

Perhaps this expression of reluctance to deal with clients with a mental health problem was associated with one of the major themes to emerge being related to feelings of confusion and lack of control many students reported:

I'm so confused and mixed up,
I feel like I could admit myself.

This was a difficult position for students to find themselves in. They expect to come to a new rotation with associated clinical area to learn, acquire new skills and gain control. Now students often felt that they had little to offer, feeling helpless because the lack of control. These feelings of helplessness were identified as resulting from a lack of skills and experience in dealing with this particular client group:

On the unit, I feel helpless and out of control.
I don't know what to say, can I help a single soul?

The lack of control and resultant confusion led to negative feelings towards the experience for some students. On one occasion this was strongly worded as:

I hate this
I want to help so badly
But I don't understand how.

As the clinical experience drew to a close after seven or eight weeks confusion still remained unresolved. There was a realization that even after several weeks working with mental health clients, students were still left with many unanswered questions that personally challenged them:

I feel like I keep asking questions
That no one will answer
I don't understand what I'm seeing or hearing
Am I going crazy myself?

This environment of confusion was recognized as being an integral component of dealing with this client group:

The more I learn the more I realize
I am never going to fully comprehend
The people I am to help.

d) Moving on: "Sad because…"

Eventually there came a time to move to the next clinical rotation and students were quick to acknowledge their feelings of advancement, often comparing their position to the fate of the clients who remained behind in the units:

Ready to move on
But sad to leave
For relationships I did shape
And conversations will be remembered.

And often feeling,

Sad that I will never see these patients again?
Sad because I am leaving 'new' friends?
Sad because I liked this rotation?

The students reflected on feelings of having accomplished something, having learnt something that was of value to them in the future. Tinged with these positive feelings were feelings of sadness at terminating the relationships they had developed with clients:

Then a feeling of accomplishment
creeps over our group
We're finished! we triumphantly cry
and hold our heads high
And we smile at the future.

Students were appreciative of the opportunities to learn that had been presented to them:

The knowledge I have gained
Will follow me anywhere.

Often they articulated gratitude to the clients for providing them with a learning experience. This was expressed forthrightly by one student in her last poem:

I will never forget the lessons you have taught me.

In summary, students experienced a range of emotions as they moved through the clinical experience. Initially they had many fears and uncertainties regarding their role and safety issues. These were gradually replaced with personal challenges about the work they were expected to carry out and their relationships with the clients. They often developed empathy for the clients and expressed doubts concerning their own motivation and abilities to work in this particular environment. As they neared they end of their clinical experience the students began to focus on what they had learnt and how they would feel about leaving the clinical area they had been in for the past seven or eight weeks.

Student Evaluation of the Project

Following the end of the clinical experience the students were asked to fill in an anonymous questionnaire comprised of open questions to evaluate the use of poetry and to provide feedback to the faculty involved in the project. The students also joined in a group session where they were able to express opinions concerning the use of poetry within the mental health clinical experiences.

From these evaluations the poems allowed the students "to grow in an area you did not want to grow in." This was reported as meaning that participation in reflective exercises, and expressing emotional feelings, did not come easily. The use of poems allowed the students to reflect in novel ways and examine feelings they might not have otherwise been able. The students appreciated the fact that the writing of poems is 'short and concise," not involving the prolonged labor they associated with producing a reflective paper.

Although being "easier' than writing a paper, the poetry exercise was time consuming in that students reported they "had to return to it," and therefore they could "not just do it in one go." Through this process of thinking about the content and returning to the themes they were writing about, the students reported that they could "unwind and spend time on it," thereby using the reflective process to debrief themselves from the clinical experience.

Some students viewed the process almost as a recreational activity, many reporting they had "fun" writing the poems. One student reported that her strategy for writing was to think of a well known tune and use that to inspire her to write her poem. For example, she used the tune of the song "I will survive" to compose a poem that began:

First I was afraid,
I was petrified.
Thinking I could never go in without a guard right by my side
But then I spent some time in prayer,
Thinking about how I could help
I grew strong
I learned how to get along
And so I'm back
In the psych ward
I just walked in to find them there
And love them like the Lord.

When asked about the negative aspects of carrying out this project most students reported that there were none. A few students did however express that they did not initially feel very confident in carrying out this reflective project as they did not feel they were very "good" at creative writing. One student complaining that "I always felt I was doing it wrong."

Yet when asked, anonymously, if they preferred the poetry writing as a reflective exercise or whether they would prefer to write a traditional reflective paper, the students unanimously agreed that they preferred the poetry project. In fact some students commented that they were inspired by the process enough that they intended to use poetry as a tool for self reflection in future clinical experiences.

Although they might have initially been intimidated somewhat by the prospect of writing poetry, most of the students reported that "poetry is not as bad as we thought." They acknowledged that the experience had helped to "review improvements in attitude" as the clinical experience in mental health settings had progressed.

The students reported that it was useful to be able to journal and reflect on each week of clinical experience, allowing time and space to think about their own challenges and performance. Some reported enjoying the challenge they presented themselves in writing form the point of view of a client, reporting that this helped to develop insight into the issues clients face.

Students were in agreement that the mental health clinical was "The best clinical to do this [poetry] with," as there were many "abstract concepts" to deal with in this rotation. Students could link theoretical perspectives taught in the mental health course with the reality of the clinical environment, and tie these in with the process of acquiring new knowledge along with their own related feelings. It was also a suitable environment in which to explore their own mental health and some students did so buy comparing themselves to the clients. But there was a lack of self disclosure of physical/emotional abuse or mental health problems as suggested by Kidd and Tusaie (2004, p413). Perhaps this was because the students were aware that a clinical instructor in mental health was reading their poems every week. Yet in the anonymous evaluation forms several students commented that they forgot they were writing the poems to be read by anyone else as they became engrossed in the process of producing a poem each week.

DISCUSSION

This study did differ from previous studies employing the use of poetry as a reflection tool with nursing students undertaking mental health clinical experiences. For example, it differed from the work of Olsen (2002) in that he used the poetry as an assignment for students to reflect on their mental health experience as a whole by writing "a poem about their experiences with one or more patients some time during the semester," (2002, p49).

The study conducted by Kidd and Tusaie, was similar to the present study in that students were "required to write a weekly journal reflecting on their experiences," (2004, p403), with the intention of facilitating learning and the processing of what was held to be meaningful to the students. Kidd and Tusaie reported that the students felt frustrated by not being able to provide appropriate information and faculty were disappointed by the lack of meaningful comment in the journals Therefore, Kidd and Tusaie modified their reflective exercise and had students "create an original poem about their clinical experience or about the experience of mental illness from the client's perspective," (2004, p404). In so doing it was noted that the students were "able to express themselves more freely using poetry" (2004, p404).

Students in the present study also reported that, although the production of a weekly poem might be a challenge, they were able to express themselves more freely than had they been writing a reflective journal. The study sought to provide the vehicle for students being able to express their own feelings and opinions, and from the content analysis of the poems produced, this appears to have been the case. Unlike previous studies, this study asked the students to produce poems on a weekly basis as a means for students to record a chronological log of their feelings and progress within the clinical setting. Student emotions and on-going professional development were monitored weekly by the clinical instructor. Poem content was often used as a springboard for the discussion of issues relating to incidents the students were involved with in the clinical area or feelings they were dealing with as they progressed through the clinical experience.

Olson noted in his study that the students' "initial doubt about writing a poem often seemed to match their skepticism about the usefulness of working with patients with mental illness,"(2002, p50). In the present study students never really expressed open skepticism regarding the production of a poem each week, in fact the authors were surprised at the lack of dissent or questioning of the project. Perhaps the novelty value of the project was intriguing for students who normally have to write 'paper.' However, many students, in class sessions and in their poems, did express doubt about the future usefulness and relevance of the information that was taught in the mental health course. When students do not perceive value in learning then they are more vulnerable to fear. Some students expressed a clear lack of interest in mental health either as an experience or a career option. Just as Kidd and Tusaie noted that "initial beliefs were challenged and altered," (2004, p406), so too in the present study as the clinical experience progressed over the seven or eight weeks, the students began to empathize more with the clients, many in fact reflecting on their own experience through the perspective of the client. At the end of their clinical rotation most students expressed some sadness, mostly due to the termination of relationships they had developed with the clients and not knowing what the outcomes would be for these individuals. They also expressed an appreciation for the learning they had gained and acknowledged that this knowledge would be of use to them in their future clinical experiences, as well as their nursing careers.

As in Kidd and Tusaie's study, many of the poems produced in the present study were found to be "profound, sensitive, and somehow universal" (2004, p412). Also, as was the case in the study by Olsen, students gained "valuable insights" (2002, p50) into the world of the client, giving them a "deeper and more complete sense of humanity." Olson suggested that the students' awareness of themselves grew as their awareness of the patients grew (2002, p50). In the present study the opposite dynamic was observed. As the students explored their own feelings so their awareness of the clients grew and became more recognized. Their own feelings, for example of being in a locked environment, were compared to those of the client, the student might feel afraid and cut –off from society, but they were going home each evening. The environment and approaches to treatment were explored more thoroughly in the poems as the students settled into the clinical environment and could begin to look beyond their own fears to the experiences of the people they were expected to deal with. The students began to view the system as somewhat unjust and uncaring and they often expressed feelings of wanting to care for, and help the clients. Often they did this in the form a prayer to ask for assistance in increasing their own insight and professional skills to be able to be more understanding and effective with the clients. Empathetically they viewed clients as someone "who was created by God."

God, fill me with Your perfect love
Help me to love the patients as you love them,
Help me to be able to help them and listen to.

The four themes identified in the present study were:

a) Initial uncertainty and fear
b) Coming to terms with the clinical environment
c) Confusion and control
d) Moving on.

These four themes appear to confirm, and can be matched with, the five themes identified by Kidd and Tusaie (2004), in that the students in the present study:

1) Expressed fears about personal safety and personal competence, especially at the beginning of the clinical experience when these fears were the major focus in most of the poems
2) Had empathy for the lived experience of clients, sometimes writing their poems from the perspective of the client.
3) Attempted to normalize the mental heath status of the client, questioning what was 'normal' and the way in which clients should be treated by society.
4) Expressed openly feelings of being the wounded healer, confused about their role, doubting their own abilities and even their own mental health

5) Expressed metamorphosis in terms of personal change and growth, altering their view of mental health clients and recognizing the knowledge they have gained.

Perhaps the most valuable outcome was the self realization developed by the students. At the end of the clinical rotation they were asked to collate their poems and submit them as one file to be archived as the reflective exercise for that clinical experience. This allowed the students to review their poems and chart their own progress through the mental health clinical experience. The students were able to read their own feelings as they progressed from nervous newcomer in the clinical area to a more confident and insightful student who had develop relationships with some of the clients.

The experience of using student poems in practice was also challenging and instructive for the clinical instructor. Having read the weekly poems, he sought to identify themes he thought were apparent, and, when appropriate, would tactfully raise issues that were identified during discussion time spent with the student group. As he carried out this process on a regular basis with different groups of students he noticed recurring feelings being expressed. Common in every rotation of students were the feelings of fear, identification with the clients, and recognition of the cathartic effect the poems were having with the students. The instructor was able to, as Kidd and Tusaie describe, view clients "through naïve student eyes" (2004, p412). In so doing he was able to remember the anxiety associated with new clinical experiences, recognize the potential disappointment of failed interventions and share the joy of limited successes and steps forward witnessed in the clients.

During group discussions in the clinical area with the clinical instructor the students discussed the experience of a cathartic type of reaction whereby they would not only be able to identify submerged emotions, but also be able to examine these emotions in relation to the experience of being a student nurse. This is similar to Raingruber's description of "poetry is itself an experience rather than a description of an experience." (2004, p18). The act of creating a poem was part of a different and new clinical experience for the students, an integral part of the experience and, therefore, part of the emotion associated with the experience. The emotion was indeed becoming part of the voice, the voice became a poem for the students (Coudriet, 2004). As Hunter notes, "Hermeneutics is the study of words, and poetry uses words to express the innermost thoughts of a being… Most nursing studies using poetry as data are hermeneutical in nature," (2002, p146). The use of poetry in this study allowed for the study of the innermost thoughts of the student nurse. The words written allowed for "processing, reflecting on, and gaining understanding about personal and human meanings," (Raingruber, 2004, p19). The insights so provided were made available through the poems not just to the student nurse, but also to their clinical instructor, therefore self knowledge was developed through the shared aesthetic of healing encounters with others (Olson, 2004, p50).

CONCLUSION

This study sought to build upon previous approaches using poetry as a means of reflection for undergraduate student nurses experiencing a clinical rotation in mental health settings. Unlike previous studies this study utilized poems produced on a weekly basis to chart the emotional and professional development of the students as they progressed through a seven or eight week clinical rotation. Through poetry the students were able to express their feelings. They detailed insights into clients' conditions and the way clients were dealt with by the mental health system, as well as society at large. The students were also able to express their feelings when terminating the clinical experience, reflected upon the value of knowledge gained through the clinical rotation.

The present study was conducted in areas where the client population were, demographically, relatively stable. Clients in the forensic unit did not usually change during the course of a seven or eight week student placement. The clients in the admission unit did move in and out of that environment but, with an average length of stay of several weeks, there was usually a cohort of patients with whom the students had the opportunity to develop relationships. It may be of interest to extend this study to use poetry with students in other clinical rotation sites in mental health where the client length of stay is only a few days duration. In settings, such as district hospitals with mental health units, the group of clients that the students meet often changes from week to week. It could be interesting to discover if students in these clinical environments had similar feelings to the students in clinical locations where the present study was conducted and where the client population was more 'stable' in terms of length of stay.

The clinical instructor involved with the present study was also one of the researchers and authors of this chapter. It would be of interest to discover if other clinical instructors, not associated with designing the project, were able to gain the same insights into the students and themselves as had occurred in this study. It is anticipated that this would be the case as this study has suggested that "the use of metaphor and emotive language provides the opportunity to gain new meaning and truth about lived experiences and nurse-patient relationships." (Hunter 2002, p146). Clinical instructors should therefore be better able to chart the progress of students, and identify problems students are faced with but maybe reluctant to discuss. Student poetry writing provides educators with an opportunity "to be challenged and to grow," and "provide a freshness of perspective in the clinical setting." (Kidd and Tusaie, 2004, p412). In this study the use of poetry has provided an excellent reflective tool to be shared by the students with their instructor.

Although poetry has been widely used with clients in mental health settings to explore experiences and feelings, this is a relatively untapped approach for use as a reflective tool for student nurses. The authors, like Kidd and Tusaie, were struck by "the paucity of nursing research that has been completed that takes advantage of poetry as a unique way of knowing" (Kidd and Tusaie 2004, p405). Remembering Hunters (2002) remarks on students reflecting on starting an intravenous line on a patient for the first time, it is suggested that the use of poetry by nursing students in a variety of clinical experiences is appropriate. Hunter suggests that "poetry is a rich, untapped source of meaning especially suited to qualitative nursing inquiry. ... little research has been conducted with poetry as text." (2002, p146). Studies across the range of clinical experiences in student undergraduate programs could help provide deeper reflection and awareness of the emotional dimension of nursing. In so doing this would provide an avenue to explore the affective domain usually ignored within Bloom's taxonomy of learning behaviors (Bloom, 1956).

The authors suggest that poetry should be considered as a viable and vibrant tool for use in nursing courses for reflection. Acknowledging that the journey through various clinical experiences is an emotional experience for student nurses, we should acknowledge that reality and employ the means to explore in depth the experiences and associated emotions that students are facing, and dealing with, on a regular basis. In doing so the education of nurses will demonstrate that an holistic approach to dealing with fellow humans is a reality in theory and practice.

REFERENCES

Akhtar, S. (2000) Mental pain and the cultural ointment of poetry. *International Journal of Psychoanalysis,* 81, 229-243.

Anthony, M.L. (1998) Nursing students and haiku. *Nurse Educator,* 23(3), 14-16.

Barilan, Y. M., Hertzano, R., and Weintraub, M. (2000) Bedside humanities: A vision from the renaissance and two case reports from the present. *Israel Medical Association Journal,* 2, 327-331.

Bastable, S.B. (2003) *Nurse as Educator: Principles of Teaching and Learning for Nursing Practice. Second Edition.* Sudbury, MA: Jones and Bartlett Publishers.

Benner, P. (1984) *From novice to expert: Excellence and power in clinical nursing practice.* Menlo Park, CA: Addison-Wesley.

Bloom, B.S. (1956) *Taxonomy of Educational Objectives. Handbook 1: Cognitive Domain.* New York: David McKay.

Carper, B. (1978). Fundamental patterns of knowing in nursing. *Advances in Nursing Science,* 1. 13-23.

Carty, L. (1988) The group dynamic and poetry: a support source for hospitalized patients. *Small Group Behavior,* 19, 127-131.

Chinn, P.L., and Kramer, M.K. (1999) *Theory and nursing: Integrated knowledge development* (5th ed.), St.Louis: Mosby.

Connelly, J. (1999) Being in the present moment: Developing the capacity for mindfulness in medicine. *Academic Medicine,* 74, 420-424.

Coudriet, D. (2004) Constellation of Suffering: Poetry's Role in Nursing. *Clinical Nurse Specialist.* Volume 18, number 2. 100-101.

Chouvardas, J. (1996) The symbolic and literal in Schizophrenic Language. *Perspectives in Psychiatric Care,* 32, 20-22.

Denzin, N.K. and Lincoln, Y.S. (1998) *Collecting and Interpreting Qualitative Materials.* Thousand Oaks, CA; Sage Publications, Inc.

Field, P.A. and Morse, J.M. (1991) *Nursing Research: The Application of Qualitative Approaches.* London; Chapman and Hall.

Friedrich, M. J. (1999) Passion for poetry: Compassion for others. *JAMA,* 281, 1159-1161.

Holmes, V. and Gregory, D. (1998) Writing Poetry; a way of knowing. *Journal of Advanced Nursing,* 1998, 28(6), 1191-1194.

Hunter, L.P. (2002) Poetry as an aesthetic expression for nursing: a review, *Journal of Advanced Nursing,* 40(2), 141-148.

Jeffries, P.R. and Norton, B. (2005) Selective learning experiences to achieve curriculum outcomes. In D.M. Billings and J.A.Halstead (2005). *Teaching in Nursing: A Guide for Faculty. Second Edition.* St Louis, Missouri: Elsevier Saunders.

Kidd, L., I. and Tusaie, K., R. (2004) Disconnecting Beliefs: The use of poetry to know the lived experience of student nurses in mental health clinicals. *Issues in Mental Health Nursing,* 25; 403-414.

Linney, B. J. (2000) Can you take your soul to work? The Physician Executive, 26(2), 59-62.

Madden, P. (1990) Rhymes and reasons. *Nursing Times,* 86, 64-65.

McArdle, S. and Byrt, R. (2001) Fiction, poetry and mental health: expressive and therapeutic use of literature. *Journal of Psychiatric and Mental Health Nursing,* 2001, 8, 517-524.

Melies, A, I. (1997) *Theoretical Nursing: Development and Progress, Third Edition.* Philadelphia, PA: Lippincott-Raven Publishers.

Miles, M.B. and HubermanA.M. (1994) *Qualitative Data Analysis.* Thousand Oaks, CA; Sage Publications, Inc.

Ogden, T. H. (1999) The music of what happens in poetry and psychoanalysis. *International Journal of Psychoanalysis,* 80, 979-994.

Olson., T. (2002) Poems, patients and psychosocial Nursing. *Journal of Psychosocial Nursing,* Vol. 40 , No. 2, February 2002, 46-51.

Peck, S. (1993) Monitoring student learning with poetry writing. *Journal of Nursing Education,* 32, 190-191.

Polit, D.F. and Hungler, B.P. (1997) *Nursing Research Methods. Appraisal and Utilization,* (4th Edition). Philadelphia: Lippencott.

Priest H., M. (2000) The use of narrative in the study of caring: a critique. *NT Research,* 2000 Jul-Aug; 5(4): 245-52.

Raingruber, B. (2004) Using Poetry to Discover and Share Significant Meanings in Child and Adolescent Mental Health Nursing. *Journal of Child and Adolescent Psychiatric Nursing, Volume 17, Number 1, 13-20.*

Read, J. and Reynolds, J (eds.) (1996) *Speaking Our Minds: An Anthology,* London; MacMillan Press Ltd.

Reichhold, J. (1996) Another Attempt To Define Haiku. Written for and first posted on the *Shiki International Haiku Salon,* April 16, 1996. Accessed on 14th Dec 2006, at http://www.ahapoetry.com/haidefjr.htm

Richardson, L. (1992) The consequences of poetic representation: Writing the other, rewriting the self. In C. Ellis and M.G. Flaherty (Eds.), *Investigating subjectivity: Research on lived experience* (pp125-140). Newbury Park, CA:Sage.

Schuster, S. (1994) Haiku poetry and student nurses: An expression of feelings and perceptions. *Journal of Nursing Education,* 33, 95-96.

Simms, J. (1993) Creative and expressive approaches. In H. Wright and M. Giddey, (eds.) (1993) *Mental Health Nursing. From First Principles to Professional Practice.* Chapman and Hall, London.

Smith, M. (1996) The use of poetry to test nursing knowledge. *Nurse Educator,* 21(5), 20-22.

Smith, K. and Sweeney, M. (1998) *Beyond Bedlam. Poems Written Out of Mental Distress.* Anvil Press Poetry, London.

Stowe, A. (1996) Learning from literature: novels, plays, short stories, and poems in nursing education. *Nurse Educator,* 21, 16-19.

Strauss, A. and Corbin, J. (1998) *Basics of Qualitative Research.* Thousand Oaks, CA; Sage Publications, Inc.

Taylor, J. (1985) Haiku: a form to air feelings about aging. *Geraiatric Nursing,* 6, 81-82.

Treistman, J. (1986) Teaching nursing care through poetry. *Nursing Outlook,* 34, 83-87.

Van Maanen, J. (1988) *Tales of the field: On writing ethnography.* Chicago: University of Chicago Press.

Watson, J. (1994) Poeticizing as truth through language. In P. Chinn and J. Watson (eds.) *Art and Aesthetics in Nursing,* National League for Nursing, New York, (pp3-17).

In: Nursing Education Challenges in the 21st Century
Editor: Leana E. Callara, pp. 195-219
ISBN 1-60021-661-7
© 2008 Nova Science Publishers, Inc.

Chapter 7

DEVELOPING PROFESSIONAL IDENTITY: A STUDY OF THE PERCEPTIONS OF FIRST YEAR NURSING, MEDICAL, DENTAL AND PHARMACY STUDENTS

Susan Morison[1] and Ailsing O'Boyle[2]

[1] Centre for Excellence in Interprofessional Education (NI), Queen's University
[2] School of Education, Queen's University, Belfast, Northern Ireland, UK.

ABSTRACT

Background: Working in a team has become a significant component of modern healthcare practice and pre-qualification education must prepare students for this role. Interprofessional learning is increasingly regarded as key to achieving this although there remains considerable debate about the value of it. In particular there is concern that students need to develop their own professional identity before they can learn to work with others.

Aim: To use social identity theory as a vehicle to examine and compare nursing, dental, medical and pharmacy students' perceptions of the professional identity of their discipline and to consider the implications for developments in interprofessional education.

Method: Focus groups were carried out with pre-qualification students from four healthcare professions in the first semester of the first year of their course in order to gain an insight into the shared understandings, attitudes and values of becoming a healthcare professional. Focus group data were analysed using an ethnographic approach where interaction is analysed as being negotiated through sequenced talk.

Results: Some common themes emerged with all groups indicating that their knowledge of the identity of their discipline, and their motivation to join the profession, came from contact with professionals in healthcare settings or having a member of their family involved in healthcare. Analogies were made between the process of becoming a professional and the developmental process of moving from childhood to adulthood. Differences emerged between the professions with regard to students' perceptions of their future professional role, of other healthcare professionals and others' perceptions of them. In-group and out-group identities were apparent with nursing students located in the out-group of the other professions and also placing themselves in this group. The focus group process itself reinforced the group identity.

Conclusion: A greater understanding of students' perceptions of their professional identity and the processes involved in becoming a professional can help to inform developments in pre-qualification healthcare education. Pre-qualification interprofessional learning should be developed to encourage students to have an inclusive rather than an exclusive professional identity if effective team workers are to emerge.

INTRODUCTION

Working collaboratively as part of a team has become a significant component of modern healthcare practice and pre-qualification education should be key area where students can begin their preparation for this role. Traditionally, healthcare students have been educated separately rather than together, and teamwork and communication skills were not recognised in the core curriculum. However, this picture is slowly changing and it is important to understand what has brought these changes about, some of the difficulties associated with developing pre-qualification shared learning, and how social identity theory can help us to understand more about the role of group interaction in this process.

Background

In the UK the healthcare professions' regulatory bodies and the Government have recognised a need to provide pre-qualification students with opportunities for shared learning or interprofessional education (IPE) (GMC 2002, GDC 2002, NMC 2001, and RPSGB 2004). Additionally, reports that resulted from a series of high profile cases of medical failures (Department of Health 2001, Laming 2003) have added impetus to the desire to ensure that healthcare students and professionals learn together to improve their teamwork and communication skills. Similarly in the US acknowledged failures in the healthcare system include a significant number of medical errors (Institute of Medicine 2003) and reforms are being introduced in healthcare education aimed at improving quality of care and limiting such errors. Again, like the UK, policy makers in the US have suggested that educating all healthcare professionals to work in teams and communicate effectively is one answer to this problem (Institute of Medicine 2001 and 2003, Kelch and Osterweiss, 2004). Other bodies such as the American Council on Pharmaceutical Education, the Accreditation Council for Graduate Medical Education, and the National League for Nursing Accreditation Commission have all developed some interprofessional competency statements (Rafter et al 2006) designed to help improve communication and teamworking skills.

Other drivers of change include the changing expectations of patients who are generally much better informed, less deferential and with more diverse needs (Barr et al 2005 and Institute of Medicine 2003). Concomitantly, the healthcare workforce is under pressure to work flexibly, adapt to the demands of changes to clinical practice and governance issues in the workplace, and respond to the changing expectations of patients (Department of Health 2000).

Developing Pre-Qualification Shared Learning

Reports of interprofessional interventions in healthcare education to develop teamwork and communication skills are increasingly common, but a recent systematic review of the evidence base for interprofessional education (Barr et al, 2005) found that only 19% of the studies reported concerned pre-qualification courses. It is evident that although the provision of shared learning opportunities for pre-qualification healthcare students is now a requirement in the UK there is limited published evidence under-pinning this. Similarly in the US there is recognition that funding must be provided to evaluate developments in interprofessional education if it is be accepted as a way forward (Rafter et al 2006). Advocates of IPE remain divided on some important issues, such as the optimum time to introduce shared learning into healthcare curricula (Barr et al 2005 and Morison et al 2003) and this has implications for the planning and introduction of future initiatives.

The issue of when to introduce shared learning is worth further examination. There is clearly a role for shared learning at post-registration level and in continuing healthcare education. Healthcare professionals should already understand and be secure in their own role and will probably have some practical experience of teamwork. Interventions can also be evaluated directly in relation to clinical practice and patient outcomes. This is not the case for pre-qualification shared learning. Arguments in favour of pre-qualification shared learning suggest that it should be embedded throughout curricula to provide continuity and progression for learning with and about other healthcare professionals (Tope 1999, Areskog 1998 and Harden 1998). However, arguments against suggest that pre-qualification students may not have acquired an understanding of their own professional role or professional identity, both of which are prerequisites for shared learning (Oandasan et al 2004 and Solomon et al 2003). The issue of identity is particularly pertinent to any discussion about the appropriate time to introduce shared learning as the future professional identity and attitudes to other healthcare will be determined throughout the learning experience and the early stages of professional learning may have a particularly significant role.

Shared learning aims to enable participants to understand more about their own and other professionals' roles and responsibilities, and to encourage the development of teamwork and communication skills, which should ultimately improve the care a multidisciplinary healthcare team provides to patients. However, the barriers to its success include professional identity, rivalry, history and culture, professional status, prejudice and lack of trust (Miller et al 1999 and Headrick et al 1998). Participants in shared learning events bring with them preconceived ideas that potentially can harm rather than improve working relationships and this includes stereotypes of the 'other' profession (Mandy et al 2004). Additionally participants may have a distinct group identity (Barr et al 2005) that includes group knowledge, attitudes, skills, and expectations of other healthcare professionals. Shared learning is likely to encourage students to compare their own groups' qualities with others (Carpenter and Hewstone 1996) and it is thus important that developments in interprofessional education consider the potential impact of these attitudes.

Professional education enables the development of an identity that is acceptable to that profession and defines for students and practitioners how they must behave and what they must know in order to be perceived as professionally acceptable to their teachers and fellow professionals (Slotnick 2001 and Cavenagh et al 2000). In other words it enables students to develop an appropriate professional identity. Members of the profession become role models from whom students learn their profession's values, attitudes and beliefs and how to approach the professional world (Paice et al 2002 and Slotnick, 2001). Developments in shared learning need to consider what impact these professional and educational differences may make and at what stage 'identities' begin to develop. Social identity theory would appear to be a suitable vehicle for examining this phenomenon (Hean et al 2006, Adams et al 2006 and Mandy et al 2004).

THE SOCIAL IDENTITY APPROACH

Organizations work most effectively when roles, values, norms and purpose are understood by individuals working collectively (Smith 1995). Yet an "awareness of membership, or self-categorization is critical" (1995:425). Development of a professional identity or membership of a particular group has been investigated through social identity theory (Tajfel and Turner, 1979) and self-categorization theory (Turner, 1985; Turner, Hogg, Oakes, Reicher and Wetherell, 1987). While the former is broadly concerned with intergroup relations and conflict, self-categorization theory examines the processes involved in group formation and those processes which result in the belief of individuals that they share membership of the same group, and how this affects their behaviour and perceptions (Haslam, 2004).

Social identity theory contains three major tenets; categorization, identification and comparison. In order to understand the world, people categorize objects and each other. The process of categorization specifies the particular features of the object/person, and the functions that they carry out. Objects and people in different categories therefore carry out different tasks. Categorization also creates expectations about the functions and tasks of the behaviour of the people who have been categorized. Belonging to a particular group involves the perception of similarity. Members of the same group are perceived as identical, while members outside the group are perceived as dissimilar. However, while maintaining a group identity, individuals also perceive themselves as holding a 'personal identity', unique within the group. It is the operation of these levels of identity of self-categorization, which Turner et al. (1987) argue is important in the social self-concept (Turner with Hogg, Oakes, Reicher and Wetherell, 1987:45). Tajfel and Turner (1979) suggest that a positive self-concept is necessary to operate effectively. In order to evaluate the self, it is necessary to compare with others. Individual members of the group compare themselves with each other and identify themselves as being members of a group which is positively perceived. However when groups minimize the differences between their group and another group they do so in order to minimize perceived negative qualities which may be attributed to their group. This negative distinction again produces an effect so that the group can be viewed positively.

Self-categorization theory (Turner with Hogg, Oakes, Reicher and Wetherell, 1987) is concerned with how people move from identifying themselves as individuals to identifying themselves as members of a group with a shared identity. The theory pursues the notion that there are more than three levels of identity (levels of abstraction); a superordinate level in which members identify themselves as sharing the basic characteristics of being human as opposed to other members of other species; a social level, based on social similarities and differences using ingroup and outgroup categorizations (e.g. nursing students and medical students); and a subordinate level, a personal level which operates using individual characteristics separate form those members within the same group (e.g. within a group of nursing students, individuals may perceive themselves as different as they hold an identity different from others within the group, such as being a mature student or a mother).

A social identity approach to investigating nursing, medical, dental and pharmacy students' perceptions of the professional identity of their discipline is one way of viewing how students self-stereotype and present an idea of their self-concept as understood at the social level of abstraction where they are becoming members of their profession. Of particular interest to the study described below is the degree of identity present in students who have just entered training for a healthcare profession.

Aim of the Study

The aim of this study was to use social identity theory as a vehicle to examine and compare first year pre-qualification nursing, dental, medical and pharmacy students' perceptions of the professional identity of their discipline and to consider the implications of this for developments in interprofessional learning.

Method and Analysis

Method

Focus groups were chosen as an appropriate method to collect data on the experiences, opinions and views of participants as revealed through group interaction and on-going talk. Essentially, focus groups are a type of group interview but rather than discussion moving between interviewer and group the participants are encouraged to discuss ideas between themselves and share their different perspectives (Cohen et al 2000). By their make-up, the formation of focus groups results in a collective activity where participants talk to one another, ask questions, exchange stories and comment on others' views and experiences. The development of the discussion appears to be determined by the participants and not the researcher and ideas emerge from the interaction. Focus groups allow the researcher to explore the way the group and individual's opinions are presented, challenged and developed during this interaction (Barbour and Kitzinger 1999).

This study was not concerned to determine social attitudes, as other instruments of data collection would be more suitable for this purpose, nor did it aim to present a report of static attitudes linked to traits and behaviours. Again, these can be measured by other means. Rather, the study aimed to present the opinions of students produced in specific situations through the production of talk that occurs within focus groups to examine the perceptions which first year students hold about the professional identity of their discipline.

Sampling has been identified as a major key to the success of a focus group and care must be taken to ensure that participants share relevant common characteristics, or background or experience (Morgan 1988 and Kitzinger and Barbour 1999). In this case participants were randomly selected from the first year pre-qualification healthcare student population in the first month of the first semester of their course of study. Focus groups are also known to be more successful where participants are not known to one another (Cohen et al 2000) and the random nature of the selection process for this study and the stage of the students in their course made it less likely that students would know one another well prior to their attendance at the focus group discussion. However, the researchers were aware that students might have had some prior interaction.

Focus groups were carried out separately with each of the four disciplines (Nursing, Medicine, Dentistry and Pharmacy) with the number of participants ranging from four to eight, typically the number preferred by social sciences researchers (Kitzinger and Barbour, 1999). The focus groups took place in non-teaching areas of the academic institution attended by the participants and participants were provided with refreshments in order to ensure an informal and non-threatening atmosphere. Before the discussion was initiated all participants were asked to complete a consent form and the purpose of carrying out the focus groups was made explicit to all participants.

The level of moderator involvement was low-moderate as the purpose of the research was to investigate the interaction within the group through the production of opinions and responses to their experiences and those of others within the group. Open methods of moderation were preferred as these should result in participants own efforts to establish relations with one another (Ryfe, 2006). Topics were managed by the moderator (AOB) who intervened to elicit responses on particular topics and to back-channel in order to mark the discourse, extend turns, or display listenership. Additionally, the moderator tried to ensure questions were not perceived as having a right or wrong answer, nor that participants' knowledge was being tested. It was also important that the moderator was not regarded as an authority on the subject under discussion (Puchta and Potter 2004).

Particularly in a study designed to examine professional identity, the moderator's professional identity, and the students' knowledge of this, was relevant to the interaction of the focus group. The moderator was not a healthcare professional but worked within the area of healthcare education and participants were informed of this. In this way the identity of the moderator allowed the participants to speak at ease with shared knowledge of the discipline without hierarchical barriers (Puchta and Potter 2004).

The topics for discussion were chosen following detailed interviews carried out with professionals in each of the disciplines and a review of literature on professional identity. Broadly, the topics were students' perceptions of their own disciplines, of other healthcare disciplines, and of how other disciplines perceived them.

Discussion and review of the literature, conducted by the moderator, also afforded the opportunity of becoming familiar with the language, terminology and cultures of the different healthcare professionals. This can help to ensure that lack of understanding would not lead to misinterpretation of the data being collected (Puchta and Potter 2004).

Analysis

The focus groups were audio recorded and transcribed using conventions appropriate to conversation analysis of spoken English (Wray et al 2006, Puchta and Potter 2004). As well as transcribing what was spoken, behaviours such as pauses in discussion, interruption of speech, corrections, and turn-taking were also marked. The resulting transcripts were examined by the moderator and independently by another researcher (SM) to determine how the points of view were constructed, expressed and evaluated by participants and what key themes emerged as a result of this process.

The researchers independently identified and coded the themes common to all focus groups (Cohen 2000, Frankland and Bloor 1999) and then met to agree these and thus ensure the consistency and authenticity of interpretation (Guba and Lincoln 1989). Next, as with the identification of themes, the researchers independently examined the text for evidence of how these themes were constructed through the talk that was produced and how identities were negotiated as part of this process (Silverman, 2000). The utterances were regarded as specific to the context in which they were expressed (Putcha and Potter 2004, Myers and Macnaghten 1999, Potter and Wetherell 1987). The researchers then met to discuss and agree interpretation.

A table and text will be presented in the results section. The table will provide a simple summary of what was said and the text will illustrate *how* this was said. Stretches of text have been used to provide a transparent view of the course of the interaction (Myers and Macnaghten, 1999).

Results

Five common themes emerged from the focus group discussion and these were:

1. Motivation to study for the profession
2. The profession
3. Learning to become a professional
4. Perceptions of other healthcare professions
5. Perceptions of 'others' about the profession

1. Motivation to Study for the Profession

The discussion around this theme highlighted commonalities and differences between the healthcare professions. Comments are summarised in Table 1, 1.1. The motivations of medical and nursing students were similar with both groups stating that they had always wanted such a career and that they were influenced by personal experience, role models and family.

Nursing Students
   1.1
   Female 3: Most people just seem like they just want to be a nurse you know that kind of thing you know they've just have always wanted to .. to be a nurse
   1.2
   Female 4: I had wanted to do it since I was a child … aam my mother is a nurse so she would have told me .. a wee bit about it
   1.3
   Female 2: You know .. the kind of person that I am .. I have a wee boy and I love.. you know even though you are meant to be encouraging them to be more independent I enjoy doing things for people .. okay there is a side where you have to encourage people to maintain their independence especially an elderly person .. but aam at the

same time like a lot of nursing is doing stuff for people cos they're too ill to do it themselves .. and I enjoy that I get a .. you know get something out of that

1.4

Female 3: Any time I was looking after .. a grandparent or something .. like when I was a wee girl .. am .. even just lift their feet or rub their feet for half an hour or something they would just always say to me God you should be a nurse

Table 1. Summary Of Comments On Focus Group Themes

1.1. Summary of comments on motivation
Nursing
Always wanted to be, a part of my personality
Personal experience, role models and family
Range of opportunities but about more than money
Want to be part of things – saving lives and helping others
Medicine
Always wanted this career
Personal experience, role models and family
Working with people and not in an office
Dentistry
Got the grades (also considered pharmacy, science, teaching)
Good hours, good pay (for women), hands-on and variety of specialisms
Medically-related but not medicine
Personal experience
Pharmacy
A job guaranteed when you finish
Variety of areas to work in, flexible hours, good for women
Didn't get into dentistry and interested in the medical side
Science results were important - wanted to use the chemistry side
1.2 Summary of comments on profession
Nursing
A sense of belonging
Care, help, work closely with patients
Satisfying, rewarding
Medicine
A vocation – more than just a job
Cure, help and serve patients
Doctors are: responsible, compassionate, hard working, knowledgeable, respected, clever and high achievers
Dentistry
Not like Medicine – no life/death decisions, problems not taken home
Physician of the mouth
Dentists are: friendly, clean, respected
Pharmacy
Not just working behind a counter, build up a relationship with customers
Not like medicine - do not have to work nights and long hours
Scientific - white lab coat and smart clothes symbolise the professional role
1.3 Summary of comments on learning to be a professional
Nursing
Culture shock of practice – realising the meaning of illness
Chance to bond, observe, respect, help and care for patients
Tough, making progress with a clear goal and sense of achievement

Table 1. (Continued)

Medicine
On the road - a process of change, maturity and inclusion in a professional group
Lot to learn, hard work, slog and exciting
Making friends
Dentistry
Moving from childhood to adulthood – transformational
Gain professional identity, older students as role models
Hard work, exciting with an end product
Pharmacy
Learning to be more independent - think for yourself, look after yourself
Gain professional identity - older students as role models
Hard work, but job for life at the end
Making friends
1.4 Summary of comments on 'other' healthcare professions
Nursing
Therapists and doctors not as directly or emotionally involved as nurses
Doctors very responsible early on
Doctors dress well
Medical practice, like nursing, is tiring
Dentistry is boring
Pharmacists understanding of drugs is interesting but being a chemist is boring
Medicine
Useful to know pharmacists and dentists for future practice
Nurses are caring
Dentistry
Doctors, pharmacists and opticians are like dentists – make lives better
Medicine is more emotionally demanding – life/death decisions
Pharmacy is boring
Nurses get the dirty jobs
Pharmacy
Medics are smartly dressed, intimidating
Dental students have no particular characteristics
Nursing students usually girls
Medicine and nursing more stressful
1.5 Summary of comments on 'other' professionals' views of their profession
Nursing
Doctors viewed as higher status than nursing – nurses commonplace
Looked down on or excluded by some doctors Nurses are less respected than other healthcare professionals
Medicine
Superior, clever, nerdy
High expectations
Dentistry
Lonely, repetitive and respected (like Doctors, vets, pharmacists and opticians)
Different from medicine
Pharmacy
Not the sort of people who wear bright clothes or look 'arty'

Medical Students

1.5

Female 1: I never really pictured myself being anything else so aam like I think I've always been able to picture myself being a doctor

Male 3: There was never anything else for me it was always .. since primary school I've always.. that was it I never remember it coming into my head .. its just that was just it

1.6

Male 2: There's so many new things like everybody's got a different ailment and if you are sitting in an office you are doing the same thing constantly over and over again but with medicine everybody comes in with different things like different people and things

Although dental students also indicated they were motivated by personal experience, the dental and pharmacy students were motivated more by the promise of a guaranteed, well-paid and flexible career, particularly for women. They also identified themselves as being motivated by the medically-related nature of the job.

Dental Students

1.7

Female1: I think that dentistry is probably a better option like for women anyway because its much more flexible in time and stuff if you're having children and stuff and like .. its not .. you know .. as sort of mentally demanding

Male 1: I have a lot of personal experience being at the orthodontist with braces and stuff

Male 2: I was going to do teaching for a long time before I chose dentistry

Mod: Umhmm … what made you change

Male 2: Well my my my grades made me change cos I never …I never considered myself you know the way you get the top people that get all the As I never would put myself in that bracket and neither would me teachers

Female: When I was young I wanted to do medicine but I think that was mainly because that was what both my parents did then .. when I fainted that put me off a whole lot .. and I was basically looking for another sort of medical related career cos I still found it all really interesting and stuff .. so that's why the reasons I chose dentistry

Pharmacy Students

1.8

Female 1: I also think it's a really good degree cos you're actually once you've finished it there's there will be a job waiting for you you know and there is all these degrees people finish and they have no job [..] I think yeah it is a really good job for women as well so it's so well paid and ..you can do your locum work and .. you know if you want to work in a community pharmacy you can basically choose when you want to work

Mod: Umhum

Female 1: so it is you know flexible and .. if you were doing medicine you know you're working your long hours and night shifts whereas in pharmacy you have the opportunity not to do that

1.9

Female 2: I tried to get into dentistry but didn't get in so this degree was my second choice really but I just wanted to do something medical

2. Professional Role

Comments are summarised in Table 1, 1.2. The medical and nursing students were again similar in describing their profession as a vocation. However, their perceptions of what that role is were very different and this is reflected in the language used to describe this.

Nursing Students

2.1

Female 4: It's difficult to articulate but .. you just .. going into work every day it's just it's .. what's today gonna be like what are we gonna do .. and .. you get through the day and you know when your lunch breaks are and that kind of thing as any job .. but .. don't know it's just really hard to put into words..

Mod: Umhum

Female 4: The feeling that you get maybe .. like for example a stroke patient last week was able to say to me that her dinner was tasty and that was the first word I'd had out of her in three weeks but I'd been feeding her nearly every day for three weeks and that was just like .. and just .. aam like to me that's a a sense of achievement for me that you've got that relationship so far but as well .. asking them questions and trying to interact with them rather than just seeing that person as .. no she's too low to even be bothering with just get the food into her and away you go

Mod: Umhum

Female 4: You know to me it takes a nurse to recognise that that person needs to be spoken to what kind of questions you need to ask how you need to ask them like if they their clothes and that kind of thing

Medical Students

2.2

Female 1: Its all about either making people better or making people comfortable or seeing people go through life and death .. its just because certain people in society need to know .. how to deal .. with all those its its mostly interaction .. with people .. medicine

2.3

Male 3: Medics are really like responsible for you so it's a responsible thing to like be a doctor because you are responsible for so many people

2.4

Male 4: if your intelligent enough to get into medicine you'd probably make a lot more money doing a different kind of job with not as much work and not as much responsibility so I think it's a kind of it's a vocation you know more than a job

Both dental and pharmacy students defined their profession by explaining what it was *not* and particularly that it was *not* like medicine.

Dental Students

2.5

Male 1: What is dentistry I don't know

Female 2:Its teeth there's so many different+

Male 1: physician of the mouth I suppose [..] I mean the difference between a dentist and a doctor is between life and death and there's not many ethical issues as well so its not its more .. plus .. you're guaranteed a job at the end of your degree as well .. and you work your own hours .. whereas a doctor he works long hours as junior doctor and its not as good a pay as dentists

Pharmacy Students

2.6

Male 1: It's just .. the white coat that you wear in the lab [laughter] you just you can just see yourself in it you know

2.7

Female 3: Pharmacists are kinda like nine to five but doctors are going twenty four hours

3. Learning to become a professional

Comments are summarised in Table 1, 1.3. All students considered the task of learning to become a professional as something that involved hard work and perseverance. All students perceived the process as transformational, like moving from childhood to adulthood or like encountering a new culture. The medical, dental and pharmacy students described the process as becoming part of a professional group and learning to take on the identity of that group.

Medical Students

3.1

Female 2: There's a lot just what we've been learning already and realizing there are so many things that I just don't know

Male 2: Yeah before you think that there is a lot of work to be done but you didn't know what had to be done what you had to learn what essays you had to write and stuff like that

Mod: Umhmm...

Male 1: I think its really exciting though to be on its really really ..we're actually doing like like kind of mediciney things .. you're on the road you know you're kind of in medicine alright so

Dental Students

3.2

Male 1: I suppose like in terms of being a dentist we're kind of like the child stage at the minute its we're just sort of learning everything and then eventually we'll learn everything and be like I suppose we'll be like an adult type of thing just starting off off from scratch really so its exciting its like the first sort of step along the way now for the rest of your life its quite ..you know

In addition, medical and pharmacy students described making friends as a part of the learning process, and dental and pharmacy students viewed older students as role models.

Pharmacy Students
    3.3
    Female 7: But that was probably only natural .. they [older students] would be keep saying like you know actually that it gets easier as you go along a lot of people have told me that first year was your hardest .. they found anyway and then they found it easier from then on so I kinda ..bit of encouragement I suppose [laughter]
    3.4
    Female 3: I'm so used to following a syllabus with just going on with it
    Female 2: I suppose maybe they're going to tell us
    Female 3: That's what you get for not being at school ..more independent than school like looking after yourself

The nursing students were unique in describing the learning process from a practical, ward-based perspective.

Nursing
    3.5
    Female 4: The ..first couple of days were just ..
    Female 3: very tough
    Female 4: a complete culture shock
    3.6
    Female 4: You don't really see .. the nitty gritty
    Mod: Umhum
    Female 4: But .. yeah it was …quite admittedly very distressed I felt very upset at the end of the first day just cos
    Mod: Umhum
    Female 4: Cos it was such ..a culture shock you just forget how ill people are

4. Perceptions of 'other' healthcare professions
Comments are summarised in Table 1, 1.4. Nursing students identified doctors in particular as being different from them in the way they interacted with patients, their appearance and responsibilities. However, they thought the professions were alike in being demanding, and the pharmacy students also commented on this.

Nursing Students
    4.1
    Mod: How do you see them as being different from you I mean you are both students
    Female 2: Probably more knowledgeable
    Female 3: a lot more
    Female 2: because [..] they've just qualified they're working as doctors and I was just sitting thinking the other day actually..God imagine if you were training to be a doctor you would really have to know your stuff you know you would have to do the

studying and all whereas you couldn't just try and get out try and bluff your way because when you are actually making diagnosis for people you have to know exactly what's wrong with them and I thought that would be a very responsible thing I think

Female 4: Yeah

Female 3: Well no well I wouldn't put it down to just being more than ..I would put it down it is a different type of knowledge it is a different

Mod: How is it different

Female 4: Aam ..

Female 3: It is more medical based it's not

Female 4: It's more medical based whereas Nursing is more care based for example if you give somebody .. antibiotics and within hours they'd come out in a rash it is up to the nurses to say to the doctor she's come out in a rash it only happened two hours after you gave her antibiotics .. try a different one .. you know you are there twenty four seven . well .. but the d= it's up to the nurses to feed that information through to the doctor and if the doctor's only there for an hour a day on the ward and maybe maybe not doesn't see the irritation but doesn't notice that where the irritation comes from rather than saying look put a cream on it

Mod: Umhum umhum

Female 4: Small things like that or .. I don't know you think right well that rash has cleared up you can take them off that cream or take them off the antibiotic it might be the doctor that legally has to put the signature there but then .. they're learning as well they know for the future that that drug doesn't correlate with that drug and whereas a nurse might not know that

Female 2: It must be really tough for them actually coming up to patients seeing patients on their own saying what's wrong with them and that you know when they have just come out of .. you know

Mod: umhum

Female 4: Training I mean I think that would be really scary having to diagnose someone [laughter]what was wrong with someone

4.2

Female 4: It must be difficult for the other students that are coming on to wards as well like .. the doctors that maybe aren't long qualified cos they know the teamwork that is there between nurses

Female 2: Yes I know and it must be hard for them

Female 4: Yeah

Female 2: I was thinking that the other day coming up on to the ward

Female 4: Coming on to an unfamiliar .. culture environment as well

Female 2: And nobody really talks to them it's all just sort of like .. hello under your breath but there's not really a lot of communication going on there

Female 4: No

Mod: Why do you think that is

Female 2: You see it all the time .. I don't know if it's just .. like a barrier thing they're doctors and we're nurses and you know it's that status thing again where .. you know .. we don't really have the same kind of banter with doctors as you would but ..I don't know I think it's the discipline and that

Female 4: I asked one of them the other day what was his name was and he just looked at me as if I was in

Female 2: Yeah exactly

Female 4: something that came off his shoe and I just said to him well you're up here every day I just gave it back to him I said you're up here every day what's your name … and he was like oh right it's .. whatever it was like

Female 2: Yeah

Female 4: Pleased to meet you

Female 2: It's almost as if they haven't

Female 4: there's a pot of tea ready if you want a cup [..] but … maybe it was shock that somebody spoke to him

Medical, pharmacy and dental students all identified a relationship between their three professions but did not make this association with nursing students.

Medical Students

4.3

Female 2: And they [dental students] will be useful later on to if you had a patient came in with a tooth problem and you weren't specialized in that area you could phone your friend up and ask them for their advice it's the same with other courses like Pharmacy

4.4

Male 2: If you think of nurses and all that there they're really caring like you know whenever you meet them

Dentistry Students

4.5

Male 1: The same cos you go in there is never any such thing as an ignorant doctor they're all very welcoming .. reassuring .. just and you know some doctors I know are maybe more thorough than others but you get the same treatment you know they're all you know typical doctor or dentist its like they've been trained to be that way

4.6

Female 2: Nurses get the dirty jobs do you know what I mean if the man .. wets the bed or whatever the nurse has to clean him up sort out that bed or whatever its not .. wouldn't like that

Pharmacy Students

4.7

Female 1: If you see them oh you say that looks like one [medical student]

Mod: What is it about them that makes it makes them look

Female 6: I really don't know like

Female 2: They're smart [laughter]

4.8

Mod: Would you like to do something like that in your own course..you as pharmacy students working with medical students would you like to be in that kind of a situation

Male 1: [laughs]

Female 3: its like oh no don't listen to me

Female 4: I'd kind of feel a bit intimidated

4.9

Mod: What about a nurse

Male 1: [inaudible]

[laughter]

Mod: What did you say there

Female 1: A large group of girls

[laughter]

Female 1: A large group of girls right

Female 3: And one boy even

[laughter]

5. Perceptions of 'others' about their profession

Comments are summarised in Table 1, 1.5. Medical students described 'others' as seeing them as superior whereas nursing students saw themselves as being viewed as inferior. Dental and pharmacy students spent very little time discussing others' perceptions of them.

Medical Students

5.1

Male 1: I think you can get like a God like you know what you were saying earlier like a God mentality

Male 4: Aye

Male 1: about being a doctor

Male 2: Yeah

Male 1: You'd need to get rid of that pretty soon wouldn't you

Male 4: Aye... it seems that there is a stereotype .. definitely from people looking out aam towards doctors doctors have an air of superiority and they think that they're the top dogs about the place so I think that .. straight off from first weeks its definitely a good idea that they mix with other people who are doing ..uh you know just normal three year degrees and whatever because after they graduate you'll still be like a student so its good having friends in all different areas .. of jobs I think

Female 1: But even whenever you start to tell people that you are doing medicine they all go [both hands raised and palms open with a loud intake of breath]

Male 1: Yeah

Male 3: You're right

Male 2: I deliberately don't tell them

Female: I only tell them if they ask

Male 4: Naa I say .. because I think whenever you they say ah they're doing for example Ancient Philosophy and then they ask you .. if unless they ask you I wouldn't go well I'm doing medicine cos people straight away would think he's up he's up himself or whatever

Male 2: Yeah but would you not think the same like say for somebody doing English or doing like some essays real essay-based thing .. I'd be going .. you're mad like cos I really can't do that all the essays

Male 4: Mmmm

Male 2: like history and stuff like that like impressed that they are doing that there as well

Female 3: I don't like to telling people I'm doing medicine because they relate then something about you are really really smart or something

Male 4: Yeah I know

Female 3: You just need three As to get in .. like they think well they must be super intelligent and they do like stereotype you

Male 1: Its like this thing ahh well you must be really smart but it's not like a compliment its like a kind of .. like .. insult

Mod: And do you think that say for example dentistry students or pharmacy students they don't get that

Male 2: No

Mod: reaction

Male 2: Not so much

Female 2: No

Male 4: Not as much not as much

Nursing Students

5.2

Female 2: Yeah they have you know .. something that they would perceived as having a higher status than nurses and that's just the way life is and I don't think it will ever really change do you I think that's just the way it is

Female 4: I don't think it'll ever really change but you can see why it's there I mean years ago people always put the doctors aye doctors and lawyers and .. eh clergymen on a pedestal and they were godlike .. whereas but I think that was more to do with the fact that you never really saw them and it was like… nudge nudge there's the doctor oh my God you know and bow down whereas .. maybe just resources-wise for every one doctor there could be ten nurses so you see more of nurses so it's not such .. they're not such a flash in the pan if you like

5.3

Female 3: A lot of the patients appreciate the nurses appreciate the work they're always you know saying oh the nurses are great you know they really help me whereas .. my boyfriend his dad's a doctor and my boyfriend told him I was doing nursing .. and he goes oh dear .. you know why did she chose that he has been a doctor for thirty years and I think there's the .. you know a lot of people perceive nurses as sort of ..

Female 4: Just wiping mouths or something

Female 3: Yeah

Female 4: every day..I think there's a lack of understanding from other professions as well

Female 3: Definitely

5.3

Female 3: Well there was a doctor up in the ward about three weeks ago [..] and he said to one of the nurses .. you know I think you should be weighing her since she mustn't be eating properly and one of the nurses became very defensive because .. this is one of the continuing care patients who they you know if she's not gonna eat properly obviously they're gonna be putting her on something else you know like a build up drink or something ..and he was ..he was being very ..I don't know how to say …you know I think .as if they didn't as if they didn't know the patient as if they hadn't been taking care of them for weeks months

DISCUSSION

The aim of this study was to examine and compare first year nursing, medical, dental and pharmacy students' perceptions of the professional identity of their discipline and to consider the implications of this for interprofessional education. Using focus groups as a research method to capture participants' views provided the opportunity to scrutinise the linguistic interaction between participants to further illuminate the process of developing a professional identity.

The data suggest that all groups entered their professional training with preconceived ideas of their discipline's professional identity and the groups with the strongest idea of, commitment to and belief in, their professional identity were nursing and medical students. For both of these groups motivation to join the profession was similar. Motivations were described as originating in childhood and were regarded as intrinsic to their idea of themselves in future. In respect of medical student this concurs with the findings of Cavenagh et al (2000) who concluded that medical students had a strong commitment to their career choice and a strong professional identity even at the outset of training. However, both Carpenter (1995) and Adams et al (2006) have suggested that nursing students do not have a strong professional identity. This difference may be explained by the research method used here. Rather than presenting students with a check-list of questionnaire items defining professional characteristics, the focus group method provided participants with the opportunity to discuss and develop their ideas and thus to give a more considered view of how they view their profession.

The data show that the nursing students were as highly motivated as medical students by professional ideals to become a member of their professional community. Developments in interprofessional education would be helped by recognising this and building on these positive attitudes to ensure that future development of a strong professional identity is inclusive rather than exclusive in its nature. A study by Morison et al (2004) found that by the fourth year of their undergraduate programme medical students had already developed a more exclusive attitude to learning with other healthcare professionals than nursing students and the early introduction of shared learning could make a positive contribution to this potential problem.

The strength of commitment to their profession by nursing and medical students suggests that they have already begun the process of categorising themselves as a part of that professional group. An essential component of group identity is an emotional as well as actual sense of belonging (Hogg and Abrams, 1988) and this is apparent from the emotive language used by both groups to describe their motivation to join the profession (extracts 1.1 - 1.6):

And I enjoy that I get a .. you know get something out of that (NS)

There was never anything else for me it was always..... (MS)

In contrast the dental and pharmacy students described their motivations less personally in terms of a good salary and working conditions. Their discussion touched on personal issues but they did not dominate and, unlike the nursing and medical students, they were still striving to identify what makes their chosen profession distinct. They were able to identify the group they aspired to join as high status but as lower in status than medicine and therefore they needed to find other reasons why it was important to be a member of such a group (see extracts 1.7 – 1.9).

....if you were doing medicine you know you're working your long hours and night shifts whereas in pharmacy you have the opportunity not to do that. (PS)

The divide between nursing and medicine on the one hand, and dentistry and pharmacy on the other becomes more apparent when we examine the way in which the students described their perceptions of their future professional role. The nursing and medical students both had a very clear idea of what it means to belong to their group but the dental and pharmacy students struggled in their description and resorted to explaining the identity of their group by how it differs from medicine. Dental and pharmacy students had a stronger idea of what a doctor is and does than of *their* future professional role and resorted to generalisations and symbols of professionalism to describe their group (see extracts 2.5 – 2.7).

It's teeth (DS) and ....the white coat you wear in the lab (PS)

However, what is important to this discussion is that the focus group interaction offered the opportunity for the dental and pharmacy students to begin to develop their identity and in order to do this they categorised themselves as a group different to and distinct from medicine.

It is noticeable that all of healthcare groups had a strong image of the discipline of medicine and its practitioners who were regarded in some undefined, non-specific way as being a superior profession. This poses some interesting challenges for interprofessional developments and is an issue that cannot be ignored. Cavenagh et al (2000) speculated that medical students' early formation of a strong professional identity and subsequent powerful socialisation, may explain the profession's inability to adapt to changing roles and new demands including teamwork. The study described above suggests that medical students strong identity additionally includes notions of superiority, which are acceded to by the other healthcare professionals. Pre-qualification shared learning could provide a way of helping students to discuss such issues and early exposure to other professions may help to ameliorate the development of professional identities.

Although the nursing and medical students both had a very distinct idea of their future professional role, the way in which this was described was very different (extracts 2.1 – 2.4). The medical students described their group with language that included,

'Life and death,' 'you are responsible for so many people' 'intelligent' and 'it's a vocation you know'

Their views were presented as abstract ideas or stereotypes of high status professionals and are characteristics that the students admired, valued and aspired to acquire. Further, extract 2.3 illustrates the way in which the focus group interaction gave the medical students the opportunity not just to describe but also to begin to take on the identity of the group they aspire to join. Thus the introduction of the word 'you' into the discussion shows how readily the students begin to include themselves in this 'special' group.

In comparison, nursing students' concept of their identity was much more tangible and practical and their group identity included ideas of hard but rewarding work, close and caring relationships with patients and selflessness (extract 2.1). Although these were almost the opposite of the medical students' group stereotypes they were nevertheless equally aspirational qualities. This contrast illustrates one of the problems of developing pre-qualification shared learning to satisfy these equally strong but different professional expectations. Recognising this problem however is also a step towards its solution and appropriate shared learning could be used to help professions to develop an interprofessional identity as well as having a strong and distinct professional identity. In other words effective interprofessional understanding and team interaction should be as much a part of professional identity as disease diagnosis and patient care have traditionally been.

For all groups of students it would seem that at the outset of training they were anxious to define the group they belonged to and to identify the characteristics of that group even though some professional groups had more definite ideas than others. Again this has implications that may be addressed by the development of pre-qualification shared learning which could be used to begin to encourage students from an early stage to perceive their group as part of a network of different but overlapping groups who need to work together for the benefit of the patient. It is generally accepted that interprofessional education should be determined by the appropriate and complementary nature of the learning experience (Harden 1998 and Barr et al 2005) and learning in a practice (as well as a classroom) setting would enable the students to explore the different but inter-connected role of each profession in patient care. Students' discussion about their journey in learning to become a professional further highlights the opportunities provided by the early introduction of appropriate shared learning.

All of the students described the process of learning to become a professional as something transformational and there is no doubt that they found this prospect exciting and challenging. The students regarded this early stage in their career as being like the transition from childhood to adulthood and for all of them it represented an important step towards becoming the professional they wished to be in future. All groups were also conscious that this would be a time when they are strongly influenced by their student peers and by new learning experiences. Although the nursing students were the only group able to describe this experience from a practical perspective all students were aware of the significance of this early experience. From an educational perspective it would seem an ideal opportunity to introduce students to the positive benefits of groups of healthcare professionals working together in a team. Social identity theory would suggest that in order to do this it is important for groups to have a strong in-group identity, but also to have a positive view of the out-groups they interact with (Hean et al 2006). Educators need to ensure interprofessional programmes take account of possible in-group and out-group perceptions. As role models, it will also be important for the educators to exemplify the new values of teamwork and collaboration being promoted by shared learning rather than the old values of tribalism and rivalry.

The healthcare students' views on other professions and how others perceived them provide a useful means to examine further these interprofessional, group identity issues. The nursing students provided a lengthy commentary on their views of the medical profession but had very little to say about either pharmacy or dental students. Their interest is in the out-group that they will have the most contact with in their professional role. Although they appeared to present stereotypical views of doctors they were speaking about events they had experienced and as the discussion developed they identified ways in which they were different from the medical profession and recognised that there were similarities.

Extract 4.1. illustrates the way in which the focus group discussion allowed the nursing students to develop their views. The students began by describing doctors as different and in some way superior, '*more knowledgeable.*' However, the four nursing students revised this view and were able to conclude that although their role is different from that of doctors it is not necessarily inferior. Nursing, is redefined as being of equal status because it involves working closely with patients. Similarly, illustrated in extract 4.2, the students were able to identity positive attributes of their professional identity such as being part of a ward community, which the doctors are excluded from. They also suggested that doctors' remoteness might be determined by their exclusion from this community. Thus the focus group discussion provided an excellent example of the way in which the students created their in-group identity, extended this to the context of their practice as well as the practice itself, and began to gain insight into why the medical out-group might find it difficult to interact in a positive way. Interaction and discussion would appear to be powerful tools for forming opinions and shaping identities and the early introduction of shared learning might have an important role in this respect.

In contrast to the nursing students, medical students had very little to say about any of the other professions. Of interest however, is that they made an association between themselves and other 'higher status' professionals like dentists and pharmacists who might have future value to their medical practice. Nursing students were not discussed in relation to their future practice but merely described as *caring,* and all three of the higher status groups placed nursing students in a low status out-group. The pharmacy students' extracts (4.12 and 13) illustrate the complete contrast in attitude to the different professions. The medical students were given high status labels and in contrast the nursing students were a source of amusement. The evidence of this study is that medical, dental and pharmacy students entered their training with a low status stereotype of nursing students already in place. If pre-qualification interprofessional education is to be successful it must aim to tackle this problem at the outset.

An examination of the views students expressed about how they thought 'outsiders' perceived their profession supports the argument that professional identity is an issue that must be considered by interprofessional education developers. The dental and pharmacy students did not enter training with a very strong idea of their professional identity and consequently did not have strong views about how other groups might perceive them. The most interesting groups were the nursing and medical students who each recognised the high and low status respectively associated with their profession. In contrast to having little to say about other professions, a high status behaviour in itself, the medical students had much to say about how others perceived them. The tight development of the discussion itself (extract 5.1) illustrates how the students bonded together on this issue.

In extract 5.1 the signals of agreement between the students describing shared experiences of negativity from others towards the medical profession are evidenced through rapid exchanges of conversation. There are many occurrences of words of agreement such as 'yeah' and 'you're right' and although initiating disagreement in turn twelve, Male 4, completes his response agreeing with the others in the group and giving an additional idiomatic example of the negative features attributed to their group "he's up himself". Throughout these exchanges this and other metaphors used negatively by 'others,' enable the members of the group to demonstrate their shared experiences. Once the negative attributes have been exposed the speakers seek to minimize these negative characteristics, "you *just* need three As to get in" and then agree that those who attribute such qualities are unjust, "its not like a compliment its [..] insult".

In contrast to the medical students, nursing students (extracts 5.2 and 5.3) acknowledged that their profession was not highly regarded by many outsiders but that patients appreciated what they did. Their discussion also created a strong group identity through a shared acknowledgement of their low status but also agreement that this view was mistaken and the result of a 'lack of understanding.' Like the medical students' discussion the use of words like 'yeah' and 'definitely' confirm the group's shared experiences and utterances are taken up and completed readily by another speaker. Doctors are used as an example of a highly regarded profession but there is implied disagreement in the explanation for this – that they are highly regarded because they are rarely seen. Doctors are also used to illustrate examples of professional prejudice and the practical example provided by Female 3 supports the nurses implied view that doctors neither understand what actually happens on the ward nor do they appreciate the daily care of patients carried out by nurses.

The views presented by nursing and medical students very clearly help to illustrate the underlying prejudices present in the different professional groups at the outset of their training and demonstrates the need to deal with these issues in the development of pre-qualification interprofessional learning.

The group interaction and linguistic behaviours displayed by the nursing and medical students are consistent with theories of self-categorisation (Tajfel and Turner 1979). This study suggests that the process of sharing experiences with other trainees itself encourages the development of a group or professional identity. It is therefore important to consider how powerful a tool this might be for developments in interprofessional learning. Understanding students' interaction through social identity theory allows us to see that interprofessional, interactive, patient-focused learning opportunities should be introduced early in pre-qualification healthcare curricula to help ensure that positive in-group and out-group identities are promoted and a better understanding of other professionals' roles and responsibilities is encouraged.

CONCLUSION

The results from this study suggest that nursing, medical, dental and pharmacy students all entered training with preconceived stereotypes of their own and other healthcare students' professional identities. Nursing and medical students had a much stronger idea of their professional identity than did dental and pharmacy students but these latter two groups nevertheless wanted to create a strong identity for themselves. All groups of students used the focus group process itself as a means to begin to create this identity. Medical, dental and pharmacy students all viewed nursing as a lower status profession and although the nursing students were aware of that others held this view the focus group interaction enabled them to perceive this as mistaken.

Appropriate pre-qualification shared learning, led by educators who exemplify good collaborative and team working skills, could provide a vehicle to encourage discussion and exploration of professional stereotypes and prejudice to help students develop an interprofessional identity within a distinct professional one.

A greater understanding of students' perceptions of their professional identity and the processes involved in becoming a professional is a highly valuable tool to inform developments in pre-qualification healthcare education. Pre-qualification interprofessional learning should be developed to encourage students to have an inclusive rather than an exclusive professional identity if effective team workers are to emerge.

REFERENCES

Adams, K., Hean, S. Sturgis, P., and Macleod Clark, J. (2006). Investigating the factors influencing professional identity of first-year health and social care students. Learning in Health and Social Care, 5, 2, 55-68.

Areskog, N. (1988). The need for multiprofessional health education within undergraduate studies. Medical Education, 22, 251.

Barbour, R.S. and Kitzinger, J. (Eds.) (1999). Developing focus group research: politics, theory and practice. London: Sage Publications.

Barr, H., Freeth, D., Hammick, M, and Koppel, I., and Reeves, S. (2005). Effective Interprofessional education: Argument, Assumption and Evidence. Blackwell Publishing, London.

Carpenter, J. (1995). Doctors and nurses: stereotypes and stereotype change in interprofessional education. Journal of Interprofessional Care, 9, 151-161.

Carpenter, J. and Hewstone, M. (1996). Shared learning for doctors and social workers: evaluation of a programme. British Journal of Social Work, 26, 239-257.

Cavenagh, P., Dewsbury, C., and Jones, P. (2000). Becoming professional: when and how does it start? A comparative study of first-year medical and law students in the UK. Medical Education, 34, 897-902.

Cohen, L., Manion, L., and Morrison, K. (2000). Research methods in education. 5th Edition. London: Routledge Falmer.

Department of Health (2000). The NHS Plan: a plan for investment, a plan for reform. London: TSO.

Department of Health (2001). Learning from Bristol: The Report of the Public Inquiry into Children's heart Surgery at the Bristol Royal Infirmary 1984-1995. London: TSO.

Frankland, J., and Bloor, M. (1999). Some issues arising in the systematic analysis of focus group material, In: Barbour, R. and Kitzinger, J. (Eds.) Developing Focus Group Research: Politics, Theory & Practice, London: Sage Publications.

General Dental Council (2002). The First Five Years. London: GDC.

General Medical Council (2002). Tomorrow's Doctors. London: GMC

Guba, E.G. and Lincoln, Y.S. (1989). Fourth generation evaluation. Newbury Park, CA: Sage Publications

Harden, RM. (1998). Effective multiprofessional education: a three-dimensional perspective. Medical Teacher, 20, 5, 402-408.

Haslam, S.A. (2004). Psychology in Organizations: The Social Identity Approach. 2nd Edition. London: Sage Publications.

Headrick, L., Wilcock, P., and Batalden, P. (1998). Interprofessional working and continuing medical education. British Medical Journal, 316, 771-774.

Hean, S., Macleod Clark, J., Adams, K., Humphris, D., Lathlean, J. (2006). Being seen by others as we see ourselves: the congruence between the ingroup and outgroup perceptions of health and social care students. Learning in Health and Social Care, 5, 1, 10-22.

Hogg, M. A., and Abrams, D. (1988). Social Identifications: A Social Psychology of Intergroup Relations and Group Processes. London: Routledge

Institute of Medicine of the National Academies (2001). Crossing the Quality Chasm: a New Health System for the 21st Century. Washington: The National Academies Press.

Institute of Medicine of the National Academies (2003). Health Professions Education: A Bridge to Quality. Washington: The National Academies Press.

Kelch, R., and Osterweiss, M. (2004). Health professions and quality care: the promises and limitations of interprofessional practice. Washington: Association of Academic Health Centres.

Kitzinger, J., and Barbour, R.S. (1999). Introduction: the challenge and promise of focus groups in Barbour, R.S. and Kitzinger, J. (Eds.) (1999) Developing focus group research: politics, theory and practice. London: Sage Publications.

Laming, L.J. (2003). Inquiry into the death of Victoria Climbie. London: TSO.

Mandy, A., Milton, C., Mandy, P. (2004). Professional stereotyping and interprofessional education. Learning in Health and Social Care,3,3,154-170.

Miller, C., Ross, N. and Freeman, M. (1999). The role of collaborative shared learning in pre and post registration education in nursing, midwifery and health visiting. London: ENB.

Morgan, D.L. (1988). Focus groups as qualitative research. Newbury Park CA: Sage Publications.

Morison, S., Boohan, M., Jenkins, J.and Moutray, M. (2003). Facilitating undergraduate interprofessional learning in healthcare: comparing classroom and clinical learning for nursing and medical students. Learning in Health and Social Care, 2, 92-104.

Morison, S., Boohan, M., Moutray, M. and Jenkins, J. (2004). Developing pre qualification inter-professional education for nursing and medical students: sampling student attitudes to guide development. Nurse Education in Practice, 4, 20-29.

Myers, G., and Macnaghten, M.(1999). Can Focus Groups be analysed as talk? In Barbour, R.S., and Kitzinger, J. (Eds) (1999) Developing focus group research: politics, theory and practice. London: Sage Publications.

Nursing and Midwifery Council (2001). Fitness for Practice and Purpose. London: NMC.

Oandasan, I., D'Amour, D., Zwarenstein, M., Barker, K., Purden, M., Beaulieu M., et al (2004). Interdisciplinary Education for Collaborative, Patient-Centred Practice: Research and Findings Report. Toronto: Health Canada.

Paice, E., Heard, S., and Moss, F. (2002). How important are role models in making good doctors? British Medical Journal, 325, 707-710.

Potter, J., and Wetherell, M.S. (1987). Discourse and social psychology: beyond attitudes and behaviour. London: Sage Publications

Puchta, C., and Potter, J. (2004). Focus group practice. London: Sage Publications

Rafter, M., Pesun, I., Herren, M., Linfante, D., Mina, M., Wu, C., and Casada, J. (2006). A Preliminary Survey of Interprofessional Education. Journal of Dental Education, 70, 4, 417-427.

Royal Pharmaceutical Society of Great Britain (2004). Making Pharmacy Education Fit for the Future. London: RPSGB.

Ryfe, D.M. (2006). Narrative and deliberation in small group forums. Journal of Applied Communication Research, 36, 1, 72-93

Silverman, D. (2000) Analyzing talk and text. In Denzin, N.K., and Lincoln, Y.S. (Eds.) Handbook of Qualitative Research (2nd Edition) Sage: USA

Slotnick, H.B. (2001). How doctors learn: education and learning across the medical school-to-practice trajectory. Academic Medicine, 76,10, 1013-1026.

Smith, P.M. (1995). Organizations. In Manstead, A.S.R., and Hewstone, M.R.C. (Eds.). The Blackwell Encyclopedia of Social Psychology. Oxford: Blackwell

Solomon, P., Salvatori, P. and Guenter, D. (2003). An interprofessional problem-based learning course on rehabilitation issues in HIV. Medical Teacher, 25, 4, 408-413.

Tajfel, H., and Turner, J.C. (1979). An integrative theory of intergroup conflict. In Austin W.G., and Worchel, S. (Eds.) The social psychology of intergroup relations. Chicago: Nelson-Hall.

Tope, R. (1999). A Literature Review Prepared for the NHS Executive South West. Bristol: NHS South West.

Turner, J.C. (1985). Social categorization and the self-concept: A social cognitive theory of group behaviour. In Lawler E.J. (Ed.) Advances in group processes. Greenwich: JAI Press.

Turner, J.C., Hogg, M.A., Oakes, P.J., Reicher, S.D., and Wetherell, M.S. (1987). Rediscovering the Social Group: a self-categorization theory. Oxford: Basil Blackwell.

Wray, A., Trott, K., and Bloomer, A. (2006). Projects in Linguistics (2nd Edition). London: Arnold.

In: Nursing Education Challenges in the 21st Century
Editor: Leana E. Callara, pp. 221-242

ISBN 1-60021-661-7
© 2008 Nova Science Publishers, Inc.

Chapter 8

ENCOURAGING ACTIVE PARTICIPATION IN TUTORIALS BY HEEDING STUDENT VOICE: AN ACTION RESEARCH APPROACH

Helen Chapman and Ruth Elder

School of Nursing, Queensland University of Technology, Queensland, Australia

ABSTRACT

This chapter reports on an Action Research study, conducted at a university based school of nursing in Brisbane, Australia, with the aim of improving interaction in tutorials and subsequently encouraging intellectual growth and social and personal development in learners. The study was directed by the following two questions: 1) from a student perspective, what constitutes a useful learning experience in a tutorial context and what factors contribute to that usefulness? and 2) what strategies can be incorporated into tutorials to encourage student attendance and active participation? Composite pictures of what makes a useful learning experience and what factors contribute to that usefulness were developed from information gathered from students. The information – the students' voice - was then used to direct quality improvement and curriculum development within the tutorials of a large undergraduate mental health nursing unit. Strategies developed and used to enhance teaching and learning within the tutorials of this unit are described along with the pragmatic, pedagogical and professional reasons that supported the innovations. Outcomes for both teachers and learners are detailed and some recommendations made for future thinking and planning for encouraging the intellectual growth and social and personal development in learners.

INTRODUCTION

In order to meet society's changing aspirations, universities worldwide have attempted to clarify the nature of the education they offer (Barnett 1990). Many have chosen to do so through a description of the generic qualities and skills of their graduates (Barrie, 2004; 2006). Thus, the development of generic qualities and skills in students has become increasingly important to universities.

Graduate attributes are the qualities, skills and understandings a university community agrees its students should develop during their time with the institution. These attributes include but go beyond, the disciplinary expertise or technical knowledge that has traditionally formed the core of most university courses. They are qualities that also prepare graduates as agents for social good in an unknown future (Bowden et al., 2000)

Arguments put forward for university courses to include the development of generic capabilities include the rapid rate of knowledge development and changes in professional practice, the requirement by employers for employees with employment related skills as well as disciplinary expertise, and that the end-product of higher education should be more than disciplinary expertise (Bowden et al., 2000). The acquisition of generic capabilities is clearly consistent with the notion that university education is about more that getting a degree; that a university education goes beyond acquisition of disciplinary content knowledge. According to MacIntyre (2002) the aim of education should be the development of students' intellectual powers, not merely the passing of examinations. Educated people, according to Cronon (1998) know how to pay attention, how to talk, how to write persuasively and movingly, and how to solve puzzles and problems; educated people love wisdom even more than they love learning; they are open to perspectives different from their own, they know how to get things done, and understand they belong to a community; above all else "being an educated person means being able to see connections that allow one to make sense of the world and act within it in creative ways (Cronon, 1998, p. 78). From this perspective, a university education is not only about the acquisition of discipline specific knowledge but also about intellectual growth and personal and social development. In the interests of promoting the acquisition of generic capabilities and broadening higher education outcomes beyond disciplinary expertise, it is essential that learning experiences and opportunities conducive to the development of generic skills are provided during a course of study (Bowden et al., 2000).

Walker (2001) argues that university classroom practices should be located in "landscapes of possibility" (p.17) associated with, for example, new ideas, risk, openness, dialogue, trust, and respect. According to Hassel & Lourey (2005, p. 5), "knowledge is not just about reading the book and being tested on it; it is the conversations we have about that knowledge that give it meaning". Dewey (1966, p. 4) claims that "Men [sic] live in a community by virtue of the things which they have in common: and communication is the way in which they come to process things in common". Janhonen and Sarja (2000, p. 107) claim the purpose of dialogue is to build a gradual mutual and reciprocal understanding". This is in accord with the argument that learning through dialogue promotes the growth of understanding and tolerance between people (Darbyshire, 1995; Higgins, 1996; Porter, 1995).

Learning experiences and opportunities for making connections, sharing ideas and discussing issues through dialogic learning is usually provided in small class – tutorial - settings. However, the usefulness and efficacy of tutorial discussion is dependant on the presence and participation of learners; a situation that is made problematic by not only absenteeism but also disengaged students.

Decline in attendance or class absence has been the subject of much debate and research in recent years. For example, cases for and against compulsory class attendance policies have been put forward and subsequently been the topic of correspondence or letters to journal editors (see for example, Brauer, 1994; Marburger, 2006; Romer, 1993; St Clair, 1999); reasons for why students attend or do not attend class have been investigated (see for example, Friedman, Rodriguez, & McComb, 2001; Gump, 2004; Launius, 1997; Wyatt, 1992); and the relationship between attendance and grades has been both investigated and debated. Despite numerous studies confirming a positive relationship between attendance and grades (see for example Clump, Bauer, & Whiteleather, 2003, Durden & Ellis, 1995; Gump, 2006; Gunn, 1993; Marburger, 2001, 2006; Romer, 1993) the issue remains equivocal. Regardless of findings related to student attendance (such as that of Marburger (2001) who found that on any given day, one-third of the class was absent, 79% of students agreed that up to six absences a semester was acceptable; and among students with a high rate of absenteeism, only about 25% bothered to familiarise themselves with the missed information) there is growing concern that even when students attend classes a large number of them are not engaging with the academic experience.

The problem of disengaged students has been addressed by a number of scholars (see for example, Hassel & Lourey, 2005; Sacks, 1996; Shilling & Schilling, 1999; Trout, 1996) and the topic has been connected with a decline in academic standards, lack of student accountability, and decreasing student expectations for academic effort. Trout (1996) claims that students who are disengaged (or detached, indifferent, or alienated) display a frustrating number of behaviours including failure to read assigned books, avoidance of participation in class discussions, expectations of high grades for mediocre work, resentment of attendance requirements, inadequate preparation for class and tests, and moreover, they regard intellectual pursuits as boring. According to Hassel & Lourey (2005), despite society requiring more of graduates, students seem to give less and apathy, absenteeism, and grade inflation all contribute to a lack of student accountability. However, as Hassel & Lourey (2005, p.3) ask: "how can we instil accountability when we cannot even get students to the classroom"? Schilling and Schilling (1999, p.8) found that "actual work fell short of faculty expectations not only in the amount of time invested but also in the kinds of activities in which students engaged". For example, while faculty believe two to three hours of work outside of class is necessary for success, students expect to spend about a third of that time; while faculty expect students to engage in activities such as using primary source materials, students emphasised texts or used passive study strategies rather than higher-level thinking skills. As Shilling and Shilling (1999) maintain, "if students don't spend time and effort studying and engaging in other learning activities, the learning just won't happen".

Only a limited number of papers in nursing journals could be found that acknowledged or addressed the above issues in any way. Some of the papers concentrated on attrition (see for example, Glossop, 2002; Last & Fulbrook, 2003; Lynn & Redman, 2005); others investigated the predictors of, or influences on, academic performance (see for example, McCarey, Barr, & Rattray, 2006; Salamonson & Andrew 2006). However, it is more and more apparent through observations and discussions with colleagues that the issues described above are present within Bachelor of Nursing programs. Nevertheless, it was not the primary purpose of this study to contribute to the debates or specifically add to knowledge about these issues. Rather, the primary purpose of this study was to bring about a change is a specific situation; a change that was driven by student voice.

THE STUDY

This study was directed by the following two questions: 1) from a student perspective, what constitutes a useful learning experience in a tutorial context and what factors contribute to that usefulness? and 2) what strategies can be incorporated into tutorials to encourage student attendance and active participation? The study was conducted at a large, university based, school of nursing in Brisbane, Australia. All students enrolled in undergraduate nursing courses were invited by email to complete a self-administered questionnaire eliciting general opinions and perceptions about their learning experiences within tutorials. True figures for this population are difficult to determine, however, there were 1136 equivalent estimated full-time student units (EFTSUs) enrolled during 2003 - the year of the study. A total of 111 students completed the questionnaire. While this number was small in terms of completion, the numerous responses by each student to each statement provided rich information that gave insight into aspects of the subjective world of participating students.

The primary purpose of the project was to change and improve a specific situation. Therefore Action Research, with its emphasis on improving practice through the creation of solutions to identified problems and on reflective and collaborative processes (Kemmis & McTaggart, 1988), was determined as the most appropriate methodology – the body of knowledge - to guide the change. Action Research is a useful methodology in today's rapidly changing environments because it "provides the mechanism for changing practice and simultaneously evaluating the success of change" (Jenks, 1999, p. 255).

Information Gathering Strategies and Procedures

A questionnaire of three sections was specifically designed to generate and gather both quantitative and qualitative information. Section 1 sought demographic information across 10 response areas. Section 2 comprised quantitative information. Section 3, the focus of this chapter, consisted of five incomplete statements soliciting general opinions and perceptions about the following five statements:

1. I find tutorials USEFUL learning experiences when:
2. I find tutorials ARE NOT USEFUL learning experiences when:
3. I like to ATTEND tutorials when:
4. I DO NOT like to attend tutorials when:
5. My ideal tutorial is when:

While these questions were structured to promote response to predetermined categories, no restrictions or limitations were placed on the feedback that could be given. This strategy was intended to indicate not only a valuing of student opinion, but also a true desire for student feedback. Asking for responses to each of the categories in terms of both strengths and shortcomings was a strategy aimed at capturing as many perceptions as possible and thus providing optimal insight into aspects of the students' subjective world.

Students were invited via email to participate. The purpose of the study was explained as follows:

We wish to find out what you and other undergraduate nursing students think about tutorials. Your opinions will greatly assist staff within the QUT School of Nursing to provide better learning experiences for BN students.

Respondents were asked not to put their name on the questionnaire to allow anonymity of response. Confidentiality was assured with responses to be used only for research and quality assurance purposes. Consent was signified by return of the completed questionnaire in hardcopy form to the school of nursing Student Information Centre. Initial emails were followed a month later by a reminder email. Ethics approval was granted by the University Human Research Ethics Committee. The gathered information was transcribed onto a computerised data base in order to facilitate organization for examination and interpretation.

Examining the Information

Each student responded with a number of opinions about each statement giving a total of 847 responses. The responses to each of the five statements were searched for emerging concepts, themes, or issues. Essentially, the themes were inductively derived from the data. Responses to each of the statements were examined independently of the other statements. No attempt was made to analyze difference or relationship between perceived strengths or shortcomings in any category. Rather, the good and the bad aspects of each category were integrated to form composite pictures of what makes a useful learning experience and what factors contribute to that usefulness. Eighteen themes emerged across the five response categories. Working descriptions of these themes were inductively derived from the responses and are described below:

Themes from Student responses:
Assessment: notions related to assessment
"Turnout": notions related to cohort attendance at tutorial
Conduct: notions related to how the tutorial is conducted, run, managed, carried out
Format: notions related to the pre-set or planned framework/structure of the tutorial– student or tutor led, case studies; role play; debates, presentations
Learning quality: notions related to acquisition of knowledge/understanding, skills - relevant content, not wasting time, includes motivation/attitude
Preparation: notions related to preparation for tutorials – homework, research, SDL; readings
Professionalism: notions related to the behaviour expected of a professional including agreement and consistency between staff (collaboration)
Relationships: notions related to psychological security
Relevance to Workplace: notions related to nursing, the real life/world etc
Resources: physical resources such as parking facilities
Sharing of Ideas: notions of active participation, interaction, voicing of opinions, chatting, discussing
Size: notions related to student numbers allocated to a tutorial
Teaching quality: notions related to how teaching is delivered including attitude – how the teacher teaches

Time: notions related to times at which tutorials are held

All the identified themes or issues for each question were subsequently subsumed within five clusters:

A. **Tutorial teaching:** Subsumed within this cluster are themes related to Teaching quality; Conduct; and Professionalism
B. **Tutorial atmosphere:** This cluster is concerned with Relationships
C. **Tutorial framework:** Subsumed within this cluster are themes related to Format; Size; Time; and Resources
D. **Tutorial learning:** This cluster included themes of Learning quality; Sharing of ideas; and Relevance to the workplace
E. **Tutorial attendance:** Subsumed within this cluster are themes related to Assessment, Marks; Preparation; and "turnout

The assigned number was inserted onto the data base beside the response that corresponded to the cluster. (Essentially, this manner of organizing the unstructured data is a modification of content analysis methods well described by, for example, Burns, 1994; Field & Morse, 1985; Miles & Huberman, 1984). Finally, in order to provide a visual representation of the information, the clusters from each category were organized into frequency distributions.

Student Voice

Each of the five response categories is introduced separately. The constructed frequency distribution is presented first. The clusters for each of the five response categories are presented in the same sequential order each time (A to E); this was done for consistency and ease of interpretation; ranking provides a useful way of presenting the data, it does not indicate level of importance. Each response from each participant has significance for someone. Each cluster is briefly described and illustrated with a compilation of excerpts transcribed from the responses. By using the natural language of the students' own terms, it is hoped a vicarious experience for the reader will be generated.

Statement 1: I find tutorials USEFUL learning experiences when:

The 185 perceptions or responses to this question were organized into the five clusters:

A. Tutorial teaching   34
B. Tutorial atmosphere   10
C. Tutorial framework   24
D. Tutorial learning   89
E. Tutorial attendance   28

A. How the teacher teaches was identified 34 times by the respondents as a contributing factor to the usefulness of tutorials and related to three themes. **Teaching quality**

(26): [I find tutorials useful learning experiences]: when they are conducted by experienced tutors [43]; when tutors present important information in ways that are easy to understand [55]; when the tutor is a gifted teacher [80]; Tutorials are very useful but dependent on the teacher [37]; **Conduct (6):** tutor guides and corrects; **and Professionalism:** when the tutor is organised and prepared for tutorial [44].

B. The atmosphere within the tutorial was identified 10 times as having an important impact on tutorial usefulness. All were associated to relationship themes. [I find tutorials useful learning experiences when]: the environment is comfortable to ask question in [63]; tutor is approachable and helpful [84]; [there is] a safe environment for answering even if a guess [75].

C. Twenty four responses identified the framework of the tutorial as a contributing factor to the usefulness of the learning experience in tutorials: Themes related to **Format (21):** there is purpose to the tutorial, ie practice questions, not just going through readings [6]; there is planned structure to the lesson, with chapters or reading explaining the concepts [24];teacher led [25] [this opinion was expressed 9 times]; **Size (1), and Time (2).**

D. Issues related to tutorial learning were identified 89 times. There were three recurring themes. **Learning quality (42):** Increases my understanding [13]; Help us to think about how and when to apply our knowledge [26]. **Sharing of ideas (35):** all students are actively participating in discussions and sharing ideas [4]; **Relevance to the workplace (12):** areas of discussion relate to nursing prac and care [38].

E. Twenty nine responses identified issues related to attendance as contributing factors to the usefulness of the tutorial learning experience. There were four recurring themes **Assessment (13):** content of tute relates to exam [38]; topics discussed relate directly to assessment material [107]; **Marks (1)** should be an incentive to attend – maybe marks awarded so that people will attend [17]; and **Preparation (14):** having background work to do allows me to understand the subject matter more and I can actively participate [39].

Statement 2: I find tutorials ARE NOT USEFUL learning experiences when:

The 162 perceptions or responses to this question were organized into five clusters:

A.	Tutorial teaching	47
B.	Tutorial atmosphere	5
C.	Tutorial framework	39
D.	Tutorial learning	43
E.	Tutorial attendance	28

A. Tutorial teaching was identified 47 times by the respondents as a contributing factor to the ineffectiveness of tutorials and related to three themes. **Teaching quality (24):** [I find tutorials ARE NOT USEFUL learning experiences when] students not challenged/invited to think [75]; tutor waffles through several loosely linked topics [110]; **Conduct (4):** students are disruptive[71]; **and Professionalism (7):** tutor does not turn up [7]; tutors unprepared/not fully understand the content[71]; tutor rushes through things to leave quicker [89].

B. The atmosphere within the tutorial was identified five times as having an important impact on tutorial usefulness. All related to relationship themes. [I find tutorials ARE NOT USEFUL learning experiences when] tutor is unapproachable [12].

C. Thirty nine responses identified the framework of the tutorial as a contributing factor to the ineffectiveness of tutorial. Themes related to **Format (28):** when they are student directed [19]; when I have to sit and listen to a video [24]; **Size (1):** Class has over 20 in it – classes should be limited [80]. **Time (6):** sometimes too short, not much time for questions [27].

D. Issues related to tutorial learning were considered contributing factors to the lack of usefulness of the tutorial learning experience 43 times. There were three recurring themes. **Learning quality (21):** not much learning encouraged [54]. **Sharing of ideas (20):** students sit there and say nothing [8]; and **Relevance to the workplace (1):** nothing is covered that is useful/relevant to nursing [83].

E. Twenty eight responses identified themes related to tutorial attendance as contributing factors to the lack of usefulness of tutorials as a learning experience. There were four recurring themes. **Assessment (4):** has no bearing on assessment [73]; **Marks (1):** no marks for participation (8); **Preparation (15):** when I have to read irrelevant readings [93]; **Turnout (8):** when they are poorly attended – should be compulsory? [79].

Statement 3: I like to ATTEND tutorials when:

The 164 perceptions or responses to this question were organized into five clusters:

A.	Tutorial teaching	24
B.	Tutorial atmosphere	14
C.	Tutorial framework	28
D.	Tutorial learning	61
E.	Tutorial attendance	37

A. Tutorial teaching was identified 25 times by the respondents as a contributing factor to the usefulness of tutorials as a learning experience and related to four themes. **Teaching quality (16):** [I like to ATTEND tutorials when] information is presented so it is interesting [15], tutor has done their homework and knows the subject [37]; **Conduct (5):** focused, task oriented tutes that stay on topic [45]; **Professionalism (3):** tutor turns up [7]; tutor on time [23].

B. The atmosphere within the tutorial was identified fourteen times as having an important impact on the usefulness of tutorials as a learning experience. All related to relationship themes. [I like to attend tutorials] when it is a good environment where I feel comfortable sharing ideas and asking questions [13].

C. Twenty eight responses identified the framework of the tutorial as a contributing factor to the usefulness of tutorials as a learning experience. Themes related to

Format (10): [I like to ATTEND tutorials] when tutor led [47]; Size (1): small groups [76]; Time (17): when they are conveniently timed [20].

D. Issues related to tutorial learning were considered contributing factors to the usefulness of tutorials as a learning experience 61 times. There were three recurring themes. **Learning quality (40)**: [I like to ATTEND tutorials] when going helps me understand the material [30]; **Sharing of ideas (16)**: when all students actively participate in discussion and share ideas [4]; **Relevance to the workplace (5)**: when we go through topics of interest or relevant issues to the real world/clinical setting [71].

E. Thirty six responses identified tutorial attendance as a contributing factor to the usefulness of tutorials as a learning experience. There were three recurring themes. **Assessment (19)**: [I like to ATTEND tutorials] when it is vital (ie contributes to the final mark) [73]; when I need help with assignment [73]; when I know they directly relate to assessments [106]; **Attendance (5)**: when everyone attends [61]; when others turn up[97]; when marks for attending [79]; **Preparation (12)**: when some work is to be done before class for discussion in class [26]; when I know the work we will be covering [35];when I am prepared [51].

Statement 4: I DO NOT like to attend tutorials when:

The 143 perceptions or responses to this question were organized into five clusters:

A.	Tutorial teaching	26
B.	Tutorial atmosphere	4
C.	Tutorial framework	44
D.	Tutorial learning	52
E.	Tutorial attendance	17

A. How the teacher teaches was identified 26 times by the respondents as a contributing factor to the usefulness of tutorials as a learning experience and related to three themes. **Attitude (5)**: [I do not like to attend tutorials when] tutor is not interested [12]; tutor don't care about what they are teaching; **Conduct (3)**: tute is unstructured [75]; **Teacher ability (18)**: tutor expects you to understand everything already [26]; tutor has no idea on the topic or very limited knowledge [89]; tutor has made no effort and time is wasted [10].

B. The atmosphere within the tutorial was identified four times as having an important impact on the usefulness of tutorials as a learning experience. All related to **relationship** themes. [I do not like to attend tutorials when the] atmosphere is intimidating [17]; tutor is condescending [74].

C. Forty four responses identified the framework of the tutorial as a contributing factor to the usefulness of tutorials as a learning experience. Themes related to **Format (21)**: [I do not like to attend tutorials when] sit in on a video [24]; students are presenting [68]; tutes are entirely self-directed – prefer tutor input [101]; **Size (1)**: two tutes are combined – can hardly fit into room [23]; **Time (20)**: they are scheduled at inconvenient times [26]; at bad times – either late or not near lecture times [72.

D. Issues related to how the learner learns were considered contributing factors to the usefulness of tutorials as a learning experience 52 times. There were three recurring themes. **Learning (38)**: [I do not like to attend tutorials when] I don't get something out of them [2]; I am not learning something new [36]; general activities for fun do not help me understand – I would rather spend time on further readings [41]. **Sharing of ideas (12)**: just sitting "listening" to someone talk [18]; tutor sits and dictates – participation helps me understand [42]; I only have to sit and listen [96]; **Relevance to the workplace (2)**: tute is not practice related [35].

E. Seventeen responses identified incentives for learning as contributing factors to the usefulness of tutorials as a learning experience. There were three recurring themes. **Assessment (4)**: [I do not like to attend tutorials when] tutorials are not focussed on helping us pass exams [5]; don't contribute to final exams [65]; **Attendance (5)**: few students attend [9]; no students turn up[12]; **Preparation (8)**: pre reading not done by fellow students [49]; allotted 30-50 pages of reading [51]; have to read pages and pages of material prior to tute [107].

Statement 5: My ideal tutorial is when:

The 193 perceptions or responses to this question were organized into five clusters:

A.	Tutorial teaching	24
B.	Tutorial atmosphere	8
C.	Tutorial framework	38
D.	Tutorial learning	88
E.	Tutorial attendance	35

A. How the teacher teaches was identified 24 times by the respondents as a contributing factor to the usefulness of tutorials as a learning experience and related to five themes. **Attitude (7)**: [My ideal tutorial is when] tutor is enthusiastic [79]; everyone is there to gain the most they can [74]; **Collaboration (1)** tutors are all on the same wave length and there has been some discussion about what is needed to be taught between tutors, lecturers and unit coordinator [40] **Conduct (1)**: tutorial is directed [75]; **Professionalism (1)**: tutor is on time, organised and get straight into tute [51]; **Teacher ability (14)**: questions are posed and tutor constructively comments on answers given [76]; tutor is easy going but informed about what we are learning and willing to explain anything students do not understand [68];... tutor challenges students . . . exercises students brains [24].

B. The atmosphere within the tutorial was identified eight times as having an important impact on the usefulness of tutorials as a learning experience. All related to **relationship** themes. [My ideal tutorial is when] atmosphere is relaxed [17]; tutor is interested in students and helpful [84].

C. Thirty eight responses identified the framework of the tutorial as a contributing factor to the usefulness of tutorials as a learning experience. Themes related to **Format**

(15): [My ideal tutorial is when] (group discussion) led by tutor [34]; teacher led with group presentations as a basis [65]; activities not readings [98]; **Size (6):** size is about 16 people [28]; smaller groups (15-29) [53]; **Time (17):** interaction with the people and the tutor is longer than 1 hour [16]; 1hour or less [65]; follows lecture on same day [84].

D. Issues related to how the learner learns were considered contributing factors to the usefulness of tutorials as a learning experience 88 times. There were three recurring themes. **Learning (43):** [My ideal tutorial is when] I come away feeling I have benefited from attending [19]; I have learnt something/gained new knowledge – difficult points made clear through good explanation [27]; pushed to think critically and in new ways [35]. **Sharing of ideas (37):** students actively participating in discussions/activities [18]; all contribute constructively to tute [37]; discussions are enjoyable and relevant [42]; **Relevance to the workplace (8):** tutor provides real life scenarios to relate to [25]; tutor relates material to experience [51].

E. Thirty five responses identified incentives for learning as contributing factors to the usefulness of tutorials as a learning experience. There were three recurring themes. **Assessment (8):** [My ideal tutorial is when] tutor runs the session with the view to helping students pass exams [5];it includes info on assignments or exams[47; tutor helps with tests/essays [111]; **Attendance (8):** tute attendance and participation is rewarded with marks [97]; participation marks (10%) not just showing up [42]; get % for attending [32]; **Preparation (19):** pre readings to do but not too much [25]; some minimal preparations to enhance understanding [26]; practice questions and a short reading to go through [86].

Table 1. Summary of the frequencies

CLUSTER	Q1	Q2	Q3	Q4	Q5	Total responses per cluster
Tutorial teaching	36	51	25	26	24	162
Tutorial atmosphere	10	5	14	4	8	41
Tutorial framework	21	36	28	44	38	167
Tutorial learning	89	42	61	52	88	332
Tutorial attendance	29	28	36	17	35	145
Total responses	185	162	164	143	193	847

REFLECTING ON THE COLLECTIVE VOICE

The respondents valued purposeful tutorials with a planned structure with input from the tutor. They appreciated enthusiastic, interested, and knowledgeable tutors who challenged them to think, guided and corrected them in an organised, professional manner, and did not who "waffle" through loosely linked topics. They valued a safe, respectful, and relaxed environment in which they could ask or answer questions and share ideas. They did not want to just sit and listen to someone talk – they wanted to participate, to share ideas and be encouraged to think critically, and in new ways. They wanted everyone to contribute constructively. They valued tutorials in which everyone attended and actively participated and they recognised the value of reading and preparing in advance so they could better participate in informed discussion. The respondents wanted to increase their understandings, and gain new knowledge in tutorials. They wanted to feel they had benefited from attending. The respondents wanted their learning to be related to the workplace and to their assessment items, and they wanted attendance and participation to be rewarded with marks.

Clearly, issues related to learning were important to this group of students. They expected to learn and they knew what mattered to them in terms of their learning. The category of Tutorial Learning received the largest number of responses and their concerns about learning were clearly connected to the categories of Tutorial Teaching and Tutorial Framework. This suggests that issues such as class absence and apparent disengagement can be attributed to what happens in the classroom rather than to student apathy or lack of responsibility or accountability. Indeed, the voices resonate with the claim by Hassel & Lourey (2005, p. 6) that "If we want students to come to class, we have to make what occurs in the classroom matter – to their learning, their grades, and their understanding of education".

Shilling and Shilling (1999) claim that "expectations shape the learning experience very powerfully" (p. 5) and they call for academics to clarify "those activities students must pursue in order to achieve desired ends" (p.9). While we concur with these sentiments we also suggest that the expectations of students equally shape the learning experience. The voices from this study clearly demonstrate that students expect their teachers to be knowledgeable and enthusiastic, and they expect to be challenged to think critically and to engage in classroom discussions. They do not expect, or want, didactic teaching methods within their tutorial sessions – rather, they want to actively participate and share ideas.

These student expectations are consistent with contemporary thinking about teaching and learning in higher education which not only recognizes that students are responsible adults and capable of self-direction and that their motivation and independence is diminished by authoritarian, directive actions (Musinski, 1999; Schaefer & Zygmont, 2003; Weimer, 2002), but also recognizes that adult learners do better with less direction and more participation (Knowles, 1990). The call for students to be perceived as active participants rather than passive recipients or empty vessels waiting to be filled is manifest in the notion of student centeredness. Within a student-centered approach to teaching and learning, the focus is on student learning rather than on what the teacher teaches; the teacher is a facilitator of learning with responsibility for creating and maintaining the conditions and interactions that make understanding possible. The student is an active constructor of meaning, and it is the student's responsibility to take advantage of learning opportunities or activities (Biggs & Moore, 1993; Laurillard, 1993; Schaefer & Zygmont, 2003; Weimer, 2002).

There is evidence of significant pedagogical shifts toward student-centred approaches (Hubball & Burr, 2004), likely underpinned by the arguments that teachers' conceptions of teaching is one of the most significant elements affecting the outcomes of student learning (Biggs & Moore, 1993; Kember, 1997; Gow & Kember, 1993; Kember & Gow, 1994). Understanding teaching in terms of facilitating learning rather than transmitting knowledge is more likely to promote deeper and more meaningful approaches to learning (Gow & Kember, 1993; Kember & Gow, 1994; Saroyan & Snell, 1997; Trigwell et al., 1999However, there were voices within the responses that suggested that the shift toward student-centred approaches had not occurred in many classrooms.

Voices reported that in some classes students were not invited, much less challenged, to think. Even more troublesome were the reports of tutors who "waffled" through several loosely linked topics, did not turn up, were unapproachable, condescending, unprepared, did not understand the content, or rushed through things to get away. There were voices that claimed tutors were not interested and did not care about what they were teaching. Some classroom atmospheres were seen as intimidating; in others students sat listening to someone else talk or watched a video.

That student-centred learning is not the reality of some classrooms is problematic given the arguments outlined earlier for classroom practices be located in "landscapes of possibility" (Walker, 2001, p.17) and for learning experiences and opportunities conducive to the development of generic skills to be provided during a course of study (Bowden et al.. 2000). For some academics the rhetoric may have remained just that because "faculty may know the language of student-centred teaching [but] do not understand the language" or are frustrated by barriers such as "large class sizes, type of course, expected outcomes and curriculum mandates" (Scharfer and Zygmont, 2003, p. 242). As Smith (1993) cautions, merely changing understandings - the way we name reality - is not to change reality.

As teachers, we are both convinced of the need to focus on the process of learning rather than the process of teaching. Following our reflections on the student voices we began to think of ways to incorporate their expectations into our classes and transform our tutorials into learning experiences that were valued by students.

Heeding Student Voice

This section of the chapter describes the development and application of a curriculum change carried out in response to the student voices. The unit selected for the change was Mental Health Nursing - a compulsory subject in the second year of a three year Bachelor of Nursing course in Queensland, Australia. One of us is the unit coordinator and both of us teach in the unit.

The unit is driven by the conviction that nurses need to be able to identify and care for people experiencing mental health problems. Mental disorders represent nearly 30 per cent of the national disease burden (Commonwealth Department of Health and Aged Care, 2000) and mental health is now recognised as a major health issue for the whole Australian community. Mental health care is no longer provided solely by a specialised psychiatric service, but in a variety of general health and community settings. The aim of the unit is to provide fundamental knowledge about mental health and mental disorders across the lifespan and the role of the nurse in providing mental health care. The unit also facilitates development of professional competencies and generic attributes related to: knowledge/problem solving abilities; ethical/attitudinal characteristics; and social/relational qualities.

The mental health component of the Bachelor of Nursing course consists of nine lectures each of two hours; eight tutorials of two hour duration; and two weeks clinical placement in a mental health unit or agency. Tutorial sizes range from 16 to about 20 students. Tutors and the unit coordinator are available to provide direction and/or feedback on progress in person, or via phone or email. Unit assessment is essentially summative and at the beginning of this cycle of change consisted of a tutorial oral group presentation and a multiple choice examination. The oral group presentation assessment item was seen as an appropriate place to intervene. We decided to keep this assessment item but to change the format from a presentation with limited discussion into a discussion with limited presentation and to also introduce strategies to promote student engagement with learning, thinking and reasoning.

In their original format the oral presentations were given by groups of two or three students who were expected to work together to prepare an integrated presentation. They were expected to last for 15 - 20 minutes, followed by a five minute question and discussion period. Selection to a group was by mutual consent, usually driven by proximity of seating on the day or a pre-existing friendship. Group-work abilities were not assessed, only the product. Presentation was based either on a direct question that required investigation of a contemporary problem (e.g., changes in ideas about the ideal female body shape) or a case scenario. The scenarios were brief (60-100 words) and followed by two to four questions. These dealt with a range of nursing activities (e.g., assessing clients, describing appropriate interventions, or evaluating goals). The scenarios were based on either a psychiatric condition (e.g., depression or post-traumatic stress disorder); or a psychiatric treatment (e.g., electroconvulsive therapy). Each group chose and presented a different topic. If two or more groups chose the same topic students were expected to negotiate a resolution.

The decision to keep the group presentation assessment item was made for a number of pragmatic, pedagogical and professional reasons. The pragmatic reasons relate to the large number of students (350->450) and the small number of academic staff (3-4) qualified to teach or practice psychiatric nursing.

Pedagogically, the unit assessment items are matched to the unit learning goals and instructional methods. The unit clearly sets out what learning is expected, how the teaching and learning will be approached, and what has to be done in order to achieve the expected learning. In other words "assessment tasks address the objectives, so that you can test to see if the students have learned what the objectives state they are learning" (Biggs, 2003, p. 64). The group presentation assessment item is matched specifically to the unit objective that a completing student has the ability to 'demonstrate proficiency in communicating orally with peers about mental health issues'. This ability is fundamental to mental health nursing, and as such is a very important learning outcome. We believed that engaging students in a presentation activity would promote their proficiency in communicating orally with peers about mental health issues. This belief is in accord with the argument by Shuell (1986) that:

If students are to learn desired outcomes in a reasonably effective manner, then the teacher's fundamental task is to get students to engage in learning activities that are likely to result in their achieving those outcomes (p. 429).

A pedagogical influence for group presentations rather than individual presentations was related to the obligation in group work to co-construct knowledge – a requirement that is consistent with the argument by Vygotsky (1978) that interacting with others is likely to produce new understandings. The discussion and debate advanced by group work encourages the "justification of ideas, resolution of disagreements and understanding of new perspectives" (Webb, 1995, p. 244).

Professionally, it is an expectation that nurses employed within a mental health context will work in a multi-disciplinary team. Registered nurses in the mental health setting require professional skills such as collaborating with other members of the multidisciplinary team and the ability to discuss patients' mental status at shift handovers, in ward rounds and in clinical team meetings. Indeed, as Kneisl (2004, p. 685) claims "much of the nurse's professional life is spent in groups". There is also an expectation that mental health nurses have the ability to facilitate group work within a mental health context. While mental health nurses have long been involved in leading therapeutic groups it is argued that these skills will become increasingly important as the need to provide cost effective treatments becomes greater (Leff, 2000; Ormont, 2000; Taylor, Burlingame, Kristensen, & Fuhriman, 2001).

These pedagogical and professional reasons for using group presentation as an assessment item follow the counsel that assessment should help prepare students for life (Rowntree, 1987). The professional life of a nurse is closely connected to group processes and thus this assessment item has the added value of helping to develop a professional competency. While the decision to keep group presentation as an assessment item was validated by these reasons, in its present format it allowed for limited discussion and this was usually curtailed by the presenters asking "any questions?" We wanted to modify this assessment item so that would better promote student interaction. The students had clearly voiced their dissatisfaction with merely sitting listening to anyone talk and we wanted to encourage a higher degree of learner activity by increasing interaction among students and between students and tutors during the tutorial periods.

After much reflection, deliberation, and critical debate between ourselves and other interested members of the teaching team we decided to adapt the group presentations as student-led discussions. The discussion was still to be led by students in groups of two or three. However, any actual "presentation" was to last only about five minutes in order to set the scene and be followed by a 15 minute discussion facilitated by the designated group of students. Group selection was to remain the same, and as before group-work abilities would not be assessed. The case scenarios were to be used again, but this time as topics for discussion rather than presentation.

We were aware that leading a discussion would be a "big ask" for second year undergraduate who had limited knowledge or experience of either the content area or the process. However, a tutorial discussion was expected to occur after the lecture on the particular topic and guidelines for facilitating discussion were developed and explained. The guidelines included suggestions such as: ask questions that are non-threatening, open ended, and probing; allow time for response; actively listen to the response and then clarify or elaborate if appropriate; refocus the discussion if necessary. The skills associated with discussion were to be modelled by the tutors in any preceding teacher-led discussions.

In order to better enhance student engagement with learning and to develop critical thinking and reasoning abilities we introduced a modified form of peer assessment using a criterion referenced assessment matrix for this assessment item. Given the small number of full time academics qualified to teach mental health nursing and the subsequent need to employ casual tutors, we had previously developed a matrix composed of criteria and standards based on an earlier reproduction (Brown, Rust, & Gibbs, 1994). Initially only tutors used the matrix to provide feedback to students about their presentation and to establish an assessment mark. We now intended to use the matrix for a modified form of peer assessment of the student-led discussions. There were a number of reasons influencing this decision.

We wanted the students to more actively engage with the subject matter and with their own learning, but we also wanted to position assessment as an integral part of the learning process, rather than something separate that assumes primacy. The critical influence of assessment methods on learning has been well argued (Biggs, 2003; Boud, 2000; Ramsden, 2003). Regrettably, for many students assessment tasks identify what is important in a unit – what is important in terms of 'what am I supposed to learn in this unit'? It has been claimed that "from our students' point of view, assessment always defines the actual curriculum" (Ramsden, 2003, p. 182). Peer assessment offered some possibilities.

The notion of peer assessment is of course not new. According to the literature, debate about, and evaluation of, this method of assessment has existed for over 30 years (Dann, 2001). Research in the area of peer assessment is largely inconclusive with strong arguments for and against the process. For example on the positive side peer assessment is seen to develop responsibility and enterprise, maturity and confidence (Goldfinch, & Raeside, 1990); to act as a socialising force and enhance relationships and relevant skills (Earl, 1986). It is also argued that peer assessment helps students learn to justify their ideas (Brew, 1999); to listen & reflect critically (Somervell, 1993); to become more autonomous (Brindley, & Schoffield, 1998) and essentially to think more, learn more and become more critical (Falchikov, 1986). These are clearly very positive features of peer assessment.

Negative features include challenges in terms of accuracy & reliability (Oldfield & Macalpine, 1995; Stefani, 1992), and ethical issues such as student comfort with assessing their peers and even overt or covert peer pressure to be given a good mark (Falchikov, 1986, 1995; Heylings & Stefani, 1997). There are also negative features related to adequate preparation or learning about how to assess others or how to construct an assessment matrix - when and how is this learning to take place?

The negative outcomes were largely responsible for the modifications we devised for both the matrix and for peer assessment. Peer assessment ideally involves students in three practices: determining evaluation criteria and standards; making judgements and comments about each others work; and awarding a grade. Peer assessment of the presentations was first modified in terms of matrix construction. Initially students were invited to participate in the construction of the matrix. This was not successful. Students mostly had very limited experience with criteria or standards. Indeed this was so for most of the academic staff within the school at this time. 'Marking guides' without standards and written in terms of what the student must do to pass a unit had mostly provided the answer to the student question of 'what does he/she want'? The unit matrix has continued to be constructed by academics not students throughout all its revisions.

Peer assessment was also modified in terms of grading. Peer grades were not to be considered in the overall grade. The groups would receive only the grade allocated by the tutor. It was intended that the modifications would encourage students to use the matrix and peer assessment for learning rather than assessment.

At this point we also considered it necessary to simplify the matrix for student use. The matrix was reduced to five criteria: addressing the question; understanding of topic content; use of literature; and presentation and discussion. The five standards were reduced to three: unsatisfactory (<40%); satisfactory (50% to 75%) and excellent 76% to 100%). The decision to simplify the matrix was based on not only student inexperience with both criteria and standards but also their inexperience with assessing the work of others.

To help familiarise students with the discussion requirements and the assessment matrix, a tutorial was specifically allocated to detailed explanation of the criteria and standards, and the discussion topics. A brief discussion based on an unused scenario was then given by the tutor. Students were asked to attend to the strengths of the tutor-led discussion across the criteria according to the standards, and make suggestions for improvement. At the end of a tutorial the scenario topic for the following tutorial and the relevant chapter in the text book were drawn to students' attention.

Copies of the matrix were distributed each tutorial, and each student was asked to assess each group discussion according to the matrix. The student assessor remained anonymous. Only the names of the students leading the discussion were evident. Peer assessment sheets were collected at the end of the tutorial and are later perused by the tutor. During the next tutorial student assessment sheets as well as the graded tutor assessment sheet were returned to the relevant students.

OUTCOMES

There was a noticeable increase in interaction and participation during tutorials. The student-led discussions were somewhat stilted at first but the students quickly adapted to the idea of being encouraged to interact in class. This is not to suggest that the discussions were exemplary or even good – but there was more discussion – more sharing of ideas - than there had been before the format of this assessment item was changed. We cannot be certain that this change in itself advanced new understandings. However, it is highly probable that the increased tutorial interactions together with the discussion and debate required to work effectively as a group to prepare for the discussion, encouraged the "justification of ideas, resolution of disagreements and understanding of new perspectives" (Webb, 1995). The discussions also facilitated the learning of content – the propositional knowledge of the unit, only now content was being used to advance generic skills such as critical thinking, reasoning and reflection.

As the criteria and standards for making decisions about grades become more transparent, students became more aware of the assessment requirements. Following the introduction of peer assessment we agreed that there were less disputes about marks and that the students seemed to be engaging more deeply with the unit topics. While the matrix was previously available to students, possibly it was not seen as important and merely skimmed over or not read at all.

There was an increase in the creativity level of the group work - possibly promoted as students strived together as a team to think of ways to promote discussion and to meet the criteria and standards. The increased creativity was arguably accompanied by its complementary process – critical thinking. Certainly, critical thinking was encouraged through engagement with the matrix to assess peers. As the students assessed the group discussion item the activity required them to engage in at least four of the core characteristics of critical thinking namely, interpretation, inference, analysis, and evaluation (Facione, 1998).

The matrix proved to be an efficient and effective marking system. It was efficient in terms of being easy to use and in the way the standards tended to make the writing of copious feedback notes redundant. This became even more apparent as the semester proceeded and the students became more familiar with the criteria and the standards. Intra and inter-rater reliability between tutors became much less of a problem. This outcome was not unexpected with all of us marking for the same standards. The use of the matrix by students provided yet another way to verify consistency.

In order to develop and promote more interactive tutorials the teaching team in the mental health unit fell into more collaborative practices almost by default. Each of us willingly contributed our time, thoughts and ideas to all aspects of the unit, including the scenarios and the matrix, and advanced other suggestions for improving interaction. As a group we moved our teaching practices beyond what has been censured by Hargreaves (1992) as presentism (short-term planning for the present situation), conservatism (avoiding fundamental change and clinging to the status quo), and individualism (consistently working alone and avoiding judgements and criticism) and truly became a collaborative teaching team. This collaboration, in turn, became a type of collective "reflective practice" as we spent time individually and also collectively, thinking and talking about our practice in order to make a difference

CONCLUSION

In this Action Research study we compiled composite pictures of what makes a useful learning experience in a tutorial context and what factors contribute to that usefulness from the students' perspective. By listening to the student voices we were enabled to successfully direct quality improvements and curriculum development within a large undergraduate mental health nursing unit. The changes we introduced into tutorials resulted in positive outcomes for both learners and teachers. The students actively engaged with their learning and participated in classroom activities enthusiastically and creatively. The changes we introduced arguably resulted in an increase in generic skills such as critical thinking and social qualities, and thus encouraged intellectual growth and social and personal development in learners. The positive outcomes for the teachers lay in the development of more collaborative practices. Because we worked together rather than alone our planning became more strategic and we became more open to change and to others' perspectives and values.

The unit continues to undergo transformations, especially in relation to the tutorials. For example, the matrix has gone through a number of iterations with the criteria and descriptors for the standards being continually refined, and the scenario questions have been reviewed to make them more conducive to discussion.

While at its most basic level the function of nurse education is to produce competent practitioners who can carry out competent and direct 'hands-on' clinical nursing care, a university education is intended to advance nursing education past such simplistic levels toward the highest possible level of achievement. Undergraduate nurse education is expected to produce graduates who have acquired not only discipline specific knowledge but also generic capabilities. It is essential therefore, that experiences and opportunities conducive to such learning and development are provided during university courses.

We advocate continuous monitoring of the curriculum to ensure that it is being equally responsive to the interests, concerns and expectations of the students; that there is a balance between the development of discipline specific knowledge and the encouragement of social and personal development – a balance between the content and process of learning; and that propositional knowledge be used to advance generic capabilities. We also advocate the building of collaborative teaching teams in which teachers talk together and reflect, individually and collectively, about their practice in order to make a difference.

REFERENCES

Barnett, R. (1990). The idea of higher education. Buckingham: Society for Research into higher Education and Open University Press

Barrie, S. (2004). A research-based approach to generic attributes policy. Higher Education Research and Development 23(3), 261-275

Barrie, S. (2006). Understanding what we mean by generic attributes of graduates. Higher Education, 51, 215-241

Biggs, J. (2003). Teaching for quality learning at university, 2nd edition, Buckingham, SRHE and the Open University Press.

Biggs, J., & Moore, P. (1993). The process of learning. New York, Prentice Hall.

Boud, D. (2000). Sustainable assessment: rethinking assessment for the learning society, Studies in Continuing Education, 22(2), 151-167

Bowden, J., Hart, G., King, B., Trigwell, K., & Watts, O. (2000). Generic Capabilities of ATN University graduates. http://www.clt.uts.edu.au/ATN.grad.cap.project.index.html

Brauer, J. (1994). Should class attendance be mandatory? Correspondence section of Journal of Economic Perspectives, 8(3), 205-215

Brew, A., 1999, Towards autonomous assessment: using self assessment and peer assessment, In Brown, S., and Glasner, A., Assessment matters in higher education: Choosing and using diverse approaches, Buckingham, SRHE and the Open University Press.

Brindley, C. & Schoffield, S., 1998, Peer assessment in undergraduate programmes, Teaching in Higher Education, 3(1), 78-89.

Brown, S. Rust, C. and Gibbs, G. 1994 Strategies for Diversifying Assessment in Higher Education Oxford: Oxford Centre for Staff Development. Retrieved August 2005 from: http://www.londonmet.ac.uk/deliberations/ocsld-publications/div-ass2.cfm

Burns, R. (1994). Introduction to research methods (2nd ed.). Melbourne: Longman Cheshire

Clump, M., Bauer, H., & Whiteleather, A. (2003). To attend or not to attend: Is that a good question? *Journal of Instructional Psychology,* 30(3), 220-225.

Commonwealth Department of Health and Aged Care (2000), National Mental Health Report 2000: Sixth Annual Report. Changes in Australia's Mental Health Services under the First National Mental Health Plan of the National Mental Health Strategy 1993-1998, Canberra, Commonwealth of Australia.

Cronin, W. (1998). "Only connect . . .": The goals of a liberal education. American Scholar 67 (4): 73-80.

Dann, K. (2001). Peer assessment: a missing link between teaching and learning? A review of the literature – Commentary, Nurse Education Today 21, 513-515

Darbyshire, P. (1995). Lessons from literature: Caring, interpretation and dialogue. Journal of Nursing Education, 34(5), 211-216

Dewey, J. (1966, c1916). Democracy and education: an introduction to the philosophy of education. New York: Free Press.

Durden, G., & Ellis, L. (1995). The effects of attendance on student learning in Principles of Economics. The American Economic Review; 85(2); May, 343-346.

Earl, S. (1986). Staff and peer assessment – measuring an individual's contribution to group performance, Assessment and Evaluation in Higher Education, 11(1), 60-69.

Facione. P. (1998). Critical thinking: what it is and why it counts. Retrieved August 2005 from http://www.insightassessment.com/pd

Falchikov, N. (1986). Product comparisons and process benefits of collaborative peer group and self assessments. Assessment and Evaluation in Higher Education, 11(2), 146-166.

Falchikow, N. (1995). Peer feedback marking: Developing peer assessment. Innovation in Education and Training International, 32(2), 175-187.

Field, P., & Morse, J. (1985). Nursing research: The application of qualitative approaches. Beckenham: Croom Helm Ltd

Friedman, P., Rodriguez, R., & McComb, J. (2001). Why students do and do not attend class. College Teaching 49 (4): 124-33.

Glossop, C. (2002). Student nurse attrition: use of an exit-interview procedure to determine students' leaving reasons. Nurse Education Today, 20(5), 375-386

Goldfinch, J. & Raeside, R. (1990). Development of a peer assessment technique for obtaining individual marks on a group project. Assessment and Evaluation in Higher Education, 15(3), 210-231.

Gow, L., & Kember, D. (1993). Conceptions of teaching and their relationship to student learning. British Journal of Educational Psychology, 63(1), 20-33.

Gump, S. (2005). The cost of cutting class: attendance as a predictor of student success. College Teaching, 53(1), 21-26.

Gunn, K. (1993). A correlation between attendance and grades in a first year psychology course. Canadian Psychology, 34, 157-160

Hargreaves, A. (1992). Cultures of teaching: A focus for change. In A. Hargreaves, & M. Fullan, (Eds.). Understanding Teacher Development, New York, Teachers College Press.

Hassel, H., & Lourey, J. (2005). The dea(r)th of student responsibility. College Teaching 53(1), 2-13.

Heylings, D. & Stefani, L. (1997). Peer assessment feedback marking in a large medical anatomy class. Medical Education, 31, 281-286.

Higgins, B. (1996). Caring as a therapeutic in nursing education. Journal of Nursing Education, 33(3), 134-136

Hubball, H., & Burt, H. (2004). An integrated approach to developing and implementing learning-centred curricula. International Journal for Academic Development, 9(1), 51-65.

Janhonen, S. & Sarja, A. (2000). Data analysis method for evaluating dialogic learning. Nurse Education Today, 20, 106-115.

Jenks, J. M. (1999). The action research method. In H. J. Streubert & D. R. Carpenter (Eds.), Qualitative research in nursing: Advancing the humanistic imperative (2nd ed., 251-264). Philadelphia: Lippincott.

Kember, D. (1997). Teaching beliefs and their impact on students' approaches to learning. In B. Dart & G. Boulton-Lewis (Eds.). Teaching and Learning in Higher Education. Camberwell, Vic.: Australian Council for Educational Research.

Kember, D., & Gow, L. (1994). Orientations to teaching and their effect on the quality of student learning. The Journal of Higher Education, 65(1), 58-74.

Kemmis, S. & McTaggart, R. (1988). The action research planner. Geelong: Deakin University Press.

Kneisl, C. (2004). Group and Family interventions, In Kneisl, C. Wilson, H. & Trigoboff, E., Contemporary Psychiatric-Mental Health Nursing, Chapter 29, New Jersey, Pearson Prentice Hall.

Knowles, M. (1990). The adult learner: A neglected species. Houston, Gulf Pub. Co.

Last, L., & Fulbrook, P. (2003). Why do student nurses leave? Suggestions from a Delphi Study Nurse Education Toda, 23(6), 449-458

Launius, M. (1997). College student attendance: Attitudes and academic performance. College Student Journal 31, 86-92

Laurillard, D. (1993). Rethinking university teaching. London, Routledge.

Leff, J. (2000). Family work for schizophrenia: Practical application, Acta Psychiatric Scandinavica, 102(supplement 407), 78-82

Lynn, M., & Redman, R. (2005). Faces of the Nursing Shortage: Influences on Staff Nurses' Intentions to Leave Their Positions or Nursing. Journal of Nursing Administration,35(5), 264-270.

MacIntyre, A. (2002). Alasdair MacIntyre on Education: In dialogue with Joseph Dunne. Journal of Philosophy of Education, 36(1), 1-19.

Marburger, D. R. (2001). Absenteeism and undergraduate exam performance. Journal of Economic Education 32(2), 99-109.

Marburger, D, R, (2006), Does mandatory attendance improve student performance? Journal of Economic Education, 37(2), 99-109.

McCarey, M., Barr, T., & Rattray, J. (2006). Predictors of academic performance in a cohort of pre-registration nursing students. Nurse Education Today Available online 17 August doi:10.1016/j.nedt.2006.05.017.

Miles, M., & Huberman, A, (1984). Qualitative data analysis: A sourcebook of new methods. Beverly Hills, Sage.

Musinski, B. (1999). The educator as facilitator: A new kind of leadership. Nursing Forum, 34(1), 23-29.

Oldfield, K. & Macalpine, M. (1995). Peer and self-assessment at a tertiary level: an experimental report. Assessment & Evaluation in Higher Education, 20(1), 125-132.

Ormont, L. (2000). Where is group treatment going in the 21st century? Group, 24(2/3), 185-192.

Porter, E. (1995). Fostering dialogical community through a learning experience. Journal of Nursing Education, 34(5), 228-234

Ramsden, P. (2003). Learning to teach in higher education, 2nd edition, London: Routledge.

Romer, D. (1993). Do students go to class? Should they? Journal of Economic Perspectives, 7(3), 167-174.

Rowntree, D. (1987). Assessing students: How shall we know them? 2nd edition, London, Kogan Page.

Sacks, P. (1996). Generation X Goes to College. Chicago: Open Court.

Salamonson, Y., & Andrew, S. (2006). Academic performance in nursing students: influence of part-time employment, age and ethnicity. Journal of Advanced Nursing, 55(3), 342-349.

Saroyan, A., & Snell, L. (1997). Variations in lecturing styles. Higher Education, 33(1), 85-104.

Schaefer, K. M., & Zygmont, D. (2003). Analyzing the teaching style of nursing faculty: Does it promote a student-centered or teacher-centered learning environment? Nursing Education Perspectives, 24(5), 238-245.

Schilling, K. M., & Schilling, K. L. (1999). Increasing expectations for student effort. About Campus 4(2), 4-10.

Shuell, T. (1986), Cognitive conceptions of learning. Review of Educational Research, 56, 411-436.

Smith, R. (1993). Potentials for empowerment in critical education research. Australian Educational Researcher, 20(2), 75-93.

Somervell, H. (1993). Issues in assessment, enterprise and higher education: The case for self, peer and collaborative assessment. Assessment and Evaluation in Higher Education, 18(3), 221-233.

St. Clair, K. L. (1999). A case against compulsory class attendance policies in higher education. Innovative Higher Education 23, 171-180.

Stefani, L. (1992). Comparison of collaborative self, peer and tutor assessment in biochemistry practical. Biochemical Education 20(3), 148.

Taylor, N., Burlingame, G., Kristensen, K., Fuhriman, A. (2001). A survey of mental health care provider's and managed care organization attitudes toward, familiarity with, and use of group interventions, International Journal of Group Psychotherapy, 51(2); 243-264.

Trigwell, K., Prossner, M., & Waterhouse, F. (1999). Relations between teacher's approaches to teaching and students' approaches to learning. Higher Education, 37(1), 57-70.

Trout, P. 1997. Disengaged students and the decline of academic standards. Academic Questions 10(2), 46-56.

Vygotsky, L. (1978). Mind in society: The development of higher psychological processes, Cambridge, Harvard University Press.

Walker, M. (2001). Mapping our higher education project. In M. Walker (Ed.). *Reconstructing professionalism in university teaching: teachers and learners in action (3-20).* Buckingham: The Society for Research into Higher Education & Open University Press

Webb, N. (1995). Group collaboration in assessment: Multiple objectives, processes, and outcomes, Educational Evaluation and Policy Analysis, 17(2), 239-261

Weimer, M. (2002). Learner-centered teaching: Five key changes to practice (1st ed.). San Francisco: Jossey-Bass.

Wyatt, G. (1992)Skipping Class: An Analysis of Absenteeism among First-Year College Students. Teaching Sociology, 20(3), 201-207.

In: Nursing Education Challenges in the 21st Century   ISBN 1-60021-661-7
Editor: Leana E. Callara, pp. 243-269   © 2008 Nova Science Publishers, Inc.

Chapter 9

NURSING VALUES

Insaf Altun
Kocaeli Univ., Nursing High School,
The Dept. of Fundamentals Nursing, Kocaeli, Turkey

This article are addressing bellow subjects that are also vitally important to understanding what moves the hearth of nursing

- What are values?
- What kinds of values?
- What is personal values?
- What is professional values?
- What is pprofession values?
- What are the main values that govern nurses and nursing?
- What are the kind of values that guide nursing as a profession.
- How can the values we hold and we hold and promote also ensure that nurses are and become persons of integrity, and nursing a profession of integrity?
- The kind of values nurses hold in practice, and what happens to the nurses
- Are the values we hold and promote the relevant ones?
- Are there certain values that are more valuable, more right, more desirable than others? What should this be so?
- Are nurses change their behaviours and attitudes as a result of changing values,
- Why should we challenge the values we hold?
- To what should they be changed?
- Can education change our values?
- Should we expect nurse education to change values?

In this issue the authors scrutinize the values in and of education, practice, and the very existence of nursing: those we come with, those we acquire and those we promote. Nursing educators have a professional obligation to teach and reinforce professional nursing values that are consistent with the professional nursing role. Especially today, there is a definite need for values education in nursing education programs.

VALUES IN NURSING EDUCATION

When you begin to look at why nursign exists is a health profession which is concerned with promoting and maintaining the health of individuals, families, and the public, preventing illness, helping patients with recover process, relieving suffering, and so on. The delivery of health care services is changing dramatically. Increasing longevity, shortening of hospital stays, scientific and technological advances and population mobility, social justice, equality, cultural values, poverty, discrimination contribute to the growing complexity of nursing.

Accoding to Tschudin (2003) the future for nursing lies in some distinctive areas: 1)the care the increasing population of older people, 2)Care will be in the home for people with long-term illness, 3)issues of genetics will play a major part in health care, 4) medical and nursing research will guide practice.5) nurses world wide are caring for people who are suffering the consequences of conflict and diseasters, leading them to foster non-violent ways of resolutions. These kinds of things lead to profession and professional values.

Nursing education must keep pace with these changes, which require new knowledge, skills and values. Nursing students' professional education should formalize and systematize these values, becoming the basis of their professional ethic. Then, as nurses practice good nursing, they should adhere to these values appropriately (Hall, 2006).

Nurses actions by knowing with the help of knowledge, by feeling with the help of values, and by doing with the help of skills. Values have a much wider application than feelings. There is an aspect that relates to feelings, but feelings can be quickly changing. Values also has to do with conscience, and fundamental ways of understanding something.

Nursing educators are preparing professional nurses who can think critically, use sound clinical judgment, and participate as full partners in shaping health-care delivery and policy.

Nursing education equips the student with cognitive, affective, and psychomotor competencies integral to professional nursing practice. The purpose of professional nursing education is to provide the knowledge base, values and skills necessary for the student learner to become a professional practitioner of nursing.

Learning is the acquisition of knowledge, skills, and competence that result in changes in values. To achieve these changes, nursing faculty defines the framework for acquisition of knowledge, examination of values, and application of concepts and skills.

Each student enters a nursing school with a set of values that may change during the socialization process to reflect the values that the profession holds in high esteem. Values are learned, modified, and expended through education. Values emerge over time, permeate daily operations, impact nursing practice, direct nursing behaviors, and serve as the basis for determining the means to accomplish nursing objectives.

The education for professional nursing should facilitate the development of profession values, professional values and value-based behaviors. Education for nursing must be value-focused, providing guidance for future practice, yet reality-based to prepare practitioners for the current health care system. Nursing faculty members are challenged to teach core nursing values that embody the caring professional nurse. Education for nursing role should facilitate the development of profession values, professional values and value-based behaviors. when we are aware of the professional needs can we begin to understand our real personal values. Our behaviour is the outcome of our value judgement. Nursing educators have a professional obligation to teach and reinforce professional nursing values that are consistent with the professional nursing role. If nurses are to remain central in restructuring efforts, their professional values must be at the core. Especially today, there is a definite need for values education in nursing education programs. The nursing schools respondents reported that teaching concerning the core values was woven into the curriculum as a whole.

Educational efforts and the process of socialization into the profession must build upon, and as appropriate, modify values and behavior patterns developed early in life. Nurses in any setting must be helped to identify the progressive relationship of values to philosophy and mission.

All professions largely understand their responsibilities to be tied to their professional practice. However, responsibility starts further back and reaches further out. The responsibilities to oneself and to one's values guide a person's professional values and often override these. It may be unrealistic to try to teach nursing students the kinds of values and attitudes they need to bring to their work because these values are formed when children are very young. What is more realistic is that, in group discussions and reflection on practice, set values are challenged and options presented for better ones. This is perhaps the most useful function of any teaching in values. Teachers and lecturers therefore have a crucial responsibility in how they make their students aware of issues of global professional concern in this area, and how they influence their students, especially in their understanding of values.

The development of professional values begins in formal educational programs. Students enter nursing programs with values that are modified and expanded through the educational process. Nurse educators facilitate this process in two ways: (1) by exhibiting their commitment to professional values through role-modeling behaviors related to these values; and (2) by systematically providing other value development experiences both in classroom and clinical settings that serve to socialize nursing students to the profession.

If an individual nurse values responsibility, it should be reflected in behaviors. For example, if the research component which is valued, it could be evidenced by the use of clinical practice guidelines in care delivery, evidence-based practice, as well as attending research conferences and in-service programs and consulting with experts to enhance client care. It is this internalization of values that is pivotal for initiating the sequence of thoughts requisite for making clinical judgments. Habitual response patterns imply connectedness to internalization of values. There is a continuing role for education, service, and the profession in helping to maintain professional excellence, a requisite component of which is professional values.

Values Defined

What are Values?
To talk more precisely about value, we need to operationally define the term. Dictionary.com says: "values, sociology. the ideals, customs, institutions, etc., of a society toward which the people of the group have an affective regard. These values may be positive, as cleanliness, freedom, or education, or negative, as cruelty, crime, or blasphemy." Longman

Active Study Dictionary of English says: values are principles and beliefs about what is important in life and how people should behave. According to the Concise Oxford Dictionary "value" means: "One's principles or standards; one's judgement of what is valuable or important in life." The American Heritage® Stedman's Medical Dictionary says "A principle, standard, or quality considered worthwhile or desirable". This definition, therefore, refers primarily to subjective and self-defined values, standards and principles that an individual attributes to him or herself. As regards etymological origins, the Oxford Dictionary mentions the Latin "valere" meaning "to be (of) worth". What the psychologists call "values," occultists would more typically call "true will." Dictionary.com says: "Ethics. any object or quality desirable as a means or as an end in itself." American Ethical Union says "Values are the deeply held beliefs of individuals and groups (i.e., organizations, communities, nations, schools, etc.) that drive the choices we make. İn this respect concept of the value is a ethical concepts and the principles of conduct governing an individual or a profession. As a matter of fact ethics includes values, codes, and principles that govern decisions in profession practice and relationships. Viewed within this contect, values have a standard of behavior and are ideals and beliefs that individuals, professionals and professions upholds. Values may be individual or collective or both; they embrace ethical values, but are somewhat wider. Values are guiding principles, often implicit, that inform perceptions and standards of what is right or wrong, appropriate or inappropriate, worthy or unworthy, acceptable or unacceptable in our behaviour, important or less important. Values are signals giving direction, meaning, and purpose to our lives.

PERSONAL VALUES

With regard to personal values, we refer to people's personal standards and rules of behavior. These rules deal with behaviors they feel good about and find reinforcing as proper kinds of conduct. Personal values are personal belief about worth that acts as a standard to guide one's behavior. Personal values are principles that define you as an individual. Personal values established traits that are representative of an individual's moral character. These may have an order of importance to us such as; honesty, trust, reliability, responsibility, loyalty, moral courage and friendliness. The values' people have integrated into their character are made apparent by their attitudes, beliefs and actions.

Each individual has his or her own values, which develop and form over a lifetime and are learned by observation and reasoning and through experience. Values are standards of behavior. Behavior is guided by personally held principles, beliefs, and values. Personal values are based on experience, religion, education, and culture. Personal values are reflected in individual attitudes. Attitudes, which are made up of several beliefs, are feelings towards a person, object, or idea. Personal values and beliefs that influence attitudes. İnduviduals thus think, feel, make choices and act from within well-known values, which are a person's own moral judgement about his or her morality. Others also reflect their beliefs and their acts. İnduvidual values influence choices, behaviors and actions, often serving as motivators. Moreover, the values that a person holds may determine his or her personal needs, social and cultural influences and interactions with important others.

Our values are those things, activities or qualities that are worthy, high priorities, in our lives. Values are a function of our beliefs, knowledge, and skills. People's values can only really be known by their actions. That's why so many wisdom traditions, including our own, advise us to judge others and let ourselves be judged more by actions than by words.

Values are beliefs or ideals to which an individual is committed and which are reflected in patterns of behavior. Values are standards that guide behavior, needs, and desires. Values are beliefs and considerations that are held to be true and significant. The values vary, developing and changing over time. So although a belief goes further than that which is obvious, it is at least initiated in some fact. As a result of the motivational element usually involved, values tend to be less fixed than attitudes and beliefs.

Beliefs are the assumptions we make about ourselves, about others in the world and about how we expect things to be. Beliefs are about how we think things really are, what we think is really true and what therefore expect as likely consequences that will follow from our behavior. Beliefs are a type of attitude where "the cognitive component is based more on faith than on fact." Beliefs, ideals and purposes are the basic ingredients of values.

PROFESSIONAL VALUES

In talking about professional values, on the other hand, we refer to norms and rules thought best for activities and behaviors by the prevailing professional group generally. Professional values are a word used to describe professional' moral knowledge.

The professional group determines professional values. Professional values are standards for action that are accepted by the practitioner and professional group and provide a framework for evaluating beliefs and attitudes that influence behavior. Professional values, the recognized standards for action that are embraced by members of the profession, are used to guide both education and practice..

Professional values are primarily beliefs and statements that describe practices, or established sets of behavior, that are supported by a community or group. Typically, value statements describe behaviors that the members of a community "feel good about." Value statements also describe or imply behaviors that are likely to be sanctioned or punished by other members of a group or culture. These values are the fundamental beliefs that guide our behaviors and decision-making process.

Professional values may include professional responsibility, loving interpersonal relationships, social consciousness, equality, justice, liberty, freedom, and pride in "our country." A professional value is learned. It involves one's relationship to society.

A well-developed value systems may help what a person ought to do and how one ought to be in relation to others (Altun, 2002, 2003). Values are the rules by which we make decisions about right and wrong, should and shouldn't, good and bad. Values are embedded in what it is to know the good, and are reflected in the character of the person. Values live up to what is desirable and ethically justifiable

Professional values are also standards for action that are accepted by the practitioner and/or professional group. Professional values are provide a framework for evalation beliefs and attitudes that influence behavior. Development of professional values begins upon entry into the profession education environment, continues throughout the educational experience and the professional career. Upon graduation, nurses enter a chaotic work environment. The relationship between professional values, professional education, work environment, experience, and the profesionals' personal commitment to the profession influence the perception of the significance of values in a professional's life. The development of professional values begins during the professional education experience and continues throughout the practice years. Professional values serve to guide the delivery of professional service and decision-making (Babadağ, 1998).

PROFESSION VALUES

Purposeful action requires values. Values are the motive power behind purposeful action. A profession's values -- including its ethical values -- are reflected in the degree to which its structures. Profession's values are vital to the integrity of the profession as a whole. The profession expresses its values through the decisions of the people who are members of the profession to addresses effectively barriers to access or to maintain those barriers through action or inaction.

An profession establishes its mission according to its values; it then formulates goals and aligns priorities according to those values. The values held by profession form the basis for definitions and descriptions of profession. They guide standards for action, provide a framework for evaluating behaviour and influence practice decisions. Such values provide a framework for the development of standards and expectations within the profession. Potter and Perry (1997, 310) point out that, "Because values give identity, influence actions, and sustain what is meaningful, professions are as strong as the values on which they are based". It is expected that each individual within a profession will revere the fundamental values of the particular profession.

The values of profession are found in professional codes of ethics. The Code identifies values common to profession. The Code identify the fundamental moral commitments of the profession. Institutions particularly espouse values that ideally make up their code of ethics. However, there is often a wide chasm between what is espoused and what is practiced. The code presented by professionals reflects the real practice of the profession, addressing the myriad of roles of practitioners and setting forth guidelines for ideal ethical conduct in those roles. Such detail indicates that the professional culture of professions well understood

VALUES IN NURSING

Nursing, like all professions, is based on the ideal and beliefs of service to humanity. Nursing is an inherently value-based endeavor, with a long and rich tradition. As a discipline, a science, a profession, a value nursing encompasses the complex interaction of technical skill and professional conviction with the welfare of other humans.

The essence to the practice of nursing are caring, coordination, and advocacy, and are based on the special relationship between the nurse and the patient. The practice of nursing involves altruistic behavior, is governed by a code of ethics. Therefore Nursing is by natura a moral endeavour. The moral significance of nursing is not just a matter of the objectives that are sought (i.e. the promotion of the patient's well-being), it is also a matter of the moral attitudes on the basis of which nurses carry out their tasks.

It is impossible to be a nurse without considering what is of value. Within nursing, specific values and moral requirements are necessary to maintain the interprity of the profession. Nursing values are fundamental to the practice of nursing and professional compass. Regardless of the nursing practice setting, professional nursing values influence the environment of nursing practice, nursing activity, and the development of nursing as a profession (Hendel et al, 2006).. The values of nursing are those basic assumptions about what is of value in the practice and profession of nursing: what is of fundamental importance in nursing. A value framework in nursing is essential in developing a sense of professional commitment and social responsibility. Nursing values constitute the organizational culture of nursing. The values of nursing are standards for action and responsibilities that are accepted by the practitioner and professional group. Regardless of the nursing practice setting, professional nursing values influence the environment of nursing practice, nursing activity, and the development of nursing as a profession. The values of nursing give nurses direction, guide nursing behaviors and are pivotal in decision making. In addition, values are explained to the public in a way that clarifies professional obligations to society at large. They guide standards for action, provide a framework for evaluating behaviour and influence practice decisions. Despite the importance that can be attributed to nursing values, acknowledgement of them is difficult to find in the current debate about how interprofessional working is changing the healthcare system in which nurses currently work. Professional nursing values can be traced in the discipline's history and traditions.

A Brief History of the Nursing and Nurses -A Look Back - from Virtue to Value

That values changes is welcome and inevitable; how it changes is not always easy to elucidate. By analysing over nursing history, it is possible to see the directions taken so far and the indications of future development. The trends indicate that nursing values reflects fairly closely what is happening in society in general. Nursing's roots are firmly planted in service to others - individuals, groups, and communities. Early nursing service were primarily voluntary and related to religious practice. In ancient times, when medical lore was associated with good or evil spirits, the sick were usually cared for in temples and houses of worship..In the early Christian era nursing duties were undertaken by certain women in the church, their services being extended to patients in their homes. These women had no real training by today's standards, but experience taught them valuable skills, especially in the use of herbs and drugs, and some gained fame as the physicians of their era. In later centuries, however, nursing duties fell mostly to relatively ignorant women (Fealy GM, 2004)

In the latter part of the nineteenth century the Christian virtues (good character trait) of charity, humility and compassion were important motives that prompted an occupational choice such as nursing. (Rognstad &Nortvedt et al, 2004). Altruism, or the selfness giving of oneself for the welfare of others, was a prominent aspect of nursing during this time.

For centuries, nurses have worked to help people and have served the health needs of society. The professional nursing which was pioneered by Florence Nightingale in the XlXth century, was directly influenced by the teachings of love and fraternity. As stated by Florence

Nightingale in 1860, the goal of nursing is to "put the patient in the best condition for nature to work upon him." In addition, other contributions from the religious orders / associations were the concepts of altruism, valorization of an adequate environment for the care of patients, and the division of work in nursing. Religian, the military and technology are three primary influences on the development of the profession. Religion and the military are built on loyalty and unquestioning obedience *(Manthey & Wolf et al, 2000)*.

Nursing subsequently became one of the most important professions open to women until the social changes wrought by the revival of the feminist movement that began in the 1960s. Until the beginning of the twentieth century, the prevailing virtues in nursing were, for example, benevolence, self-sacrifice, obedience, serious-mindedness, faithfulness, compassion, obendience, serious-mindedness, patriotism as well as love of humanity. These new professional values are leading to an inescapable revaluation of the patient-nurse relationship model as well as of our understanding of what nursing is. The modern nursing model has resulted in a preference for a contemporary relationship which presents mutual responsibility in place of a one-way patient-nurse relationship and patient centered nursing in place of physician-centered.

Nursing education has been subject to many changes over the years, and one educational change that has been questioned is the move into universities. They are increasingly expected to take an active role in nursing development and quality improvement by being critical, problem-solving and by using research findings. The nursing role has changed during recent decades. From being disease-oriented and subordinated to the medical paradigm and the physician, nursing has become more of an independent profession focusing on but also on holistic care. Nurses today are increasingly driven by innovations and technological transformation and by constantly changing new roles and values.(Heikkinen & lemonidou, et al., 2006).

'The Role of the ICN': A View Today and Forward

The values held by profession and professional form the basis for definitions and descriptions of profession and are outlined in Code for professional. Code for nurses are sets of standarts based on universal moral principles or values. İnternational Council of Nurses (ICN) is the body that speaks for nurses globally. ICN is the first and widest reaching health care organisation in the world, representing the millions of nurses in just 128 countries. ICN is a federation of national nurses' associations (NNAs), representing nurses in more than 128 countries. Founded in 1899, ICN is the world's first and widest reaching international organisation for health professionals. Operated by nurses for nurses, ICN works to ensure quality nursing care for all, sound health policies globally, the advancement of nursing knowledge, and the presence worldwide of a respected nursing profession and a competent and satisfied nursing workforce (İCN.2006).

Nursing's values are consistent: it is the code of ethics for Nurses. The Tenets of the Code of Ethics are based on shared values and a shared responsibility to uphold them. Members have an obligation to exercise fairness in dealing with others and to provide support and assistance when required. Members should avoid any actions or statements which can be construed as being unfairly critical of a colleague or intended to favour their own position at the expense of a colleagu. ICN codes were constructed by nurses for nurses; they therefore reflect the values of nursing in terms of the requirement to provide patient care based on the identified needs of an individual. The ICN Code of Ethics for Nurses delineates the fundamental values of professional nursing. The code for nurses provides direction for relationships of nurses to clients, the community, and the profession. The ICN Code of Ethics for Nurses, most recently revised in 2005, is a guide for action based on social values and needs. The Code has served as the standard for nurses worldwide since it was first adopted in 1953. The Code is regularly reviewed and revised in response to the realities of nursing and health care in a changing society. Nursing's professional values are articulated in the Code for Nurses.

The Code makes it clear that inherent in nursing is respect for human rights, including the right to life, to dignity and to be treated with respect. The ICN Code of Ethics guides nurses in everyday choices and it supports their refusal to participate in activities that conflict with caring and healing.

The ICN Code of Ethics for Nurses has four principal elements that outline the standards of ethical conduct. The nurse in relation to (1) people, (2) practice, (3) profession, (4) co-workers. Inherent in nursing is respect for human rights, including cultural rights, the right to life and choice, to dignity and to be treated with respect. Nursing care is respectful of and unrestricted by considerations of age, colour, creed, culture, disability or illness, gender, sexual orientation, nationality, politics, race or social status

Accoding to ICN the need for nursing is universal. ICN says: "Nursing encompasses autonomous and collaborative care of individuals of all ages, families, groups and communities, sick or well and in all settings. Nursing includes the promotion of health, prevention of illness, and the care of ill, disabled and dying people. Advocacy, promotion of a safe environment, research, participation in shaping health policy and in patient and health systems management, and education are also key nursing roles.".

According to ICN (2006) Nurses have four fundamental responsibilities:

- to promote health,
- to prevent illness,
- to holistic care and
- to alleviate suffering.

According ICN (2006) Nurses have six key roles
- Advocacy,
- promotion of a safe environment,
- research,
- participation in shaping health policy,
- in patient and health systems management,
- education

Table 1. International Council Of Nurses (Icn) Code Of Ethics for Nurses

The Icn Code

The ICN Code of Ethics for Nurses has four principal elements that outline the standards of ethical conduct.

Elements of the Code

1. Nurses And People

The nurse's primary professional responsibility is to people requiring nursing care. In providing care, the nurse promotes an environment in which the human rights, values, customs and spiritual beliefs of the individual, family and community are respected. The nurse ensures that the individual receives sufficient information on which to base consent for care and related treatment. The nurse holds in confidence personal information and uses judgement in sharing this information. The nurse shares with society the responsibility for initiating and supporting action to meet the health and social needs of the public, in particular those of vulnerable populations. The nurse also shares responsibility to sustain and protect the natural environment from depletion, pollution, degradation and destruction.

2. Nurses And Practice

The nurse carries personal responsibility and accountability for nursing practice, and for maintaining competence by continual learning. The nurse maintains a standard of personal health such that the

ability to provide care is not compromised. The nurse uses judgement regarding individual competence when accepting and delegating responsibility. The nurse at all times maintains standards of personal conduct which reflect well on the profession and enhance public confidence. The nurse, in providing care, ensures that use of technology and scientific advances are compatible with the safety, dignity and rights of people.

3. Nurses And The Profession

The nurse assumes the major role in determining and implementing acceptable standards of clinical nursing practice, management, research and education. The nurse is active in developing a core of research-based professionalm knowledge. The nurse, acting through the professional organisation, participates in creating and maintaining safe, equitable social and economic working conditions in nursing.

4. Nurses And Co-Workers

The nurse sustains a co-operative relationship with co-workers in nursing and other fields. The nurse takes appropriate action to safeguard individuals, families and communities when their health is endangered by a coworker or any other person.

This fundamental responsibilites and roles are values of the nursing profession. These values are reflected in the practice of professional nursing. Nurses delineates the fundamental values of professional nursing. This values is fundamentally the same in any society, these values give an ethical basis for nursing which is global - nurses can adopt it in whatever society and mix of cultures they find themselves. The values of the profession give nurses direction, guide nursing behaviors and are pivotal in decision making. The values of nurses would typically reflect a professional duty to provide a certain level of care. This would have to be one of the factors that should be taken in to account in the construction and application of any nuirsing care. National nursing associations should just go ahead and do it and be done with it adopt the values which are necessary for successfully fulfilling nursing's basic role and objective. Since this role is fundamentally the same in any society, these values give an ethical basis for nursing which is global - nurses can adopt it in whatever society and mix of cultures they find themselves.

The need for nursing care will grow and change in the future. Tschudin (2006) point out that, there is no doubt that nursing will change significantly in the next decade, with professional nurses taking on different roles, especially in the long-termcare of people in the community who are increasingly suffering from lifestyle illness. Such people need long-term professional contact with nurses, which demands specific skills, especially communication and building relationships. This means that individual nurses- and whole profession of nursing – put into action in far more obvious ways the "preventive" or "up-stream" responsilities and values laid on them by the ICN. Regardless of the practice setting, these value documents influence nursing activity and the development of nursing as a profession. That values can guide individual nurses toward satisfaction, fulfillment.

To Promote Health

We can trace the origins of nursing's responsibility for healthy communities directly to Florence Nightingale. Never before has health promotion beeen more important tahn is today. (Chiverton & Votava et al, 2003). The concept of the promotion of health is embedded within tenets of the ICN definition of Nursing. According to ICN promotion of a safe environment are also key nursing role *(İCN.2006)*. ICN's Vision For the Future of Nursing. "Our highest reward is the certain knowledge that our work is shaping a future of healthy people in a healthy world." The ICN's responsibilities of nurses, to 'promote health [and] to prevent illness' ICN's mission For the Future of Nursing. "Our mission is to lead our societies toward better health. Working together within ICN, we harness the knowledge and enthusiasm of the entire nursing profession to promote healthy lifestyles, healthy workplaces, and healthy communities. We foster the health of our societies as well as individuals by supporting strategies of sustainable development that mitigate poverty, pollution, and other underlying causes of illness."

Health promotion as defined by the World Health Organization is the process of enabling people to increase control over, and to improve, their health (WHO,2001).

In 1978, the Declaration of Alma-Ata, signed by nearly all member states of the World Health Organization and UNICEF, issued a bold call for "Health for All" *(Who, 2006)* Its core strategy was primary health care, comprising essential elements ranging from safe water to basic health care services.

The Ottawa Charter for Health Promotion outlines the role of Health Promotion, especially the importance of increasing people's control over their own health. According to the Ottawa Charter for Health Promotion the basic principles of health promotion are as follows:

Prerequisites for health the fundamental conditions and resources for health are peace, shelter, education, food, income, a stable ecosystem, sustainable resources, social justice and equity. Improvement in health requires a secure foundation in these basic prerequisites.

According to WHO (2001) advoncate good health is a major resource for social, economic and personal development and an important dimension of quality of life. Political, economic, social, cultural, environmental, behavioural and biological factors can all favour health or be harmful to it. Health promotion action aims at making these conditions favourable through advocacy for health.

Health promotion is the science and art of helping people change their lifestyle to move toward a state of optimal health. Optimal health is defined as a balance of physical, emotion, social, spiritual and intellectual health. It is more than lifestyle change, it is also about changing environments so they are more supportive of making healthy decisions. Lifestyle change can be facilitated through a combination of efforts to:

- enhance awareness,
- change behavior and
- create environments that support good health practices.
- Of the three, supportive environments will probably have the greatest impact in producing lasting changes.

In the purest sense, health promotion is associated with wanting to improve one's health via "behavior motivated by the desire to increase well-being and actualize human health potential." (p7) Such behavior changes might include engaging in more physical activity or getting more sleep. Health promotion, consistent with the Healthy People 2010 mandate, also includes health protection, or "behavior motivated by a desire to actively avoid illness, detect it early, or maintain functioning within the constraints of illness." (p7) (Pender.2002)

Health promotion includes the facilitation of an individual's potential and energy use, an improved quality of life, productivity and use of one's abilities regarding health. Therefore it is necessary to make people aware of their health and to provide them with sufficient information and skills.

According to this opinion, individuals have a critical role in the determination of their own health status. To reach a state of complete physical, mental and social well-being, an individual or group must be able to identify and to realize aspirations, to satisfy needs, and to change or cope with the environment. Health-promoting behaviors are an integral part of an individual's lifestyle and determinants of health status; these include taking charge of personal health responsibilities, taking part in physical activities, and maintaining good nutritional habits. A healthy individual should also have self actualization, and be able to maintain good interpersonal relations and stress-management. Self-care activities that maintain and improve functional competence, well-being, and personal development minimize health risks.

One of the most important ways to promote health is to improve the self-care agency of an individual which may be carried out through health education. Health education seeks to motivate the individual to accept a process of behavioral change through directly influencing their value, belief and attitude systems, where it is deemed that the individual is particularly at risk or has already been affected by illness/disease or disability. As more people grow in their awareness of activities that lead to good health and become knowledgeable about their own health status, the overall health of population will improve (Chiverton & Votava et al, 2003).

To Prevent Illness

The prevent illness refers to the protection of health, to prevent infection and ensure a safe, healthy environment. Health protection might include incorporating more hygienic or safer practices into daily routines, participating in disease screenings, or obtaining immunizations and vaccinations. Health protection refers to the protection of health by personal and community wide effects, such as preserving good nutritional status, physical fitness, and emotional well-being, immunizing against infectious diseases, and making the environment safe.

Prevent infection might include immunizing against infectious diseases, and making the environment safe. The goal of prevention:

1. Primary prevention - to prevent the initiation of illness through the reduction of risk factors and the promotion of wellness. Primary prevention refers to the protection of health by personal and community wide effects, such as preserving good nutritional status, physical fitness, and emotional well-being, immunizing against infectious diseases, and making the environment safe.
2. Secondary prevention - to arrest the development of illness through early detection of illness and the promotion of wellness. Secondary prevention can be defined as the measures available to individuals and populations for the early detection and prompt and effective intervention to correct departures from good health.
3. Tertiary prevention - to minimize the consequences of illness and disability through the promotion of wellness. Tertiary prevention consists of the measures available to reduce or eliminate long-term impairments and disabilities, minimize suffering caused by existing departures from good health, and to promote the patient's adjustment to irremediable conditions. This extends the concept of prevention into the field of rehabilitation. There are no precise boundaries between these levels."

Ensure a safe, healthy environment refesrs to the the reduction of risk factors, working to prevent infection and ensure a safe, healthy environment

Health challenges are constantly changing with time, due to the impact of many different factors. Considerable progress was made in the 20th century in combating infectious diseases with the development of drugs for the treatment of bacterial infections and a wide range of metabolic disorders as well as vaccines to prevent some bacterial and viral infections. Achievements included the eradication of smallpox and progress towards eradication of polio. However, major challenges now arise from new, emerging and re-emerging infectious agents. In parallel, the epidemiological transition towards noncommunicable diseases that was perceived as a characteristic of affluence is now being seen in many low- and middleincome countries, presenting a new range of challenges for prevention, diagnosis and treatment of these chronic conditions. Additional factors that are stretching the capacities of all countries, but especially those at the lower end of the income scale, include the rising tide of injuries, impacts of globalization on health and the recognition that social, economic and political determinants of health are also important and that many factors outside the health sector or system impact on the health of populations. Specific targets, whether for improvements in efficiency or cost-effectiveness or for the achievement of international goals such as the Millennium Development Goals, are also stretching the capacities of planners, managers and service deliverers—often in situations where factors such as HIV/AIDS or migration are depleting an already understrength health workforce (Martin , 2006).

All nurses are teachers, helping people learn to prevent illness and manage health problems. The nurse also protects the patient, working to prevent infection and ensure a safe, healthy environment in the hospital. Finally, the nurse teaches the patient and family about health-related matters and promotes patients' well-being in all situations, speaking for them (advocating), if necessary. The hospital nurse plays many roles on the health care team

To Care Holistically

Health, how health is perceived depends on how health is defined. The World Health organization (WHO) defines health as a "state of complete pyhsical, mental, and social well being and not merely the absence of disease and infirmity." *Preamble of the Constitution of The World Health Organization.*

Disease may be defined as the abnormal state in which part or all of the body is not properly adjusted or is not capable of carrying on all its requered functions. Disease can have a number of direct causes, such as the following: Disease-prodicing organisms, malnutrition, physical gents, chemicals, birth defects, dejenerative processes, neoplasms. Examples of predisposing causes (indirect) include the following: Age, sex, heredity, living conditions and habits, occupation, physical exposure, preexisting illness, psychogenic influences.

When a person becomes ill or is injured, generally the doctor assesses the patient, diagnoses the patient's problem and decides on the treatment needed to cure the problem or relieve the patient's symptoms.

Throughout most of medical history, the physician' aim has been to cure patients of existing diseases.

In the past only the doctor assessed and diagnosed (Breier-Mackie, 2006) Today, however, nurses play a large role in evaluating patients and detecting problems. In some rural areas, nurses admit patients to hospital and manage their care, referring only the most critical patients to distant medical centres. In every hospital nurses carry out many of the treatments prescribed for the patient. For example, the doctor may prescribe surgery orbed rest or a certain therapy. The doctor will perform some of these treatments, such as surgery. It is the nurse who gives most of the treatments.

Once a patient's disorder is known, the physician prescribes a course of treatment can be much else besides therapy. Specific measures in a course of treatment are carried out by the nurse and other health care providers under the physician's orders. If a patient needs intravenous therapy, usually the nurse sets up the intravenous line and gives the patient the fluids and drugs prescribed. If the patient needs an injection, it is the nurse who gives it. The nurse changes the patient's dressings and monitors the healing of the wound. The nurse gives medication for pain. Many physicians order medication for pain "to be given as needed". They let the nurse decide when to give the medication. The nurse also monitors the patient's progress to make sure that the recovery has no complications. Because nurses have more frequent contact with patients than other staff, they often find problems before anyone else.

Nurses care for patients continuously, 24 hours a day. Nurses play an extremely valuable role in this process by observing closely for signs, collecting and organizing information from the patient about his or her symptoms, aand then reporting this information to the physician. They help patients to do what they would do for themselves if they could. Nurses take care of their patients, making sure that they can breathe properly, seeing that they get enough fluids and enough nourishment, helping them rest and sleep, making sure that they are comfortable, taking care of their need to eliminate wastes from the body, and helping them to avoid the harmful consequences of being immobile, like stiff joints and pressure sores. The nurse often makes independent decisions about the care the patient needs based on what the nurse knows about that person and the problems that may occur. For example, the nurse may decide that, in order to prevent pressure sores, the patient needs to be turned every two hours. However, the nurse may consult the doctor about this if it is possible that turning the patient might cause some other problem. Thus the nurse uses understanding of medical conditions, as well as knowledge of nursing, in deciding on patient care. The nurse not only takes care of the patient but also gives comfort and support to the patient and his or her family. When the patient cannot recover, the nurse helps to make sure that the death is peaceful. In caring for the patient, the nurse cares about the patient. The holistic care is really the only possible type of care that nurses want to give and patients want to receive (Breier-Mackie, 2006)

To talk more precisely about caring, we need to operationally define the term. The concept of care and caring can be explained in various ways, and it can present a different meaning to each person. The American Heritage *Dictionary* says "care, attentive assistance or treatment to those in need: *a hospital that provides emergency care.* "Caring, to be concerned or interested: *Once inside, we didn't care whether it rained or not.* To provide needed assistance or watchful supervision: *cared for the wounded; caring for an aged relative at home. WorldNet* "caring" means. "feeling and exhibiting concern and empathy for others; "caring friends" n : a loving feeling " *Longman Active Study Dictionary of English says:*" caring to be worried, concerned about, or interested in someone or something". In anorher defined "caring providing care and support: the caring professions. Such as nursing."

Caring may be defined as intentional action that conveys physical and emotional security and genuine connectedness with another person or group of people (Miller, 1995).

Defined by Yancey (1995, 83), as " an action, a virtue, an ethical principles, or a way of being in the world." Caring has also been described as a basic nursing virtue and as a fundamental value that informs the nurse–patient relationship. The idea that human caring is central to nursing is certainly relevant to the role of nursing in contemporary healthcare. Caring is often seen as an admirable thing in itself and as a virtue (Skott & Eriksson ,2005). Nurse are being challenged to "ensure the ethic of caring remains a central, essential, and unique focus of nursing" (Kurtz 1991, 8; Esterhuzen, 2006). Caring is now commonly recognized within nursing as the profession's central value in all health care settings (Potter and Perry 1997, 310).

According to Gastmans (1999 "Caring as a moral attitude can be considered as a sensitive and supportive response of the nurse to the situation and circumstances of a vulnerable human being who is in need of help *(Gastmans,1999).*

The values of care as applied to nursing were addressed by reflecting on the ICN codes. Nursing is a caring profession more than any profession. Because Nursing is focused on assisting individuals, families and communities in attaining, re-attaining and maintaining optimal health and functioning. Therefore caring is described as the "essence of nursing" and the most central values. Caring encompasses empathy for and connection with people. Teaching and role-modeling caring is a nursing curriculum challenge. Caring is best demonstrated by a nurse's bability to embody the core values of professional nursing (*Fahrenwald et al, 2005*).

A nurse's training as a caring person is thus not limited to the theoretical transfer of knowledge during the period of education. The attitude to care is the result of a life of care, not of professional training or of a theoretically sound argument. As a result, it is worthwhile to direct the efforts made in developing a nurse as a caring person towards the nurse's life in its totality, and so promote the gradual growth of a caring attitude caring is a moral pursuit centred on the beneficent attention of one person shown to another. Caring can be explained as an affect, a feeling of compassion or empathy towards the recipient of care. Caring about also implies that there is a genuine concern about the well-being of the other. Care can be described as an attitude or orientation that leads to the beneficent attending, through acts or omissions, of one person towards another. Caring as a virtue and an act of ethics is from both a natural and a professional point of view inseparably related to love as a universal/ontological value. A ethic of care leads a nurse to respond to each situation with tecnical and moral knowledge, compassion, competence, and integrity. (Yancey, 1995, 85; Esterhuzen, 2006)

Nurses are increasingly aware that good nursing care consists of 'more' than the competent performance of a number of caring activities. This type of caring relationship is not limited to the nurse–patient dyad, but also comprises the relationship nurses have with other nurses, physicians and co-workers. To refer to the term 'ethical' on a theoretical level with principles and theories and apply the term 'moral' to the manifestation of what is right and wrong, good and bad in practice is an oversimplification. Caring about is characterized by the individual's ability, for example, to feel, to have insight and to be genuine in a caring situation. When a person is seen as a living being (a whole person, not fragmented into objective parts of the body) then every relationship becomes unique to both the receiver and the giver of care..

To Alleviate Suffering.

The concept 'suffering' has been central within nursing since Florence Nightingale. Rodgers and Cowles (1977), stated that "Suffering is defined as an individualized, subjective, and complex experience that involves the assignment of an intensely negative meaning to an event or a perceived threat. Kahn and Steeves (1986), stated that "suffering is experienced when some crucial aspect of one's self, being, or existence is threatened". Whether suffering occurs or not depends on the meaning that the person gives to the threat to personal integrity.

If illness, deprivation, pain, or disability obstructs one's access to the world and constricts one's horizons, suffering occurs. Suffering also attacks one's sense of meaning and purpose.

The suffering of patients can be of a physical, psychological or spiritual nature, but it is always unique to each individual. In addition to physical pain, there can be a sense of loss, especially a loss of autonomy. Other examples are feelings of loneliness, fear of death or disfigurement, and threats to the manner in which meaning and purpose are found in patients' lives.

How Can Nurses Help?

Patients need to feel supported, experience minimal symptom distress, and maintain as much control over their lives as possible (Lewis, 1982; Taylor, 1993).

Patients have reported finding meaning and thus having their suffering at least temporarily relieved when they were able to accept help, assist others, find pleasure in their environment, practice their religion, maintain an attitude of hopefulness, and if terminally ill, accept the inevitability of death (Coward, 1990; Steeves, 1992; Steeves & Kahn, 1987).

Nursing actions that address the above patient needs provide caring amid the suffering experience.

The need to experience meaning is a spiritual need that touches the core of one's being and is intensified during the illness experience. Some nursing interventions that can enhance meaning-making include listening to patients, employing insightful questioning, asking patients to tell their stories, and maintaining a compassionate presence (Taylor, 1993).

Nurses must not run from their feelings of helplessness in the presence of patient suffering. Nurses can assist patients to give voice to their suffering and expression to the ways that the suffering can be relieved and can be cahange the patient's understanding of life (Rehnsfeldt & Eriksson, 2004).

NURSES' PROFESSIONAL VALUES

Nurses' professional values are a word used to describe nurses' moral knowledge (*Yancey, 1995*). Nurses' moral knowledge may promote a reflective, ethical attitude and thereby support them in their professional growth. Kluchohn (1951) stated that a value is a 'conception explicit or imphcit, distinctive of an individual or characteristic of a group of the desirable which influences the selection from available modes, means, and ends of action' (p395). He views values as personal in nature and contributing to one's sense of identity. Kluckhohn asserted that a value has persistence over time and is organized into a system of action or a way of being for the individual. A link can be made between the action-orientation of values and the role of values in mediating the decision making of nurses. Bevis (1988) noted that all choices are made from one's value system. (Parker (cited in fawcett, 2003) said that "The values held by nurses form the basis for definitions and descriptions of nursing" (p.134). According to Raths et al (1966), determined that values are chosen freely, thoughtfully prized or cherished, and acted on.

 Professional nurses values are the foundation for practice; they guide interactions with patients, colleagues, other professionals, and the public. Profesional nurses values provide the framework for commitment to patient welfare, fundamental to professional nursing practice and critical decision making processes. Values are important in nursing care because nurses need to make decisions about value-laden practice dilemmas on a regular basis.(*Weis &, Schank, 1997,* McNeese-Smith & Crook, 2003)

The nursing code of ethics is a collective statement about the nurses' expectations and standarts of behavior *(Yancey,1995)*. The nurses' code expresses the moral commitment to uphold the goals, values, and distinct ethical obligations of all nurses. The code of ethics establishes a nonnegotiable ethical standard for the nursing profession. It demonstrates accountability and responsibility to the public, other members of the nurses team, and the profession overall. The code of ethics is the nurses' value statement. Codes of ethics define nurses' responsibilities, and provide direction for nursing obligations. The code of ethics give establish norms of behavior *(Yancey,1995)*. The Code provide professionals with a basis for professional and self reflection and a guide to ethical practice; The Code indicate to the community the values which professionals hold. The sources of professional values for nurses are the nursing profession and employing institutions. Nurse demonstrate their professional values in their attitudes and behaviors (Verpeet,& Dierckx de Carterle'. et al, 2006)

The nurse functions both as a professional and as a human being within a variety of contexts. Frequently, nurses' values are challenged, either strengthening or weakening the foundational beliefs. The socialization process in nursing education involves the modification of personal values and internalization of nursing values. At the core of professional nursing is the value that nursing practice serves to act in the best interest of the patient.

The values of the professional give nurses direction, guide nursing behaviors and are pivotal in decision making. The values central to the profession of nursing are caregiving, altruism, respect for human dignity, service to society, accountability and recognition of the client as an individual, empathetic understanding and reciprocal trust (Creasia & Parker, 2001).

Nursing Education

According to Manthey (2000) The timeless values of nursing include advocacy of the patient, intentional caring, promoting community health, awareness of the mind-body-spirit connection and a belief in the fundamental equality of people.

American Association of Colleges of Nursing (AACN, 1998) espouse that baccalaureate education programs facilitate the development of professional nursing values. The five core values embraced by the (AACN, 1998) include human dignity, integrity, autonomy, altruism, and social justice.

The American Association of Colleges of Nursing (AACN) published, in 2003, a document entitled of College and University Education for Professional Nursing in which it identified the values (as well as the knowledge and skilled practice) which were consider essential for nursing. the AACN identifies it as an attitude or personal quality, which nurses will demonstrate as a result of altruism, accountability, human dignity, integrity and social justice. These values are considered to be essential to the practice of professional nurses. These values are reflected in individual attitudes; they influence choices, behaviours and actions.

Nures, guided by these values, demonstrates ethical behaviors in the provision of safe, humanistic health care. The sample behaviors are not mutually exclusive and may result from more than one value. Conversely, the value labels provided are intended to encapsulate a core set of values and behaviors that can be elaborated in a variety of ways. The values and sample professional behaviors listed below epitomize nursing. Professional nurses values include: a) autonomy, b) human dignity, c) integrity d) responsibility /accountability, e) social justice. Usually colleges and university are evaluated by the quality of the knowledge and technical training offered to the students. Little attention is given to the acquisition of the values, behaviors and attitudes necessary to assume their professional role. Value-based nursing education appeals to the moral and character development of students. Values and behaviors are influenced by College years, studying at a College of Nursing during four years leads to a difference in values and professional behavior. Professional values are difficult to teach as part of professional education. Nevertheless, faculty must design learning opportunities that support empathic, sensitive, and compassionate care for individuals, groups, and communities; that promote and reward honesty and accountability; that make students aware of social and ethical issues; and that nurture students' awareness of their own value systems, as well as those of others (Dinc & Görgülü RS, 2002).

NURSING'S TIMELESS VALUE

Autonomy

Autonomy (Greek: Auto meaning 'self' Nomos - *nomos* meaning "law": one who gives oneself his own law) means freedom from external authority. Autonomy is a concept found in moral, political, and bioethical philosophy. Within these contexts it refers to the capacity of a rational individual to make an informed, uncoerced decision. In moral and political philosophy, autonomy is often used as the basis for determining moral responsibility for one's actions. İn nursing autonomy, defined as the right to self determination (AACN, 1998, p. 8). This nursing value is including patient autonomy. Patient autonomy focuses on respect for the patient's right to make decisions, even when those decisions conflict with the values of the nurse. Nurses have a moral obligation to the profession and to society to advocate for a patient's rights to self-determination. Autonomy is grounded in respect for patients' ability to choose, decide and take responsibility for their own lives.

Learning experiences emphasize how to facilitate the patient's right to make informed health-related choices. Autonomy has to do with personal qualities such as knowledge, realism, curiosity, honesty, rationality, inquisitiveness, responsibility, accountability, self-confidence, authenticity, and it can be explained as to document nursing care accurately and honestly. Autonomous behavior includes the provision of information so patients can make informed choices. Nurse autonomy reflects a moral obligation to provide competent care to clients and to protect clients from unsafe practice. (AACN, 1998).

Nurse autonomy takes a strong stand on the duty to respect autonomy and to keep promises. By virtue of their specialized knowledge, nurses are permitted to exercise their own judgment in the delivery of their services. Nurse who give priority to autonomy succesful in problem solving, performance positively, self-esteem highly, low levels of emotional exhaustion, high feelings of personal achievement, inquisitive and risk-taking, high in critical thinking skills (Altun, 2003, McNeese-Smith & Crook, 2003)

Human Dignity

Nurses also reflect on human dignity as applied in their own the caring attitude who is a characteristic of a nurse who is part of a network of communicative and narrative communities. Caring can be characterized in qualities such as compassion, giving of self, respectful, competence, confidence, conscience, perseverance, benevolence, sympathy, empathetic, generosity, altruism, kindness, concern, love of self and others and commitment, and can also be based on sharing and mutual respect. These feelings and characterizes are motivating elements that move the nurse to attend to and on the other; they propel the nurse into a caring mode. These foundational elements influence the caring milieu to preserve the unique nature of the human dignity. This undertaking demands a commitment to care, appropriate underpinning knowledge, and an appreciation of the possible consequences that can occur when these factors are applied. These elements illustrate that caring in nursing embraces a therapeutic ethos that can be beneficial to both nurse and patient. In professional nursing practice, is reflected by nurse's concern for the welfare of clients, other nurses, and other health care providers. Nurses demostrates altriustic behaviors such as advocates for clients, being patient, doing for another, takes risks on behalf of clients and colleagues, the welfare, protection, enhancement of the one being cared for, understanding of cultures, beliefs, and perspectives of others, recognizing another's humanity weakness and strength. Nurses also demostrates behaviors such as respect for human dignity, responding to the patient's care needs, to benefit another, a concern for the welfare and well being of others

Integrity

According to the 0nline dictionary.reference.com "Integrity are adherence to moral and ethical principles; soundness of moral character; honesty." İn addition to this integrity refers to the values of the profession, which are clarified in codes of professional ethics. Professional integrity is acting in accordance with an appropriate code of ethics and accepted standards of practice. A professional code articulates the morality or ethical conduct expected of members of the profession (ie, what ought one to do, what ought to be done for the patient). These codes articulate rules of etiquette and the responsibilities of individual members of a profession. Codes of professional ethics foster and emphasize member identification with and conformity to the core values and underlying ethical principles of the profession. The fundamental ethical principles that are the foundation for the ICN code for nurses and the explications for nursing are autonomy, which relates to a patient's right to self determination; beneficence and nonmaleficence, meaning to do good and avoid harm; justice, which relates to equity; fidelity, or keeping commitments and promises; and veracity, otherwise described as honesty.

Integrity is reflected in professional practice when nurses is honest and provides care based on an ethical framework that is accepted within the profession. Only when nurses experience the integrity of the profession can they act with personal integrity. Sample professional behaviors include: does good, avoides harm, tells the truth, respects privileged information,keeps promises,treats people fairly, provides honest information to clients and the public; documents care accurately and honestly seeks to remedy errors made by self or others;

and demonstrates accountability for own actions and those of other health care team members under the supervision of the ICN.

Responsibility /Accountability

Responsibility involves the obligation to answer for actions. Resposibility also refers to the execution of duties associated with a nurse's partikuler role. Responsibility appeared in various ways. The ICN( ) asserts that nurses have a responsibility to alleviate people's social and health needs, especially those in vulnerable populations. The fourfold responsibilities of promoting health, preventing illness, restoring health and alleviating suffering imposed on nurses by the ICN Code. In this context the nursing approach to the nursing concept can be applied internationally. It is from these values that priorities will be set, standards will be developed, resources will be allocated, and all facets of work life will be influenced. The nurse has a responsibility to be aware not only of the specific health needs of individual patients but also of broader health concerns such as world hunger, environmental pollution, lack of access to nursing and health care resources.

Nurses are also responsible for the well-being and quality of life of many people, and therefore must meet high standards of technical and ethical competence.

Responsibility includes personal qualities such as trustworthiness, courage, openness, and experience, as well as choices of empathy and love. Sample professional behaviors include: to focus on individual patients' needs, to prioritize the individual patient's needs, to accept limitations, to suit the patients' condition better

Competencies should be assessed across this continuum from entry to graduation. Each of the competencies defined can be attributed, at some level or degree, to a wide range of roles and health care providers. Nurses attains a level of competence to provide high quality, client-focused, accountable practice as a health care professional and clinical leader. In professional practice, competencie is reflected when nurses values and respects all clients and colleagues. Sample professional behaviors include: does critical thinking, does good communication, good assessment and technical skills, good teaching, gives humanistic-caring, rather well management, successful leadership, and successful integration of knowledge skills. The most common form of ethical guidance is a code of ethics/professional practice. The availability and accessibility of high quality health services to all people require both interdisciplinary planning and collaborative partnerships among health professionals and others at the community, national, and international levels. The nurse, as a professional, has responsibility to make judgments as an individual clinician responsible for quality nursing care for individuals, families, and groups (Fowler & Levine-Ariff, 1987). To be a professional requires the willing assumption of responsibility in every dimension of nursing practice. The nurse's professional responsibility encompasses a willingness to act on one's beliefs and to accept accountability for one's actions and behaviors.

Accountability is the aspects of responsibility involving giving a statistical or judicial explanation for events. Accountability refers to being answerable for one's own actions. Accountability is the capacity to decide and to exercise choice. Accountability is a concept in ethics with several meanings. It is often used synonymously with such concepts as answerability, resposibility, blameworthiness, liablity and other terms associated with the expectation of account-giving.

Accountability includes the autonomy, authority and control of one's actions and decisions. Freedom having Accountability / Responsibility is the right, power, and competence to act. Freedom involves personal qualities such as self-direction, self-discipline, confidence, hope, independence, openness, and it can be explained as to honor the individual's right to refuse treatment.

Professional practice reflects accountability when nurses evaluates individual and group health care outcomes and modifies treatment or intervention strategies to improve outcomes. Nurses also uses risk analysis tools and quality improvement methodologies at the systems level to anticipate risk to any client and intervenes to decrease the risk. Sample professional behaviors include: evaluates client care and implements changes in care practices to improve outcomes of care; serves as a responsible steward of the environment, and human and material resources while coordinating care; uses an evidence-based approach to meet specific needs of individuals, clinical populations or communities; manages, monitors and manipulates the environment to foster health and health care quality; and prevents or limits unsafe or unethical care practices.

Justice

To talk more precisely about justice, we need to operationally define the term. Dictionary.com says: "justice, the quality of being just; righteousness, equitableness, or moral rightness: to uphold the justice of a cause." *The American Heritage® Stedman's Medical Dictionary* says " justice, the principle of moral rightness; equity. Conformity to moral rightness in action or attitude; righteousness. " *On-line Medical Dictionary* says: "justice are the ethical principle that persons who have similar circumstances and conditions should be treated alike; sometimes known as distributive justice." This definition, therefore, refers primarily to subjective and self-defined justice, standards and principles that an individual attributes to him or herself. American Association of Colleges of Nursing says "justice are upholding moral, legal, and ethical principles." Let us translate its meaning into actions that will contribute to the well-being of the people whom we serve and of ourselves as members of the Nursing Professions. İn this respect concept of the justice is a ethical concepts and the principles of conduct governing an individual or a profession. Let us feel justice as a virtue of man, founded in love and respect for our own rights and obligations and those of our fellow men.

The fourfold responsibilities of promoting health, preventing illness, restoring health and alleviating suffering imposed on nurses by the ICN Code, have to be seen in the context of distributive justice and equality. The fourfold responsibilities of nurses, the need for social justice, and the advocacy role of nurses and nursing make it clear that nursing work is political work. Nurses have long believed themselves to be the patient's advocate, seeing this as a core function of nursing and a natural extension of the nurse–patient relationship. In this respect advocacy is a core value within a nurse's practice. The concept of advocacy is embedded within tenets of the ICN definition of Nursing as key nursing roles. (ICN, 2006). ICN calls on nurses and nursing organizations to promote advocacy as ' a key nursing role'. This call has been taken up internationally by regulatory organizations, many of whom have included advocacy in codes of professional conduct. ICN's Vision For the Future of Nursing "being advocates for our patients, helping people to help themselves, and doing for people what they would do unaided if they had the necessary strength, will, or knowledge."

ICN (2006) stipulates four fundamental responsibilities that nurses have: 'to promote health, to prevent illness, to restore health and to alleviate suffering'. One can apply these functions with a short-term and a long-term perspective. In the present context, it is nursing as a profession and the short-term perspective and the personal scene that are mainly considered. They apply as much to an individual nurse as to nurses collectively, as much to a single person for whom a nurse is caring as to society, with a local situation in mind or with an international and societal intention. It is increasingly evident that there is a significant ethical responsibility for nurses in the international arena. Advocacy is required on behalf of communities and societies, not only for individuals, and for the prevention of situations that are detrimental to the well-being of people. Advocacy in nursing has two components. The first is that advocacy in the nursing role implies that nurses support patients' autonomy or patients' rights to freely choose, regardless of whether the nurse agrees with patients' decisions. Second, advocacy in nursing includes the nurse's ability to take action on behalf of the patient (Schroeter, 2000; Zulfikar & Ulusoy 2001). Advocacy must be understood better. The issues in advocacy are complex and it is too easy to see only one side and identify with a person or a cause against some authority. Much has been written about advocacy, but it remains an issue that is open to abuse and frustration. It is however vital to any nursing work, in particular to the concerns of work in and with any minority groups. Hand in hand with advocacy must go ethical responsibility. That is to say the advocate includes the protection of rights, values-based decision making, to respect patients' decisions, assistance in asserting, to teach patients and enhance their autonomy (Altun, 2003).

The ICN identify that the nursing value of team co-operation should also be applied at managerial level, where nurse involvement could include a responsibility for resource allocation. Concerns about the provision of resources to support safe patient care could be articulated by nurses. These days we hear a lot about the loss of species and ecosystems, and if one such system disappears, systems further up the chain also have problems and may disappear. If you get rid of good and well qualified nurses, mental health, school health, occupational health, and such systems also collapse, simply causing problems. This is where your social justice matters (Tschudin, 2006).

Let us work for a kind of justice that will move nurses to promote the existence of adequate and fair health systems or services for all of mankind, breaking down in this way existing inequalities: A kind of justice which will be reflected permanently in nursing practice by means of respect, defense and promotion of human rights; A kind of justice that bravely defends the rights of individuals, of families and of communities to receive timely and quality health care without distinction because of social class, race, sex or religious or political beliefs.

The idea of 'justice' may not have figured large yet in the nursing mindset, let alone in the curriculum, but it cannot be avoided any longer. This must become a fundamental principle in nursing and in the kind of work in which nurses engage. All nurses everywhere have to become politically aware and act quicklybefore more people suffer. The demands of justice are pressing in two areas, *distribution* and retribution But health care has nothing to do with retribution, but distributive justice is big and needs attention. Distributive justice may require equality, giving people what they deserve, maximising benefit to the worst off, protecting whatever comes about in the right way, or maximising total welfare. Retributive justice may require backward-looking retaliation, or forward-looking use of punishment for the sake of its consequences. Ideals of justice must be put into practice by institutions, which raise their own questions of legitimacy, procedure, codification and interpretation.

Professional behaviors that exemplify social justice include "supporting fairness and nondiscrimination in the delivery of care, promoting universal access to health." *(Hirskyj, 2007)* Justice embodies personal qualities such as fairness, courage, morality, integrity, objectivity, and it can be reflected in acting as a health-care advocate, and in allocating resources fairly. This value is reflected in professional practice when nurses works to assure equal treatment under the law and equal access to quality health care. Sample professional behaviors include supports fairness and non-discrimination in the delivery of care; promotes universal access to health care; and encourages legislation and policy consistent with the advancement of nursing care and health care.

REFERENCES

American Association of Colleges of Nursing (AACN)..Working Paper on The Role of the Clinical Nurse Leader(2004).

(http://www.aacn.nche.edu/Publications/WhitePapers/ClinicalNurseLeader.htm [Accessed 1-December- 2006]

American Association of Colleges of Nursing.(AACN). The Essentials of Baccalaureate Education: For Professional Nursing Practice.. Washington, DC: Author; 1998.pp.6-9

American Ethical Union at http://www.aeu.org/.) (Accessed: November 09, 2006)

Altun İ.(2002). Burnout and nurses' personal and professional values. Nursing Ethics. 9 (3): 269-278

Altun İ. (2003). The perceived problem solving ability and values of student nurses and midwives. Nurse Education Today. 23: 575-584

Altun İ, Ersoy N. (2003). Undertaking the role of patient advocate: a longitudinal study of nursing students. nursing ethics, (9) 10: 462 - 471.

Babadağ K Nursing and Values. The Thesis of Professor, İstanbul University.1998.

Breier-Mackie S. (2006). Medical ethics and Nursing Ethics: is there really Any Difference?. Gastroenterology Nursing. 29 (2):182-183.

Cancerweb (http://cancerweb.ncl.ac.uk/omd/). (Accessed: November 09, 2006).

Chiverton PA, Votava Km, Tortoretti DM. (2003). The future role of nursing in health promotion. American Journal of Health Promotion.18 (2): 192-194

Coward, D. C. (1990). The lived experience of self-transcendence in women with advanced breast cancer. Nursing Science Quarterly. 3: 162-169

Cronqvis A, Theorell T, Burns T, Lützén K. (2004). Carıng About – Carıng For: Moral Oblıgatıons And Work Responsıbılıtıes In Intensıve. Care Nursıng. Nursing Ethics. 11 (1): 64-75

Cortis JD, Kendrick K. (2003). Nursıng Ethıcs, carıng and culture. Nursing Ethics. 10 (1): 78-88)

Dinc L, Görgülü RS. (2002) Teaching ethics in nursing. Nursing Ethics. 9(3): 259-68

Dictionary.reference.com (http://dictionary.reference.com/browse/values). (Accessed: November 09, 2006).

Dictionary reference com. (http://dictionary.reference.com/browse/altruism). (Accessed: November 09, 2006).

Dictionary.reference.com. (http://dictionary.reference.com/browse/integrity. Accessed: November 09, 2006).

En wikipedia.org. http://en.wikipedia.org/wiki/Autonomy. (Accessed: November 09, 2006).

Esterhuzen P.(2006). İs the professional code still the cornerstone of clinical nursing practice?. Journal of Advanced Nursing. 53 (1): 104-113

Ersoy N, Altun İ.(1998). Professional and personal values of nursing in Turkey. Eubios Journal of Asian and İnternational Bioethics. 8 (3): 72-75

Fahrenwald N L. (2003). Teaching Social Justice. Nurse Educator. 28 (5): 222-6.

Faithfull S, Hunt G. (2007).Exploring nursing values in the development of a nurse-led service. Nursing Ethics. 12 (5): 72-83

Fawcett J. (2003). Theory and practice: A conversation with Marilyn E. Parker. Nursing Science Quarterly. 134.

Fahrenwald N. et al. (2005). Teaching core nursing values. Journal Of Professional Nursing, 21 (1): 46–51

Fealy GM. (2004). 'The good nurse': visions and values in images of the nurse. Journal of Advanced Nursing. 46(6): 649-56.

Gastmans C. (1999). Care as a moral attitude in nursing. Nursing Ethics. 6 (3): 215-221

Hall JK. Nursing Ethics and Law. W.B. Saunders Co.,Philadelphia. 1996.

Hendel T, Eshel N, Traister L, Galon V, Baş. (2006). Readiness for future managerial leadership roles:nursing students' perceived importance of organizational values J Prof Nurs. 22: 339–46,

Heikkinen A, lemonidou C, et al. (2006). Ethical codes in nursing practice: the viewpoint of finnish, greek and italian nurses. Journal of advanced nursing. 55 (3): 310-319

Hirskyj P. (2007) An ethical issue that dare not speak its name. qaly: Nursing Ethics 14 (1): 73-82

Kahn DL, Steeves RH. (1994). Witnesses to suffering. Nursing knowledge, voice, and vision. Nursing Outlook, 42, 260-264.

Lewis FM. (1982). Experienced personal control and quality of life in late-state cancer pages. Nursing Research. 31: 113-119.

Longman Active Study Dictionary of English, new edition, Longman Group UK Limited, 1991.

Martin P, Yarbrough S, Alfred D (2003). Professional values held by baccalaureate and associate degree nursing students. Journal of Nursing Scholarship.(35) 3: 291-296 .

Matlin SA. (2006). Combating Disease And Promoting Health: Challenges For Health Research. Eastern Mediterranean Health Journal. 12 (Supplement 2), S7

Manthey M, Wolf ZR, et al. (2000). Nursing Values: A look back:A view forward. Creative Nursing, (6)1: 5-6

McNeese-Smith DK, Crook M. (2003). Nursing values and a changing nurse workforce. Values, age, and job stages. Journal of Nursing Adminstration. 33 (5): 260-270

Miller K. (1995). Keeping the care in nursing care. The journal of nursing Admiration. 25 (11): 29-52

O'Connor T, Kelly B.(2005). Bridging the Gap: a study of general nurses' perceptions of patient advocacy in Ireland. Nursing Ethics, 12 (5): 453 - 467.

Potter PA, Perry AG. Fundamentals of Nursing. Concepts, Process, and Practice. (4th ed.). St Louis: Mosby. 1997: 310

Rehnsfeldt A, Eriksson K. (2004). The progression of suffering implies alleviated suffering. Scandinavian Journal of Caring Sciences. 18:264-272

Rehnsfeldt AM, (2006). The Presence of Love in Ethical Caring. Nursing Forum. 41 (1): 1744-6198.

Rodgers BL, Cowles KV. (1977). A conceptual foundation for human suffering in nursing care and research. Journal of Advanced Nursing. 25 (5): 1048

Schank MJ. Weis Darlene, Ancona, J. (1996). Reflecting Professional Values in the

Philosophy of Nursing. Journal of Nursing Adminstration 26 (7/8); 55-60

Schank MC, Weis D. (2001). Service and education share responsibility for nurses' value development. Journal for nurses in staff development.17 (5): 226-231

Schroeter K. (2000) Advocacy in perioperative nursing practice. AORN Journal. 71: 1207-1222.

Shinyashiki GT, Mendes IA, Trevizan MA, Day RA. (2006). Professional socialization: students becoming nurses. Rev Lat Am Enfermagem.14 (4): 601-607.

Steele SM, Harmon, VM. Value Clarification in Nursing. (2nd ed.). Connecticut: Appleton-Century-Crofts.). 1983

Steeves RH. (1992). Patients who have undergone bone marrow transplantation: Their quest for meaning. Oncology Nursing Forum. 19: 899-905.

Steeves RH, Kahn DL. (1987). Experience of meaning in suffering. Image, 19: 114-116.

Skott C, Eriksson A (2005). Clinical caring – the diary of a nurse Journal of Clinical Nursing. 14: 916–921

Swanson K M. (1991). Empirical Development of a Middle Range Theory of Caring. Nursing Research, (40)3: 161-166.

Taylor EJ. (1993). Factors associated with meaning in life among people with recurrent cancer. Oncology Nursing Forum, 20: 1399-1407.

Taylor C, Lillis C, LeMone P. Fundamentals of Nursing. .JB. Lippincott Co., Philadelphia, 1989; 58-77.

Taylor C, Lillis C, LeMone P. Fundamentals of Nursing. The Art and Science of Nursing Care. (2nd ed.). Philadelphia: J.B. Lippincott. 1993.

Thompson D. The concise Oxford dictionary, 9th ed., Clarendon Press, 1995.

The American Heritage® Stedman's Medical Dictionary Copyright © 2002, 2001, 1995 by Houghton Mifflin Company. Published by Houghton Mifflin Company.

Tschudin V. Ethics in Nursing. The Caring Relationship._ (2nd ed.). Oxford: Butterworth Heinemann. 1992.

Tschudin V.(2003). The future.. Rew Latino-am Enformagem. 11 (4): 413-9

Tschudin V. (2006). Nursing Ethics. Report. Cultural and historical perspectives on nursing and ethics: listening to each other – report of the conference in Taipei, Taiwan, 19 May 2005, organized by İCNE and Nursing Ethics. 13 (3):

Tschudin V.(2006). How nursing ethics as a subject changes: an analysis of the first 11 years of publication of the journal nursing ethics. Nursing Ethics. 13 (1): 65-85.

Pender NJ, Murdaugh CL, Parsons MA. Health Promotion in Nursing Practice . Upper Saddle River, NJ. Prentice Hall. 2002

Rognstad MK, Nortvedt P, Aasland O. (2004). Helping motives in late modern society: Values and attitudes among nursing students.Nursing ethics. 11(3): 227-239.

Taylor E.J. (1993). Factors associated with meaning in life among people with recurrent cancer. Oncology Nursing Forum, 20: 1399-1407.

Importanceofphilosophy.com.   (http://www.importanceofphilosophy.com/Epistemology_ Values.html (Accessed: November 09, 2006).

International Council of Nurses. visionstatement. (http://www.icn.ch/visionstatement.htm.) (Accessed: November 09, 2006).

International Council of Nurses. Code of ethics for nurses. Geneva: ICN, 2006)(Available from: URL: http://www.icn.ch/ethics.htm [Accessed 1-December- 2006]

International Council for Nurses. Code of ethics for nurses. (http://www.icn.ch/ icncode.pdf#search=%22nursing%20values%22%22).

International Council for Nurses. Nursing definition. (http://www.icn.ch/definition.htm [Accessed 24-November- 2006]

International Council for Nurses. Ethics. (http://www.icn.ch/ethics.htm.) [Accessed 1-December- 2006]

International Council for Nurses. About İCN. http://www.icn.ch/abouticn.htm [Accessed 1-December- 2006]

International Council for Nurses. Visionstatement.(http://www.icn.ch/visionstatement.htm. (Accessed: November 09, 2006).

Verpeet E, Dierckx de Carterle' B, et al. (2006). Belgian nurses' views on codes of ethics: development, dissemination, implementation. Nursing Ethics. 13 (5): 531-45

WHO. About WHO/Policy/ottawa. Proclaimed at the First International Conference on Health Promotion Ottawa, Canada, November 17–21, 1986. Below, some portions of the Charter have been excerpted and others summarized. The full text of the Charter is available via the Internet: http://www.who.dk/policy/ottawa.htm.

WHO. Declaration almaata. http://www.who.int/hpr/NPH/docs/declaration_almaata.pdf. [Accessed 1-December- 2006]

WHO. About WHO/Policy. (http://www.euro.who.int/AboutWHO/Policy/20010827_2.. [Accessed 1-December- 2006].

http://www.euro.who.int/AboutWHO/Policy/20010827_2

Websters-online-dictionary org (http://www.websters-online-dictionary.org/definition/ALTR UISM. (Accessed: November 09, 2006).

Websters-online-dictionary.org (http://www.websters-online-dictionary.org/definition/Respon sibility). (Accessed: November 09, 2006).

Websters-online-dictionary.org (http://www.websters-online-dictionary.org/definition/Accou nt ability). (Accessed: November 09, 2006).

Weis D, Schank MC. (1997) Toward building an international consensus in professional values . Nurse ducation today 17: 366-369

Wikipedia org (http://en.wikipedia.org/wiki/Justice. (Accessed: November 09, 2006).

Yancey VJ. Values and ethics. Ed. Potter PA, Perry AG. Basic Nursing: Theory and Practice 4th ed., Mosby-Year Book.İnc. St. Louis. 1995; 74-95.83

Zulfikar F, Ulusoy MF (2001) Are patients aware of their rights? A Turkish study. Nursing Ethics. 8(6): 487-98

In: Nursing Education Challenges in the 21st Century
Editor: Leana E. Callara, pp. 271-282

ISBN 1-60021-661-7
© 2008 Nova Science Publishers, Inc.

Chapter 10

BRIDGING AN OLD DIVIDE: FORGING PARTNERSHIPS BETWEEN CLINICAL AND ACADEMIC SECTORS IN MENTAL HEALTH

Michelle Cleary[1] and Garry Walter[2]

[1]Mental Health, Faculty of Nursing and Midwifery, University of Sydney, and Research Unit, Sydney South West Area Mental Health Service
[2]Child and Adolescent Psychiatry, University of Sydney, and Child and Adolescent Mental Health Services, Northern Sydney Central Coast Health.

ABSTRACT

Background: Traditionally, health services and academia have viewed themselves as discrete sectors, with different agendas and priorities. Health services have focused on patient care, while academia has concerned itself with the advancement of knowledge through research and teaching. Although health services often incorporate research and teaching into their activities, it is generally not their primary focus.

Objectives: Using the example of a modern mental health service, this chapter sets out some opportunities for collaboration between health services and academia. These include a multidisciplinary approach, mentoring and peer support, practical steps to start bridge building, opportunities for publication, grant applications, and student supervision. The authors also briefly highlight some possible risks associated with attempting to bring the clinical and academic sectors closer together, and ways these might be addressed.

Discussion: A range of activities can help to bridge the divide between the academic and clinical sectors. These activities include: forums that promote constructive feedback and scholarly dialogue, negotiating relationships with universities to provide role orientation, positive teaching experiences and gaining insight into the realities of

---

[1] Correspondence to: Address: Research Unit, Sydney South West Area Mental Health Service, PO Box 1, Rozelle, New South Wales, 2039, Australia Tel: (02) 9556 9100; Fax: (02) 9818 5712 Email: michelle.cleary@email.cs.nsw.gov.au
[2] Correspondence to:Mailing Address: Coral Tree Family Service, PO Box 142, North Ryde, NSW, 1670, Australia Phone: +61 2 9887 5830; Fax: +61 2 9887 2941Email: gwalter@mail.usyd.edu.au

academia and the clinical setting. All these activities can be readily provided by a range of disciplines based on realistic and fair workloads. Building research capacity is not only beneficial for clinical staff, but enhances opportunity for clinically relevant academic research programs. This approach is not without risks, such as confusion among staff about roles and the time required to negotiate bureaucratic requirements; but, on balance, the advantages to staff and patients outweigh these potential disadvantages.

Conclusion: With careful planning, risks associated with forging partnerships between the clinical and academic sectors can be overcome to promote clinical and research excellence, and contribute to innovative career pathways.

Key words: Academia, Education, Evidence-Based Practice, Mental Health, Research

Key Points

- In mental health settings in recent years, there has been an increasing commitment to multidisciplinary approaches to patient care. The same approach could be used to strengthen links between academic and clinical sectors. The potential advantages of this are considerable, as it includes the sharing of philosophies, paradigms, knowledge and experiences.
- Workforce difficulties and challenges are not exclusive to the health service sector. Enhancing partnerships with academic settings may improve workplace satisfaction in both settings.
- Building a relevant research platform can be challenging for academic staff who do not have clinical links and who wish to provide post-graduate research opportunities.

INTRODUCTION

"We build too many walls and not enough bridges" – Isaac Newton

Traditionally, health services and academia are conceptualized and have viewed themselves as somewhat discrete sectors, with different agendas, priorities and processes. In essence, health services have focused on patient care, while academia has concerned itself with the advancement of knowledge, largely through research and teaching. Although health services often carry out research and teaching, they are not generally seen as "core business"; and the realities and pressures of clinical work often mitigate against their incorporation into the mainstream.

Perhaps this is becoming more difficult, when patients in mental health care settings are often more acutely unwell and in hospital for shorter periods. The resultant rapid patient turnover increases clinical and administrative demands on staff. Further, this situation may not improve in the foreseeable future as the life-span increases, chronic illnesses become more complex, and technologies proliferate (Walrath & Belcher, 2006). How, then, can "academic time" be incorporated into a full clinical schedule?

Contemporary healthcare environments require staff to demonstrate a high degree of professionalism in complex and challenging circumstances. Concern regarding access to clinical placements, limited opportunities to develop expertise, inadequate career pathways, and a dearth of positive role models are some of the factors that influence staff recruitment and retention (Cleary & Freeman, in press; Cleary & Happell, 2005a; Cleary & Happell, 2005b; Ferguson & Hope, 1999). These challenges can create dissatisfaction, especially if there is a perception that the work is not supported or appreciated (Cleary & Freeman, in press). In addition, changes in the way care is delivered (e.g. with growing attention to consumer and carer expectations, accreditation, evidence-based practice, clinical governance, etc) have contributed to new demands placed upon staff, including service evaluation, quality improvement projects, teaching and publishing (Cleary & Freeman, 2005).

One way forward is to forge stronger links between the clinical and academic sectors and narrow the divide between them. This may prove challenging if not carefully planned and performed with diligence. In this chapter, we seek to highlight, mainly from the perspective of the health sector, some of the opportunities for collaboration between health services and academia. In turn, we address the rationales for forming stronger partnerships, workforce issues, the importance of a multidisciplinary approach, mentoring and support, practical steps to get started, opportunities for publication, grant applications, bestowing of appropriate academic titles, and student supervision. We also briefly highlight some of the potential risks associated with attempting to bring the clinical and academic sectors closer together.

Rationales for Partnerships

At both organisational and staff levels, bridging the divide offers many advantages. For organisations, effective partnerships can enhance their profile and provide recognition of activities at local, national and international levels. This may lead to performance improvement through growth in research output, publications, development of innovative services, and the creation of new opportunities. Carey and colleagues (2005) argue that such collaboration can improve communication between researchers and policymakers. Potential benefits not only include mutual support of students and clinicians in their respective workplaces; but also opportunities to further develop education, research, practice and collaboration to support the growth of health professions. Partnerships can provide a means for senior clinicians to contribute to curricula through guest lectures and teaching, with students being exposed to clinical realities and "clinical wisdom" before they undertake clinical placements (Carey et al., 2005). For academic staff, particularly those currently with limited access to clinical services, new fields of research are presented by clinical settings, along with new research partners and potential students to encourage in terms of postgraduate research and academic careers.

Having stated the case for forging stronger ties, it is important that "lip service" is not paid to the notion of partnership. Indeed, clinical and academic staff need to be equal partners with both being flexible and adapting to the respective realities to demonstrate a commitment to teamwork, reciprocity and mutual benefit (Engelke & Marshburn, 2006). It is important to identify barriers which may hinder partnership processes. These can include time restraints, reluctance to purse further education and research, unfamiliarity, negative stereotypes, and complacency. Sharing information and lessons learned are essential to overcome these restraints and make bridges across organizational ghettoes (Johnson 2006).

The Workforce: Issues at the Coalface

In both hospital and community sectors there is currently an ageing workforce, staff shortages and recruitment and retention problems (Walrath & Belcher, 2006; Kenner & Pressler, 2006). To fill the gaps, there is an increased need for casual and temporary staff and this presents a myriad of challenges, especially for continuity of care (Anthony et al., 2005). Staff are increasingly forced to be task and shift driven, as well as having to manage problems that arise from systemic failures (Wiggins, 2006). All of these issues put pressure on an already fragmented healthcare system and contribute to a "silo" effect, that is, one typified by isolated services (Wiggins, 2006).

Making the work place more desirable is a priority and opportunities for staff to develop skills and expertise may assist to reduce attrition rates (Cleary & Walter, 2006). A smooth transition for new personnel, along with incentives to stay, is important for retention. Further, it is important to provide opportunities for succession planning so that staff can access information and develop skills for new roles (Woods & Craig, 2005). Continuous workplace learning can contribute to contemporary practice improvement. Incentives and rewards, for example, flexible working hours, clinical pathways for career development, financial support for conference attendance when presenting papers, can be given to staff who participate in and perform additional educational activities (Cleary & Walter, 2006).

Graduate or transition to practice programs have been promoted as a potential strategy in improving both recruitment to, and retention within, the nursing profession (Heslop et al., 2001; Owens et al., 2001). Successful completion of such programs can provide credit points towards academic courses at an affiliated university. From an academic perspective, supervising postgraduate students in higher research degrees is highly valued and is viewed favorably by prospective employers – in particular, but not exclusively, the academic sector.

Improved partnerships with universities may provide greater opportunities for nurses to engage in a range of scholarly activities to ensure education reflects the realities of requisite skills and roles. While there has been a growing emphasis on the importance of academic research in healthcare settings, partly associated with heightened awareness of "evidence-based practice", the integration of research findings into everyday work presents enormous challenges (Daly & Ferma, 2005). After all, it is difficult for many staff to meet their current demands without having additional responsibilities and pressures. Nevertheless, there are growing expectations for health staff to be involved in a range of scholarly activities and to utilize such knowledge and skills in the clinical setting. Higher research degrees are, increasingly, a prerequisite for many positions.

Workforce difficulties and challenges are not exclusive to the health service sector. An exodus from academic settings and an ageing workforce is challenging nursing education in academia (Kenner & Pressler, 2006; Walrath & Belcher, 2006). Restructuring and cutbacks in academic settings have led to increased workloads as fewer faculty try to meet the teaching load, resulting in, for example, less time to pursue other scholarly activities, such as research. This, in turn, leads to recruitment and retention problems (Walrath & Belcher, 2006).

It is against a backdrop of these complex workforce issues affecting both health services and academia that stronger partnerships between the two sectors need to be formed. The task is clearly not easy. Transitions that require professionals to step outside their "comfort zone" can bring opportunities as well as anxieties and challenges (Kenner & Pressler, 2006).

Commitment to an Interdisciplinary Approach

In mental health settings in recent years there has been an increasing commitment to multidisciplinary (or interdisciplinary) approaches to patient care. The same approach could be used to bring together the academic and clinical sectors. That is, teaching and research will have a higher chance of being incorporated into health services if the academics having input are seen to come from a variety of professional backgrounds (medical, nursing, psychology, etc) that broadly match the professional backgrounds of health service staff. In addition, it has been suggested that the identification and nurturing of individuals who are able to move back and forth between sets of institutions is an important component of effective interdisciplinary collaboration (Conte, Chang, Malcolm & Russo, 2006). There is also a need to develop integrated programs in both settings to promote and carry out multidisciplinary research. The potential advantages of this are considerable, as it includes the sharing of philosophies, paradigms, knowledge and experiences.

To this end, it is important to develop multidisciplinary resources that are accessible to staff in both settings. Examples of resources that can facilitate and support evidence based activities include information on: a) conducting surveys (Walter, Cleary & Rey, 1999), b) differentiating between quality improvement and research (Cleary & Horsfall, 2002), c) ethics and quality improvement projects (Horsfall & Cleary, 2002), d) presentation guidelines (Cleary, Hunt, Walter & Horsfall, 2003), e) apportioning time to presentations and publications (Cleary & Walter, 2004), f) publishing ethics (Walter & Bloch, 2001), and, g) a research guide (Cleary & Freeman, 2005). These aim to enhance multidisciplinary collaborations across a range of mental health settings (Cleary, Freeman, Walter & Hunt, 2005).

Mentoring and Support

For effective partnerships to be successful, mentoring is essential and must have the support of both clinical and academic sectors. Both need to make significant effort to carefully choose and develop skilled facilitators so that expertise, support and feedback can be provided. Mentors should be familiar with academic and clinical settings and be willing to spend time supporting skills development and transition into new roles. A good mentoring relationship can cultivate the feeling of being valued while protecting the protégé from excessive pressures and some competing demands and unwitting mistakes (Peters & Boylston, 2006). Experienced and appropriately qualified staff are well positioned to provide mentorship to facilitate skill development among those wishing to undertake scholarly activities.

Mentoring has been shown to be important to retaining staff as it can enhance work environments and nurture teamwork (Anthony et al., 2005; Cleary, Freeman & Sharrock, 2005; McKinley, 2004). It is very important that a culture be developed that fosters continuing supportive interaction between team members (Hoff, Pohl & Bartfield, 2004). A lack of preparatory and ongoing team building can undermine collaboration (Olsen & Neale, 2005) and result in unclear direction and poor cohesion (Shanley, 2004). Peer evaluation can also promote professional development as it provides opportunities for staff to give and receive professional support and feedback. Both peers and mentors must recognise equality and individuality whilst providing assistance, guidance and recognition (Vuorinen, Tarkka & Meretoja, 2000).

Opportunities for Collaboration

Simple enthusiasm and willingness to form a strong partnership between the health and academic sectors is insufficient for bridge building. The enthusiasm needs to be matched by an array of sustainable initiatives. There are some straightforward, practical steps that can be taken to introduce academic life and interest into mental health services. Journal clubs, research-focused grand rounds, research workshops, research bulletin boards and seminars and conferences as well as informal gatherings and forums that promote constructive consultation, feedback and scholarly dialogue are examples of some initiatives to get started (Bauer-Wu, Epshtein & Ponte, 2006; Conte et al., 2006; Fink, Thompson & Bonnes, 2005). Academics should be invited to participate in these activities, as presenters or discussants. Universities can invite health service staff to forums to discuss their academic work, gain feedback, identify potential collaborators, and establish cross-sectorial links.

Getting over the Publishing Hurdle

There is a misconception among health service staff that to publish it is necessary to be at the cutting edge of research and the recipient of large research grants. There are many written works - case reports, description of innovative services, opinion pieces, and letters to the Editor, among others - that do not depend on the author being an active researcher or the recipient of a grant (Cleary, Walter & Hunt, 2006). Some gaps between the academic and health service sectors can begin to be bridged by finding opportunities for work together on such papers.

In modern health care settings, there is an increasing expectation for employees to showcase a range of activities (for example, clinical innovations, service and quality initiatives) at forums and conferences. Although clinical nurses may be reluctant to publish because of workloads and inexperience, writing can bring considerable enjoyment and a sense of achievement by contributing to knowledge and advancing healthcare (Burnard 2001; O'Neill & Duffey 2000). Academic colleagues can be helpful for identifying the best place to submit one's work and, where appropriate, negotiating assistance with writing or review of drafts (Cleary & Walter, 2004). Publishing groups with clearly delineated timelines and responsibilities can be helpful to new and inexperienced authors to promote scholarly development and collaborative publishing (Johnson 2003; Oermann 2003; Roberts & Turnbull 2002-2003). A published paper co-written by health and academic staff will demystify scholarly writing and hopefully encourage more clinicians to become involved in similar activities.

In terms of publishing, "runs on the board" for academics include the number of articles published, an increasing rate of publication over time, publications in high impact factor journals, and publications linked to research grants. Closer ties with the health sector may help academics to improve some of these performance indicators. There are a range of untapped areas in the mental health field, such as new services and treatments being developed.

Collaborative writing is an effective way to build bridges between the two sectors, although such activities are not without risks. Projects should be constructed with integrity, with all members of the team knowing what is expected of them in relation to their roles and responsibilities, including criteria for authorship. All parties should agree on their roles and responsibilities at the outset.

Securing Grants

Just as academic writing is not predicated on securing research grants, so too successfully competing for grants does not always hinge on being a part of an established research team. Admittedly, funding for research is highly competitive, and without an established track record grants can be difficult to obtain (Cleary, Walter & Hunt, 2006). However, small grants may be provided by industry, universities, and health services. These and others are worth exploring for potential funding opportunities. Collaborative teams can enhance this process by contributing skills and expertise. Over time, the collective track record grows and one can become more ambitious and seek larger grants. A first successful grant application can breathe academic interest into a service and encourage others to seek further grants.

Not all Academic Institutions are the same

To a novice, academic institutions may appear similar, but the reality is that each has its own culture, which must be understood to some extent for collaborations to succeed. This process is likely to take a year or more (Carey et al, 2005). Administrative and organisational structures, conditions of tenure, performance indicators and promotional pathways may vary between settings and institutions. The criteria for collaborative success may differ between institutions; for instance, one institution may prefer publications, whilst another focuses on grant size. It is helpful to clarify at the outset what each is seeking from the other to increase the chances of success (Carey et al, 2005). Finally, cultivating relationships with key staff and respected leaders will increase support for the various collaborations.

At an organisational level, initiatives such as the development of Education and Research Committees can enhance collaborations by having a range of representatives from different disciplines and settings functioning in a steering or advisory capacity. A further benefit of such committees is their potential role in ensuring realistic and sustainable initiatives, and their ongoing ability to review progress.

Student Supervision

Quality placements to support student learning are essential; student dissatisfaction not only affects learning, but impacts on future recruitment opportunities (Cleary & Happell 2005a). Effective partnerships can facilitate access to continuing student placements of high quality, and perhaps, in turn, recruitment to the health service.

It is also important that a positive clinical learning experience be created to facilitate the integration of theoretical knowledge and clinical practice. Identifying learning opportunities and creating an environment that supports quality learning requires the establishment of links between clinical settings and the education sector. Further, staff in health and academic settings are often experts in their area and can assist in developing relevant and useful programmes, for example, commenting on academic curricula, treatment algorithms and clinical pathways.

Career Opportunities and Incentives

Providing new career opportunities, paths and incentives are further means for forging links between health services and the academic sector. One solution to faculty shortages offered by many academic institutions is increasing the use of adjunct faculty staff for teaching. To successfully pursue teaching responsibilities (for example, lesson plans, curricula, grading), adjunct staff need to become familiar with the university's mission, goals and policies (Peters & Boylston, 2006).

In recognition of their clinical contribution, a number of honorary titles can be bestowed on staff in these settings. The wording, and meaning, of such titles varies across, and sometimes within, countries. These clinical appointments not only provide acknowledgement of health sector staff expertise and contribution, but also are a way to build partnerships and facilitate collaboration, in part through use of a "common language". In general, clinical academic appointments are made using the same criteria as pure university appointments, but do not establish an employment relationship, that is, the appointee still reports to their health care employer.

Another option for building collaborative partnerships between clinical and academic settings is through Conjoint Appointments. These are a more formal arrangement and involve the incumbent being shared between a clinical and an academic setting. In identifying the appointment as conjoint, there is recognition and development of the partnership between the clinical setting and the university with appropriate remuneration. However, conjoint appointments are not without their problems. First, having two "masters" and reporting lines can be challenging, especially if their expectations clash. Second, the lengths of appointments vary and it can be difficult to achieve performance indicators within shorter time frames.

What are the benefits of an honorary title in the clinical setting? The title may increase access to research funding, faculty training and education. Collaboration between the university and the clinical setting via conjoint positions can, in turn, generate scholarly activities, research opportunities and knowledge development (Peters & Boylston, 2006).

For those wishing to pursue an academic career, the following are often highly regarded by decision-makers in these settings;

- An acknowledged national reputation.
- A developing international reputation.
- A record of academic achievements and collaborative research.
- Postgraduate student supervision eg; honours, masters and PhD.
- Keynote addresses and conference presentations.

- Successful grant applications.
- Research and scholarly publications in peer reviewed journals and books.
- Invitations to review manuscripts, research grants and book chapters.
- Membership of Editorial Committees and Boards.
- Evidence of professional and clinical leadership.
- A profile in the wider community.
- Risks associated with bridging the divide

In this chapter, we argue for bridging the clinical and academic divide. Although such a move is not without risks, on balance, the advantages outweigh the disadvantages. Nevertheless, the risks include weakening the identity of each sector, confusion among staff about roles, slowing of progress and initiatives due to potential increased bureaucratic hoops to negotiate joint ventures, and lack of clarity for patients and staff about their participation in research and teaching.

Collaborations between universities and healthcare providers can be difficult because both are large, complex organizations characterised by cumbersome and sometimes unclear processes. To avoid too many pitfalls, it is important to determine which organisational areas can readily share information and expertise, and benefit most from collaboration. We suggest the following to minimise risks:

- Clarify and set out roles and responsibilities.
- Begin with small initiatives and projects and build on these.
- Discuss data sharing and ownership arrangements.
- Determine authorship protocols.
- Establish if the collaboration will be named and carry an identifying logo
- Recognize and acknowledge contributions, for example, bestow academic titles and offer incentives such as funding conference travel or registration.
- Provide opportunities for continuous workplace learning, eg; guest lectures, postgraduate study.
- Establish resources to support scholarly and multidisciplinary collaborations.
- Set up mentoring frameworks to support staff and facilitate skill development, eg publishing and securing research grants.
- Determine and agree upon achievable performance indicators.

CONCLUSION

Effective partnerships between health services and academia are essential to meet the increasing expectations and higher standards required for clinical and academic excellence (Engelke & Marshburn, 2006). Certainly, a win-win situation may result from the pooling of resources to undertake an array of scholarly activities and enhanced collaborations, with both settings benefiting from the sharing of expertise to foster research, teaching and evidence-based care (Bauer-Wu, Epshtein & Ponte, 2006). From the discussion in this chapter, that there are several strategies to better forge partnerships between the clinical and academic sectors in mental health:

- Ensure realistic and fair workloads are grounded in respect and reciprocity.
- Consult stakeholders to promote awareness of and participation in partnership development.
- Recognize that it takes time to develop partnerships with different disciplines across diverse settings.
- Provide opportunities for learning that are non-hierarchical and allow constructive collaboration through peer support, coaching and mentoring.
- Build in facilities and forums to enhance interdisciplinary collaboration in both the health and university sectors.
- Start small to increase chances of success.
- Reward progress and achievements.

ACKNOWLEDGMENTS

We wish to acknowledge Dr Jan Horsfall for her helpful comments on the final draft.

REFERENCES

Anthony, M.K., Standing, T.S., Glick, J., Duffy, M., Paschall, F., Sauer, M.R., Sweeney, D.K., Modic, M.B. & Dumpe, M.L. (2005). Leadership and Nurse Retention: The Pivotal Role of Nurse Managers. *Journal of Nursing Administration, 35*(3), 146-155.

Bauer-Wu, S., Epshtein, A. & Ponte, P. R. (2006). Promoting Excellence in Nursing Research and Scholarship in the Clinical Setting. *The Journal of Nursing Administration, 36*(5), 224-227.

Burnard, P. (2001). Writing Skills – Why nurses do not publish. *Journal of Community Nursing Online,* 15(4), Available from: URL: http://www.jcn.co.uk/journal.asp?MonthNum=04&YearNum=2001&Type=search&ArticleID=337. Last accessed: 29.8.2006.

Carey, T.S., Howard, D.L., Goldmon, M., Roberson, J.T., Godley, P.A. & Ammerman, A. (2005). Developing Effective Interuniversity Partnerships and Community-Based Research to Address Health Disparities. *Academic Medicine, 80*(11), 1039-1045.

Cleary, M. & Freeman, A. (2005). Facilitating research within clinical settings: The development of a beginner's guide. *International Journal of Mental Health Nursing, 14,* 202-208.

Cleary, M. & Freeman, A. (In press). Fostering a culture of support in mental health settings: alternatives to traditional models of clinical supervision. *Issues in Mental Health Nursing.*

Cleary, M., Freeman, A. & Sharrock, L. (2005). The development, implementation, and evaluation of a clinical leadership program for mental health nurses. *Issues in Mental Health Nursing, 26*(8), 827-842.

Cleary, M., Freeman, A., Walter, G. & Hunt, G. (2005). Making evidence based practice a reality in modern mental health services. *Contemporary Nurse, 20*(2), 278-289.

Cleary, M. & Happell, B. (2005a). Promoting a sustainable mental health nursing workforce: An evaluation of a transition mental health nursing programme. *International Journal of Mental Health Nursing, 14,* 109-116.

Cleary, M. & Happell, B. (2005b). Recruitment and retention initiatives: Nursing students' satisfaction with clinical experience in the mental health field. *Nurse Education in Practice, 5*(2), 109-116.

Cleary, M. & Horsfall, J. (2002). Quality improvement projects: finding a pathway through policies. *International Journal of Mental Health Nursing, 11,* 121-127.

Cleary, M. & Walter, G. (2004). Apportioning our time and energy: oral presentation, poster, journal article or other? *International Journal of Mental Health, Nursing, 13,* 204-207.

Cleary, M., Hunt, G., Walter, G. & Horsfall, J. (2003). Guidelines for presentations and publications. *International Journal of Mental Health Nursing, 12,* 158-159.

Cleary, M., Walter, G. & Hunt, G. (2006). The quest to fund research: playing research lotto! *Australasian Psychiatry, 14*(3): 323-326.

Cleary, M. & Walter, G. (2006). Educating mental health nurses in clinical settings: Tackling the challenge. *Contemporary Nurse, 21*(1), 153-157.

Conte, C., Chang, C.S., Malcolm, J. & Russo, P.G. (2006). Academic Health Departments: From Theory to Practice. *Journal Public Health Management Practice, 12*(1), 6-14.

Daly, S. & Ferma, M. (2005). The Unique Role of Nurses in Bridging Evidence-Practice Gaps. *Australian Journal of Advanced Nursing, 23*(2), 6-7.

Engelke, M.K. & Marshburn, D.M. (2006). Collaborative Strategies to Enhance Research and Evidence-based Practice. *The Journal of Nursing Administration, 36*(3), 131-135.

Ferguson, K. & Hope, K. (1999). From novice to competent practitioner: tracking the progress of undergraduate mental health nursing students. *Journal of Advanced Nursing, 29*(3), 630-638.

Fink, R., Thompson, C. J. & Bonnes, D. (2005). Overcoming Barriers and Promoting the Use of Research in Practice. *The Journal of Nursing Administration,* 35(3), 121-129.

Heslop, L., McIntyre, M. & Ives, G. (2001). Undergraduate student nurses' expectations and their self-reported preparedness for the graduate role. *Journal of Advanced Nursing, 36*(5), 626-634.

Hoff, T.J., Pohl, H., & Bartfield, J. (2004). Creating a Learning Environment to Produce Competent Residents: The Roles of Culture and Context. *Academic Medicine, 79*(6), 532-540.

Horsfall, J. & Cleary, M. (2002). Mental health quality improvement: what about ethics? *International Journal of Mental Health Nursing, 11,* 40-46.

Johnson, J. E. (2006). Nursing Research: Thoughts on Professional Obligation, Discipline and Knowledge Management. *The Journal of Nursing Administration, 36*(5), 221-223.
Johnson, S.H. (2003). The Outcome-oriented Publishing Work Group. *Nurse Educator, 28*(6), 284-286.

Kenner, C. & Pressler, J.L. (2006). Rx for Deans: Form Follows Function or Does IT? *Nurse Educator, 31*(2), 47-48.

McKinley, M.G. (2004). Mentoring Matters: Creating, Connecting, Empowering. *AACN Clinical Issues: Advanced Practice in Acute & Critical Care, 15*(2), 205-214.

Oermann, M. H. (2003). Sharing Your Work: Building Knowledge About Nursing Care Quality. *Journal of Nursing Care Quality, 18*(4), 243-244.

Olsen, S. & Neale, G. (2005). Clinical leadership in the provision of hospital care. *British Medical Journal,* 330(7502), 1219-1220.

O'Neill, A.L. & Duffey, M.A. (2000). Communication of Research and Practice Knowledge in Nursing Literature. *Nursing Research, 49*(4), 224-230.

Owens, D., Turjanica, M., Scanion, M., Sandhausen, A., Williamson, M., Herbert, C. & Facteau, L. (2001). New Graduate RN Internship Program: A Collaborative approach for system-wide integration. *Journal for Nurses in Staff Development, 17*(3), 144-150.

Peters, M.A. & Boylston, M. (2006). Mentoring Adjunct Faculty: Innovative Solutions. *Nurse Educator, 31*(2), 61-64.

Roberts, K.L. & Turnbull, B.J. (2002-2003). Scholarly productivity: Are nurse academics catching up? *Australian Journal of Advanced Nursing, 20*(2), 8-14.

Shanley, C. (2004). Extending the Role of Nurses in Staff Development by Combining an Organizational Change Perspective with an Individual Learner Perspective. *Journal for Nurses in Staff Development – JNSD,* 20(2), 83-89.

Vuorinen, R., Tarkka, M. & Meretoja, R. (2000). Peer evaluation in nurses' professional development: a pilot study to investigate the issues. *Journal of Clinical Nursing, 9*(2), 273-281.

Walrath, J.M. & Belcher, A. (2006). Can we thrive, despite the faculty shortage? *Nursing Management, 37*(4), 81-84.

Walter, G., Cleary, M. & Rey, J.M. (1999). Want to know how to conduct a survey but too afraid to ask? - a step by step guide. *Australasian Psychiatry, 7,* 258-261.

Walter, G. & Bloch, S. (2001). Publishing ethics in psychiatry. *Australian and New Zealand Journal of Psychiatry, 35*(1), 28-35.

Wiggins, M.S. (2006). The Partnership Care Delivery Model. *The Journal of Nursing Administration, 36*(7/8), 341-345.

Woods, T., & Craig, J. (2005). Enhancing Collaboration with Academic Partners. *The Journal of Nursing Administration, 35*(12), 519-521.

In: Nursing Education Challenges in the 21st Century
Editor: Leana E. Callara, pp. 283-294

ISBN 1-60021-661-7
© 2008 Nova Science Publishers, Inc.

Chapter 11

THE NURSE AND THE MADELEINE: HOW AN EXAMINATION OF THE WORK OF MARCEL PROUST MAY SHED LIGHT ON THE PROCESS OF REFLECTION IN NURSING

Colin Griffiths[1]

The School of Nursing and Midwifery.Trinity College Dublin.

ABSTRACT

Reflective practice is generally accepted as a means of developing an individual's professional and scientific knowledge based upon how the individual observes and processes his experience, most especially his experience in his practice profession. In the nursing profession reflective practice has been incorporated into nursing curriculae and is regarded as being an integral element of the practice of nursing in the clinical setting both by students and by experienced nurses. In order to facilitate the acceptance of reflective practice it has been presented to nurses in the guise of various different frameworks. These frameworks attempt to formalize the reflective process so that it is accessible to those who are encountering it for the first time. 'In Search of Lost Time' is the magnum opus of the French writer Marcel Proust. In this book Proust tried to recapture time through the deployment of memory, in effect Proust's work constitutes a lengthy reflective essay. This paper seeks to show ways by which the process of reflection can be illuminated by examining in detail the reflective mechanisms that Proust utilised in writing his novel. The paper then explores how these mechanisms may be used by nurses who are experienced in the reflective process in order to further develop their practice.

[1] Correspondence To: The School Of Nursing And Midwifery.Trinity College Dublin.24. D'Olier Street.Dublin 2.

1. INTRODUCTION

The development of nursing practice over the past 50 years has led the discipline increasingly to a point where it is attaining a theoretical and scientific knowledge base (Retsas 1995). It would be premature to assume that nursing has developed a single conceptual structure that underpins it's knowledge base and from which hypotheses may be developed and tested which in turn would support or question the conceptual basis of nursing. It may however be assumed that the proliferation of nursing models that conceptualise how nurses carry out their work is an indicator that nursing has traveled part of the way to establishing an overarching paradigm that underpins it's knowledge base (Kuhn 1962) although it may be argued that nursing has not yet reached the hallowed ground where it may be termed a science. Nevertheless much research has been carried out in nursing and much thought has been given by nurses regarding what exactly the nature of nursing is. This is illustrated by the debate in nursing over the appropriateness of using quantative methodologies to explore a profession which focuses primarily on the human condition. Indeed it is not clear whether it is desirable that nursing should ever attain a status where it is regarded as a science because broad questions remain as to whether it is science or an art (Retsas 1995). Many nurses would deny that it is either but would assume that nursing includes the understanding of both scientific and artistic knowledge which is deployed by nurses in a personal way that can be described as an art. (Carper 1978) has examined how nurses know about nursing in her seminal paper that looked at the 'fundamental patterns of knowing in nursing'. Carper suggested that nursing knowledge has four constituent parts: scientific or empirical knowledge that is; systematically derived information that is 'controllable by factual evidence and which can be used in the organization and classification of knowledge' (Carper 1978:14). Secondly she suggests that nurses have access to an ethical understanding that is underpinned by philosophical conceptualizations of what is good and what is not good for patients and service users. This way of knowing she terms ethical knowledge. Her third element of nursing knowledge is the personal knowledge that each nurse develops in the course of a career in nursing. This type of knowledge explains who the nurse is and how he or she relates to the service user whom she cares for. Lastly Carper refers to aesthetic knowledge which she regards as the creative aspect of nursing she suggests that this way of knowing enables a synthesis of the other ways of knowing and a unique deployment of these understandings. Carper particularly emphasises that aesthetic ways of knowing bring the nurse's creativity and understanding to bear on the empirical knowledge that she possess and then allows him or her to deploy that knowledge to the benefit of the patient or service user.

This chapter will examine how nurses gain and develop these forms of knowledge in the practice environment through the process of reflecting on what they do and how they do it. Reflective practice will be examined in order to consider it's relevance to nursing and also to make some of it's major components clear. Secondly the chapter will examine Marcel Proust's novel 'In Search of Lost Time' and will offer the contention that this is a deep and thoughtful reflection on a person's life and what he has learned from it. Through looking at how Proust achieved his understanding of his life this chapter hopes to find lessons that may be of use to nurses in advancing their understanding of their professional and perhaps personal lives.

2. REFLECTIVE PRACTICE IN NURSING

2.1. History of Reflective Practice in Nursing

The history of reflective practice in nursing is a relatively short and for some nurses a contentious one. In many ways it is a history that is derived from the understandings of nursing knowledge that have been outlined in the introduction. Nightingale emphasized nurses combining theory and practice as means of developing nursing knowledge. She thought nurses should not only do but they should also think and that by observing what they are doing and thinking about it they could gain experience (Johnson and Ratner 1997). This assumption that nurses should examine the knowledge basis of what they do in their practice and should add to it through conscious examination of that practice is an important foundation for the practice of reflection. Both Carper and Benner made it clear that while empirical evidence is essential for the establishment and development of knowledge in nursing it is not the totality of that knowledge. Indeed Benner suggested that some elements of nursing knowledge are embedded in the person and are therefore difficult to articulate (Benner 1983). This intuitive or tacit knowledge is generally acquired by the experienced nurse and manifests as that information that underpins certain technical skills and also certain routines that become integrated as part of the nurse's way of being. This type of knowledge may be considered as being a double edged sword. Much of this type of knowledge is extremely powerful and relevant to the nurse's practice and of great therapeutic benefit to the service user and patient, some of it however may be learned without recourse to analyzing the evidence upon which it is based and may therefore be potentially harmful.

Reflection has been described as starting with an experience that provides the basis for the thought process. This sets in motion an exploration of the experience and subsequently this leads to a different understanding of oneself and a changed view of the situation (Boyd and Fayles 1983). Reflection implies that a critical analysis of the reflective incident is undertaken thus Fitzgerald defines reflection as 'the retrospective contemplation of practice undertaken in order to uncover the knowledge used in a particular situation, by analyzing and interpreting the information recalled' (Fitzgerald 1994: 64). So reflection may be regarded as a way of focusing in on any aspect of one's life, in this case one's professional life and looking at what happened, why it happened and what are the implications in terms of learning how to handle such a situation in the future?

The concept of reflective practice derives from the work of Donald Schon who examined the nature of professional practice and suggested that it is often concerned with situations that are not clear cut but are ill defined. He described these situations as the 'swampy lowlands' of practice (Schon 1991) he thought that frequently the solution to the problems that are thrown up in such situations is not at all clear. Schon looked at how professionals deal with such situations and suggested that they use two different types of reflection to find out what is going on, to decide what to do about it and to evaluate how things develop in the light of their actions. These two approaches he termed 'reflection in action and reflection on action'.

Schon described reflection in action as that thought that is applied to practice while one is actually carrying out the action in question. Such refection might occur when a nurse is engaged in a dialogue with a service user or patient and a disagreement becomes apparent, the nurse might see a potential conflict arising and change tack in the dialogue in order to head it off and attempt to conceptualise the disagreement in a different way so that a solution could be found. In other words reflection in action occurs during the action itself. Reflection on action is a somewhat more leisurely process, this happens when the nurse has experienced the event that provides the basis for the reflection and an approach similar to Boyd and Fayle's concept of reflection is embarked upon. Reflection on action is concerned with the conversion of raw experience in the practice area into understanding of what that experience means and consequent learning which is then incorporated into the nurse's body of knowledge. Reflection on action is thus a main source for the development of personal and aesthetic ways of knowing (Carper 1978) in nursing.

2.2. Models of Reflection

While reflection and reflective practice have largely been developed in the fields of business and education, several models of reflection have been developed in nursing. These models have been aimed at demystifying reflection and facilitating nurses to engage in reflective practice.

A popular model of reflection was developed by Chris Johns. Johns provided a series of questions for the reflective practitioner to ask (Johns 1994). He suggests that firstly the nurse should look back on the experience to find out what was going on, he or she should describe the experience then should ask 'what are the essential factors that contributed to the experience and who is involved in it? Secondly the nurse should ask what was he or she trying to achieve and how did this affect his / her feelings and those of the service user? Clarifying what factors influenced the actions that happened is an important part of this process. John's model proceeds to offer pointers to enable an analysis of the situation by asking what could the nurse have done better or done differently to resolve the situation. Lastly the nurse should ask what has he or she learned from the situation and how has that changed his or her practice?

John's model provides a road map for the novice reflective practitioner to start the process. He acknowledges that models of reflection are of necessity prescriptive and therefore may reduce the human experience to a list of answers to questions. Johns also notes that the questions he suggests may not fit every experience.

Similarly Gibbs' reflective cycle asks the nurse to describe the event and the feelings that were associated with the event. The next step is to evaluate the positives and negatives of the experience and then the nurse is asked to try to make sense of the experience in the context of considering other possible actions that he or she could have taken (Gibbs 1988). This learning Gibbs suggests then should be incorporated into the nurse's professional knowledge to broaden the nurse's understanding of what options are available should a similar situation arise in the future.

2.3. Current Understandings of Reflective Practice

Reflection in nursing can be categorized into three complementary types : technical reflection, practical reflection and emancipatory reflection (Taylor 2006). Technical reflection is used to examine scientific empirical knowledge that underpins the nurse's practice, by contrast practical reflection examines the relationship aspect of nursing. In view of the fundamental nature of relationship in nursing this can be counted as a most important part of the reflective canon. Thirdly emancipatory reflection as the name suggests is concerned with power relationships in nursing and how these may be transformed. In the context of a changing scenario where care plans and interventions for service users and patients are increasingly being negotiated with them and where power relationships between service provider and service user are being transformed this form of reflection is very relevant.

Taylor's model of reflection is framed around the nurse thinking through his or her practice systematically. Taylor emphasizes that the nurse should be in a quiet frame of mind for the process to be effective, systematic thought according to Taylor should be exercised in the context of the person being open to ideas, thinking freely but also by questioning the event under consideration in a methodical way. Out of this process insights develop which can be evaluated by the reflective practitioner. As with other approaches to reflection the insights that are derived from it can then be incorporated into the previous knowledge that the practitioner possess. Ultimately the nurse will have a changed and raised awareness that will bring about change in his or her professional or personal life.

Gary Rolfe takes a macro approach to reflection in that he is concerned with how nurses develop their personal theory of nursing or an aspect of nursing. He suggests that the nurse's personal knowledge, experiential knowledge of practice and scientific theoretical knowledge produces an 'epistemology of practice' that may form the professional judgement of the nurse. This is built up by reading theoretical journals, personal practice experience and reflecting on that experience and then on the literature and incorporating the changed understanding into the nurses' thinking. The key to this is reflecting on the experience and learning from what is gained by this process. Rolfe distinguishes reflection on practice from thinking about practice which is simply to recall information whereas reflection involves the analysis and evaluation of the information. (Rolfe 1998). The end result of this process is the development of a 'personal theory' to 'explain and predict' behaviour in the practice setting. This personal theory can then be examined and tested in the practice setting. Rolfe has collaborated with other nursing theorists to develop a very straightforward model of reflection which is put forward as a means for healthcare workers to build their personal practical knowledge and theory. This model which is termed a framework for reflexive practice (Rolfe, Freshwater et al. 2001) takes three phrases as it's basis:

What?
So what?
Now what?

The first step is the description of the event in question, what is the reason for it being noteworthy and what were the protagonists trying to achieve? This is followed by the second step which explores the implications of the event, what can be learned from it about the people involved, about nursing practice, what other information is relevant to the analysis? What could have been done differently? The final step which is termed 'action oriented reflection' asks how can the situation be resolved and what can be learned from this event?

2.4. Reflective Practice and Reflective Writing

Reflective Practice is becoming accepted by nursing theorists and more importantly by nurses in the profession as a whole as an established way in which personal practice can be developed and experience can be transformed into knowledge. The early theorists put forward fairly detailed recipes for successful reflection and each model tended to be accepted as being the way in which reflection should be undertaken by it's particular devotees.

However as the 1990's morphed into the first decade of the 21st century concepts of reflection appear to have opened out. It is becoming clear that there is no one right way to approach reflection each model has it's strengths and weaknesses however all examine the same territory; that is the relationship between the present and the past and what can be learned by analysing how things that happened in the past have influenced present events? The key elements therefore are time and the individual's mechanism for time travel which is memory. The second section of this chapter will examine understandings of these concepts. It is not the aim of the chapter to examine time and memory from scientific or psychological viewpoints rather the chapter will focus on how these are useful tools for writing. Most reflection is considered, thought about and then written down by the person who engages in it, so reflective writing constitutes both the data for the development of personal knowledge and theory and the mechanism for the analysis of it. The rest of the chapter attempts to make clear the place that reflective writing has in the literary canon and how it is informed by it's constituent parts which are time and memory and how such processes may inform the way in which nurses can engage in reflection.

3. THE NATURE OF MEMORY

"If owing to the work of oblivion, the returning memory can throw no bridge, form no connecting link between itself and the present minute, if it remains in the context of it's own place and date, it keeps it's distance, it's isolation in the hollow of a valley or upon the highest peak of a mountain summit, for this very reason it causes us suddenly to breathe a new air, an air which is new precisely because we have breathed it in the past, that purer air which the poets have vainly tried to situate in paradise and which could only induce so profound a sensation of renewal if it had been breathed before' (Proust 1992b: 221-2).

Memory according to Proust is a window on to the past, in it's purest state it enables the past to be reconstructed so that an intact picture of what was reappears; sights, sounds, smells all the accompaniments that once existed are recreated in the mind of the one who remembers. However memory is based on an interpretation of the past and it is complex because it is a composite of the relationship between the rememberer and time. That relationship is further complicated because memory contains inherent information regarding the parameters of a person's identity, history and knowledge which may become corrupted as time passes. Memory is as Toussaint states; a contested arena (Toussaint 2002).

Beckett examines Proust's description of an incident when the narrator while bending down to unbutton his boots is suddenly flooded with recollections of a similar incident when his beloved grandmother who had died a year earlier bent over him to calm him when he had been distressed as a boy. Beckett comments that the narrator is transformed, he notes that 'he has not merely extracted from this gesture the lost reality of his grandmother: he has recovered the lost reality of himself' (Beckett 1965: 41). Indeed he goes further suggesting that the narrator has switched tracks and is proceeding on a parallel track which proceeds from the memory which was buried in the past. For Beckett the acquisition and exploration of an involuntary memory has changed the rememberer.

Beckett took the view that memory is stored deep within the person and deep within the habits that each of us has formed. He contends that there are two types of memory: voluntary memory which is 'the uniform memory of intelligence; and it can be relied on to reproduce for our gratified inspection those impressions of the past that were consciously and intelligently formed' [:32]. By contrast involuntary memory is 'explosive, an immediate, total and delicious deflagration' [:33] it is the eureka moment. Involuntary memory not only restores what was forgotten, it is Lazarus in that it brings back dead things from the past. Beckett however takes the view that it is not easily to be controlled he notes that 'it chooses it's own time and place for the performance of it's miracle' [:34] a position that Toussaint aggress with as she notes that it both complex and elusive (Toussaint 2002).

To sum up it may be suggested that in his writings Proust explored the relationship between memory and the multiple layers of the self and in doing so he revealed an analytic tool that could be used to explore the culture and the life in which each person is located (Toussaint 2002). This is important for the reflective process quite simply because past experiences are important for reflection (Dewey 1933) and memory is the mechanism for the resurrection of past experiences.

4. MEMORY AND IT'S RELATIONSHIP TO TIME

Memory is dependant on the passage of time, a life lived in a constant present would prevent the formation of memories and render impossible the extraction of what had gone before.

So memory and the perception of time are related and interdependent indeed they are so intimately bound together that it is arguable that one cannot exist without the other. However in order to recognise the significance of a memory the past experience has to be identified in terms of the present.

'Merely to remember something is meaningless unless the remembered image is combined with a moment in the present affording a view of the same object or objects. Like our eyes, our memories must see double; those two images then converge in our minds into a single heightened reality' (Shattuck 1963: 47). Shatttuck goes on to suggest that the recognition of a past memory extracts it from time altogether with the effect that both the past memory and the present trigger that elicited the memory become equally accessible. Both past and present are then rendered equally accessible to conscious examination and exploration. The past is thus brought nearer by a process that Shattuck names a 'stereoscopic view of reflection' where they are both seen as different visions of a living present.

Another view of this process is that the relationship between the present self and the historical self come together at a point of equilibrium (Kristeva 1993). Kristeva contends that;

'In this case the learning process involves a return journey from the past to the present and back again. This new form of temporality, furthermore, gives an X-ray image of memory, bringing to light it's painful yet rapturous dependence on the senses' (Kristeva 1993: 3).

Kristeva's view is that we must dig down deep into ourselves and our experiences in order to gain the time of our inner lives. She regards memory as taking a picture of the past in order to understand it and to bring it to the point of equilibrium. Interestingly both authors regard memory as being essentially visual although the two main examples of the resurrection of memory in 'In Search of Lost Time' are brought about one by taste and smell and the other by a kinaesthetic jerk. However the memories that are evoked by these triggers are subsequently described by Proust in richly visual terms.

It is a fair contention that one can describe 'In Search of Lost Time' as a literary work that examined a person's past in such depth and with such a devotion to the fine detail of the life that is examined that the effect is to project the life out of time altogether and in so doing to conquer time. This process takes place through the unifying of the past and present which is perhaps the essential theme of Proust's great novel. As will become clear this is one of the essential actions that is necessary for the reflective process to take hold and allow understanding of oneself to properly develop.

5. THE REFLECTIVE PROCESS AND IT'S RELATIONSHIP TO MEMORY

The bringing together of past and present is the crux of 'In Search of Lost Time'. The archetype of this process is the recollection of the taste of the Madelaine which is an example of context dependant memory (Griffiths 2004). This type of memory is one that can be restored to current awareness by the influence of a catalyst which triggers the remembering process. This catalyst is generally a link between the person's current state and the state in which the person was when the memory was formed. This has already been described as 'involuntary memory' by Beckett. The incident of the Madeleine begins where the narrator is 'dispirited' after a dull day he tastes a piece of cake [Madeleine] that he has dipped in his tea;

'No sooner had the warm liquid mixed with the crumbs touched my palate than a shiver ran through me and I stopped, intent upon the extraordinary thing that was happening to me. An exquisite pleasure had invaded my senses, something isolated detached with no suggestion of it's origin. And at once the vicissitudes of life had become indifferent to me....this new sensation filling me with a precious essence' (Proust 1992a: 51).

At that point the narrator tries to comprehend what has happened he eventually realises that the 'vast structure of recollection' [:54 hinges on his memories of the taste of the Madelaine that has been dipped in the tea. He realises that many years ago he had been given a piece of such a cake that he dipped in his tea when he had been on holiday in his aunt's house in Combray some 50 miles from Paris and he understands 'as soon as I had recognised the taste of the piece of Madeleine soaked in her decoction of lime blossom which my aunt used to give me (although I did not yet know and must long postpone the discovery of why this memory made me so happy) immediately the old grey house upon the street where her room was rose up like a stage set ....so in that moment all the flowers in our garden.........and the whole of Combray and it's surroundings , taking shape and solidity, sprang into being, town and gardens alike, from my cup of tea' (Proust 1992a: 54-55).

Although there are at least ten other examples of the resurrection of involuntary memory in 'In Search of Lost Time' (Beckett 1965) the incident of the Madeleine and the cup of tea is perhaps the best known part of Proust's work. This incident has been termed a 'moment bienheureux' (Shattuck 1963) that is perhaps loosely translated as a happy moment. Shattuck takes the view that such moments offer a deep sense of what is real as they bring together past and present, they effectively capture and fix the experience. He also offers an analytic framework which can be used to understand and learn from such events.

The initial stage of the event is a state of mind that the person is in prior to the event, this is followed by a physical or perhaps mental sensation which is unexpected, thirdly the sensation is accompanied by inner feelings often of happiness. Next the sensation is recognised and connected to the past and linked into the person's present understanding. The fifth stage involves an understanding that what is happening and what has been learnt from it may have relevance to the future and the last stage involves the person developing a response to the sequence of events such that learning has occurred and the future is changed (Shattuck 1963).

Beckett regards such experiences as valuable because they evoke pure memory, that is memories which are not accessible to intelligent thought, he also takes the view that such memories may be derived from trivial experiences as well as more significant experiences and it is the 'encrusted elements' that facilitate the recollection (Beckett 1965: 73).

A contrasting way of viewing these episodes is that it is possible to delve down into oneself and to regain the inner life that one once had, something that evokes what can be termed felt memory (Kristeva 1993), which may be thought of as a means of reconciling and understanding time, space and their relationship to perception, emotion and desire.

Felt memory differs from involuntary memory in that while it may be triggered by involuntary events it may also be engaged in consciously whereby the person seeks to unearth what has gone before by exploring the past through the voluntary recollection of places, sights, smells, music and people. Thus although it can be argued that 'moments bienheureux' occur where the relationship between the present self and the historical self is located at a point of equilibrium. It may also be possible to achieve the recollection of the past by purposefully employing the imagination to represent the past. Subsequently the meaning that may be derived from present reflections of the past event may be brought into perspective by the imagination. The effect is that the balance between the historical self and the present self may be achieved through conscious recollection and reflection as well as through involuntary memory.

It can reasonably be argued that unearthing memories at the behest of the will does not work consistently however two points need to be made; first Kristeva's view that analogy and metaphor permit intuitive [structured but involuntary] recollection.

Metaphoric perception enables access to 'the general essence of things' and brings out commonalities this occurs beyond the reach of observation but it enables things to be stripped of their surface appearances and the underlying 'linear substratum' to become evident. Kristeva suggests that examining and describing situations through the use of metaphor enables the underlying structure of what is going on to become clear, she concludes that 'The analogical is the ontological' (Kristeva 1993:65) in other words understanding how a metaphor or analogy relates to a situation enables the essence of the situation to be made explicit. She cites the developing affair in Proust's novel of the Baron de Charlus and Jupien his tailor. Their affair is juxtaposed in the novel with the description of a bumble bee fertilising the trees in an orchard. So 'Charlus is heard to hum like a bumble bee and Jupien is implanted there like a tree' [: 63]. This use of metaphor not only explains and illustrates the event it fixes the event in a certain way in the mind enabling the memory of the event to be more easily accessed and the meaning of it to be understood more clearly during the reflective process. The second is that by recollecting an event, pondering it and dwelling on it, it is possible to engage felt memory as a tool for the reconstruction of significant past events in a conscious way. This reflection is reflection on action where it purposively acknowledges and explores memory for the benefit of understanding. Shattuck's analytic framework is another way of doing this.

The type on knowledge that may obtained as result of such a process is aesthetic knowledge, it is 'singular, particular, subjective expression of imagined possibilities or equivalent realities' (Carper 1978:16). Carper states that a fluid and open approach to the understanding of the art of nursing can facilitate 'consideration of conditions, situations and experiences in nursing that may properly be called aesthetic' [:16]. It can reasonably be contended that the mechanisms that have been explored in this chapter as ways of deepening the reflective process bear much in common with Carper's comments on Dewey's work on recognition and perception (Dewey 1933). Carper notes that recognition identifies and labels a phenomenon or an event, however perception goes beyond that. 'Perception includes an active gathering together of details and scattered particulars into an experienced whole for the purpose of seeing what is there' [:17]. That is precisely the aim of what has been outlined in this chapter. Through linking intuitive recollection, the use of metaphor, felt memory and involuntary memory reflection can be promoted and indeed developed in ways that have hitherto not been considered and may not yet be conceptualised.

6. DEVELOPING THE REFLECTIVE PROCESS

The first step in this process is understanding reflective frameworks, breaking them open and seeing how they are constituted. In order to develop a process of building on them it is necessary to go beyond indicative frameworks. This chapter suggests that one of the deepest, most insightful reflective essays of the past century was Proust's novel 'In Search of Lost Time'. A meditation on what this novel has to say about reflection has unearthed understandings of time, memory and how these may be related. If any new framework has emerged from this chapter it is that Shattuck's six point analytic framework which he applied to Proust's 'moments bienheureux' may offer a different approach to understanding how memory may be deconstructed. However this chapter really contends that reflective frameworks while of use in developing one's reflection are ultimately stifling, in fact there comes a point at which they should be discarded. 'In Search of Lost Time' is a reflective work in which the author developed his own way of bringing back to consciousness what had happened in his life and in considering what it meant to him. This chapter takes the viewpoint that this is what experienced nurses and other reflective practitioners should do also.

Kristeva's view that memory involves taking a picture which has already been alluded to very much emphasises the graphic visual nature of memory. There is a view that reflection as a term is in need of replacement and that it may be helpful to conceptualise reflection in terms of framing. Framing is described as 'the activity of processing thought' (Horan 2005: 255) and is based on the idea that the human mind thinks in pictures rather than words. Such a view is not too distantly related to Proust's view that is exemplified in his descriptions of 'moments bienheureux'. Horan's view is that pictures of practice can be 'pencil sketches, water colours, pastiches, oil paintings, ...portraits of organisational landscapes' [: 256]. He cites Donald Schon that in order to frame an experience the person who is reflecting needs to consider various factors that make up a situation: how one thinks, what strategies one might use in the situation, how one feels about the situation, how one conceptualises and frames it, what is going on in it and what is the larger context? (Horan 2005)

It can be argued that a mix of these and perhaps other pointers may be useful elements of a map for reframing reflection. This chapter suggests that these should be considered and born in mind when the nurse is engaged in reflection on an event from a professional or personal life setting. However it is contended here that the experienced nurse should be informed by such issues but not be fettered by them. Reflection is best achieved by a thorough understanding of the complex relationship between thought, memory and time. If this relationship is well understood it arguable that an approach whereby the nurse simply writes freely of what happened, how he or she felt about it and how it impacted on him or her, will free the thinking process so that intuitive recollection, metaphor, voluntary memory and felt memory will enable the nurse to examine, understand and reframe the situation so that a true understanding of the significance of the event occurs and that deep learning will be the final outcome of the process.

7. CONCLUSION

This chapter has looked at the process of reflection in nursing in some depth. It has also examined Proustian understandings of reflection in order to try to deepen nurses' comprehension of what reflection is and of what it may become for the experienced reflective practitioner. It is the hope of the author that to paraphrase (Sorrell. 1994) nurses will be able to use reflective writing to capture their professional and personal experiences through writing extensively about them and that this will allow the experiences to flow from the memory and understanding of them to develop as they are situated in the person's life and in the context of time past and time present.

REFERENCES

Beckett S. (1965). *Proust and 3 dialogues with Georges Duthuit.* London, John Calder.
Benner P. (1983). Uncovering the knowledge embedded in clinical practice. *Image. The Journal of Nursing Scholarship.* 15: 36-41.
Boyd, E. M. and A. W. Fayles (1983). Reflecting learning: key to learning from experience. *Journal of Humanistic Psychology* 23 (2): 99-117.
Carper B. (1978). Fundamental patterns of knowing in nursing. *Advances in Nursing Science* 1: 13-23.
Dewey J. (1933). *How we think: a Restatement of the Relation of Reflective Thinking to the Education Process.* Boston, Heath.

Fitzgerald M. (1994). Theories of reflection for learning in [Eds] *Reflective Practice in Nursing*. Oxford.Blackwell Science.

Gibbs G. (1988). *Learning by Doing: A guide to teaching and learning methods*. Oxford, Further Education Unit. Oxford Polytechnic.

Griffiths C. (2004). "Remembrance of things past: the utilisation of context dependant and autobiographical recall as a means of enhancing reflection on action in nursing." *Nurse Education Today* 24: 344-349.

Horan, P. (2005). Framing the new reflection. *Nurse Education in Practice*. 5 :255-257.

Johns, C. (1994). *Guided reflection in Palmer A, Burns S and Bulman C [Eds] Reflective Practice in Nursing*. Oxford. Blackwell Science. .

Johnson J. L. and Ratner P. (1997). The Nature of the knowledge used in Nursing Practice. *Nursing Praxis*. In Thorne S and Hayes V. Eds]. *Knowledge and action*. London. Sage.

Kristeva J. (1993). *Proust and the Sense of Time*. London. Faber and Faber.

Kuhn T. S. (1962). *The Structure of Scientific Revolutions*. Chicago, University of Chicago Press.

Proust M. (1992a). *In Search of Lost Time*. London, Chatto and Windus. 1.

Proust M. (1992b). *In Search of Lost Time*. London, Chatto and Windus. 6.

Retsas,A. (1995). "Knowledge and practice devleopment: towards an ontology of nurisng." The Australian Journal of Advanced Nursing. 12 (2): 20-25.

Rolfe G. (1998). *Expanding Nursing Knowledge*. Oxford. Butterworth Heinemann.

Rolfe G., D. Freshwater, et al. (2001). *Critical Reflection for Nursing and the helping profressions a user's guide*. Basingstoke, Palgrave Macmillan.

Schon,D. (1991). *The Reflective Practitioner*. Aldershot, Ashgate publishing.

Shattuck R. (1963). *Proust's binoculars: A study of memory, time and recognition in a la recherche du temps perdu*. London. Chatto and Windus.

Sorrell J. (1994). Remembrance of things past through writing: esthetic patterns of knowing in nursing. . *Advances in Nursing Science* 17(1): 60-70.

Taylor B. (2006). *Reflective Practice A Guide for Nurses and Midwives*. Maidenhead. Open University Press.

Toussaint S. (2002). Searching for Pyllis Kaberry via Proust. *Anthropology Today* 18 (2): 15-19.

In: Nursing Education Challenges in the 21st Century
Editor: Leana E. Callara, pp. 295-308

Chapter 12

LEARNING CARING SCIENCE THEORY IN NURSING EDUCATION

Margaretha Ekebergh[1]

School of Health Sciences and Social Work, Växjö University, Växjö, Sweden.

ABSTRACT

The overall aim of the present research was to describe the phenomenon of learning in nursing, and advanced nursing, education. More precisely, the aim was to better understand the integration of theoretical caring science with caring in practice in the context of nursing, and advanced nursing, education. This entailed studying how students learn caring science theory, based on experiences of and reflection on nursing care situations.

The theoretical perspective of the research was caring science and its educational approach, while phenomenology and a lifeworld perspective have formed the epistemological foundation of the method and the empirical realisation. The research data consisted of narratives and interviews.

The results of the analysis show that the student's process of learning is a solitary one. They are left with a knowledge gap and no equipment with which to bridge it. The students' need for reflection and their desire to understand caring science knowledge in both theory and practice is insufficiently met in the education. Unreflective model learning dominates the learning process, which means that a reflective dialogue together with teachers and carers in practice does not take place. The findings also show that when an intertwined, scientifically grounded approach to caring is lacking, the students are left with their unreflected "natural attitude" to caring, based in their own unreflected lived experiences.

Keywords: Nursing Education, Reflection, Teaching And Learning, Theory And Practice, Phenomenology.

---

[1] Correspondence:Margaretha Ekebergh, Växjö University, School of Health Sciences and Social work, Växjö, SE - 351 95, SwedenTel: + 46 470 70 83 01margaretha.ekebergh@ivosa.vxu.se

INTRODUCTION

It is probably well known to all those involved in nursing education that students often perceive some incongruity between theory and practice in an educational programme. Theory and practice may sometimes even appear to belong to two different worlds, according to the students. Against this background it is not surprising that students have problems trying to integrate theoretical caring science in nursing practice and that this affects their learning process in a negative way. Earlier research, both Scandinavian and international, on learning and teaching in the education of nurses also indicated that there is a state of tension between theoretical and practice-related knowledge, often described as a "gap" or "breach" (cf. Pilhammar, 1993; Rolfe, 1996; Andrews, 1996; Gassner et al, 1999; Fealy, 1999; Davhana-Maselesel et al, 2001; Brasall and Vallance, 2002; Gallagher, 2003). Such problems should not, however, from the perspective of the present paper, be ascribed to any assumed substantial difference between the knowledge of caring theory and of caring practice. The epistemological structure of caring science is the same for theory and for practice. However various contextual nuances and variations can occur depending on the situation. These can be assumed to affect the students' learning process in different ways. The question thus arises: How should the teaching of caring science be formulated in order to facilitate learning and create the prerequisites for the integration of caring science knowledge in theory and practice? This question was the overall problem for the project in focus for this article and the specific research question was; how do students in nursing education acquire caring science knowledge, which is their major subject, and how do they integrate theory with practice.

In this article the outcomes of a Scandinavian research project in nursing education will be presented and discussed. This research has previously been reported briefly in Dahlberg, Ekebergh & Ironside (2003), where the purpose was to investigate the similarities and differences between two educational perspectives in nursing education, namely Narrative pedagogy (Diekelmann, 1995, 2001) and Lifeworld pedagogy (Ekebergh, 2001).

METHOD

The aim of the present study was to explore student's experiences of learning caring science knowledge and the integration of theory with practice in nursing education. The phenomenon is illuminated from the approach of the reflective lifeworld research (RLR), based on phenomenological epistemology as described by Dahlberg, Drew and Nyström (2001). In the "RLR" approach openness is a guiding tool for the methodological work. This implies that the researchers' understanding, not least their pre-understanding, is "bridled" in relation to the studied phenomenon (Dahlberg, 2006). This striving for openness entails the researchers not letting theories or other preconceptions affect their understanding. Bridling thus means to strive towards a scientific and reflective attitude, and the challenge is to be sensitive to the phenomenon and its meanings, with the particular aim of not making indefinite meanings definite too quickly or too slowly (Dahlberg & Dahlberg, 2003).

PARTICIPANTS

Ten students in a nursing education programme as well as five students in a postgraduate nursing programme participated in the study. All the participants were women. The students from the nursing education programme were in the last year of their education, which means that they had comprehensive experience of the learning process in theory and practice and that they also had experiences from several different caring situations. These informants were recruited from two university colleges in Sweden. The students from the postgraduate nursing programme came from a university in Finland. They were all registered and professional nurses. The participants came from two different educational levels and thus the research phenomenon could be investigated and its many variations illustrated. There was no intention of comparing these two groups of students, but it was of interest to gain information about how the learning- and integration process of caring science differs at different levels.

Empirical Realisation – Narratives and Interviews

The reflective lifeworld approach was carried out with the help of written narratives and interviews. For the informant-group from the nursing education programme the study included two steps. During the first step the students were divided into three subgroups with three students in two groups and four in one group. The students were asked to write a narrative in relation to a given task, one for each group. The task was individual. One group of students was asked to write a narrative about how they had learned nursing care in a concrete and real caring situation. The task for another group was to write a narrative about how they had experienced theoretical caring knowledge as a help in a concrete caring situation and finally the third group were assigned to reflecting on a case with an ethical problem. The point with this design was to get research data that provided a number of variations and meanings. The tasks were introduced with an oral presentation of the researcher and the students had the opportunity to ask questions about their participation.

The second step of this part of the study entailed interviews based on the student's narrative. All interviews were carried out individually with the aforementioned openness, and thus the interviewees were encouraged to "tell more", to provide examples from lived events, to ponder upon, and to make explicit as much as possible the nuances of the experiences of the learning and its different aspects (cf. Dahlberg, et al, 2001). All interviews were tape-recorded and carried out by the author. The interviews were transcribed verbatim.

The study with the group of students from the postgraduate nursing programme was carried out only with interviews, because these students might be more familiar with expressing and articulating their thoughts and experiences. The informants were encouraged to describe if and how theoretical caring science knowledge had been helpful in "real" care situations. Even these interviews were carried out with the approach mentioned above. The Research met all ethical demands and had all required ethical permissions.

Analysis

The analysis of the narratives and interviews followed the guidelines of the RLR approach (Dahlberg et al, 2001; Dahlberg & Dahlberg, 2003; Dahlberg, 2006), which also relates to Giorgi's phenomenological approach (1985, 1997). The process of analysis was directed towards discovering patterns and shades of qualitative meanings that emerged from the narratives and transcriptions. The analysis was characterized by an intensive dialogue with the text. An understanding of the phenomenon was sought where the whole was understood in terms of details, as well as details in terms of whole. The challenge in this process was to be sensitive to both whole and parts of the data and the meanings of the phenomenon (Dahlberg et al., 2001). By way of differences and similarities in meaning, and by letting meanings make up for "figure" respectively "background", I tried to see a pattern of meaning (Dahlberg, 2006).

The process of analyzing entails going beyond given conditions, and avoiding linear or causal explanations, allowing the varied meaning of the phenomenon to emerge. Finally, the phenomenon's general structure was possible to describe. This essential meaning of the phenomenon, *acquisition of caring science knowledge,* is illustrated with the description of four constituents: *Lifeworld as a platform for learning, A potential of caring science in learning, Solitary learning, Model learning as the educational idea.* The meaning within the constituents is exemplified by statements from the interviews. The essential meaning can be understood as the meaningful aspect of the phenomenon's structure that binds the constituents together, and is that background against which the constituents "stand out" as figures. Therefore, the essential meaning is presented first in the results.

Result

The students' process of learning is characterised by a sense of being alone. This feeling comes when the students, as bearers of theoretical knowledge of caring, cannot share and work through it together with teachers, supervisors, or other mentors or caregivers in the clinical training. The students' need for reflection and their desire to understand caring science knowledge in both theory and practice is insufficiently met in the education. They are being left with a knowledge gap and no equipment with which to bridge it. Students could, as was found at the postgraduate level in the project, have the possibility of improving their knowledge within the framework of their educational programme, but they may on the other hand feel alone in the clinical practice, where knowledge of caring science and its theoretical base is less well developed.

The students' learning is markedly affected by their personal life, and the research results show that there is a need for them to link caring science to these lived experiences. However, this is not easily done, since this on the one hand requires a certain degree of personal maturity and insight from the student, and on the other hand presupposes that the caring science knowledge is provided in such a way that it has the power to affect the student's lifeworld. The maturity that is needed in order for caring science to be integrated into the students' lives can be developed through reflection on existential problems, and the substance and meaning of life, but this is not necessarily given in nursing education. Caring science knowledge can, in its turn, give an impetus for such reflection, which in favourable circumstances can support the students' process towards maturity. Caring science knowledge must, however, be alive and vibrant in order to be able to be developed in the students' lifeworld, something that *rigid* and *lifeless* caring theories cannot achieve. It is thus a question of the learner and the formulation of the knowledge being in a process of mutual adjustment as a precondition for caring science knowledge to become interwoven with the students' lifeworld. Particularly unsuitable conditions for learning occur when *an immature student* encounters *immature caring science knowledge*. This problem is accentuated by *learning alone* and the students' difficulty in applying theoretical caring knowledge to clinical nursing care. A central prerequisite for the integration of caring science into the students' lifeworld is individually varied guidance by a teacher, mentor, or supervisor well versed in caring science, who can support students in becoming conscious of and articulating their inner world, and their view of life, in relation to health, care, suffering and well-being. It is a question of facilitating self-reflection before being brought face to face with caring science knowledge.

The lack of confirmation of caring science knowledge in practice, together with the "solitary" learning and its consequential emphasis on unreflected "common sense", imply that the caring science's credibility is questioned. The *gap* between the theoretical abstract ideal and the concrete caring reality leads to a lack of confidence among students, which occasionally causes a rejection of theoretical knowledge of caring

Lifeworld as a Platform for Learning

The interviews show that the basis for students' learning is a "natural caring attitude", in a phenomenological sense, which already characterized the students when they began their education, including an everyday understanding of caring ethics, emphasizing general humanism. This attitude is unreflective; it is a "taking for granted" approach, a personal fundamental motive to support the other when s/he needs help. The students express that this attitude relates to their personal life, their personality:

It is a part of one's personality…to see the weak person…..It is not strange, but very natural for me, when someone has ended up in a difficult situation, then you feel concerned and feel sympathy, and you try to help the person to find solutions to the problem (3D)

The natural caring attitude is characterized by following emotional impulses in the creation of a trustful relationship with the patient. The students talk of the importance of acting as a response to emotions. In this unreflective approach the theoretical framework is not important for the learning process. The theoretical knowledge is not congruent with the students' natural attitude and they think that it is not in line with the caring reality. The theoretical knowledge idealizes the caring context with its "beautiful words" and the students think it is very difficult to conceive how the knowledge might be used in practice. One example of the tension between the ideal and reality is:

To apply them in the existing practice today, they do not work. They are not real. It is something like ideas for the future that we might believe in, that we would like it to be. In some way it seems that we have missed one phase between the real world and an ideal world in the future (1A)

Consequently, especially in relation to lived experiences from the everyday world, the theoretical knowledge lacks meaning in the students' world and is thereby insufficient for learning. The students' problem in comprehending the theoretical caring knowledge ends up in a diffuse orientation of the caring science field, which confuses more than clarifies, and one student says, that "...those theories are a mystery for me. Different perspectives on caring and nursing totally confuse me" (3D)

In this case the theoretical knowledge has no lasting value for the learning process. Theories are not important for understanding the caring situation and according to the students important knowledge is what they can recognize in practice and what is visible in the nurses' activities, for example the basic knowledge they need, such as the instruments for nursing documentation.

The interviews show, however, that there are possibilities for the theoretical caring science to encounter the student's lifeworld and thus be considered worthwhile. The most fundamental aspect for a fusion between caring science knowledge and the student's lifeworld is that the students can be "touched" by the theoretical knowledge. This aspect is clear in the interviews with the graduate students in the master programme. They express how learning is a personal process that starts in their subjective world: "It must start within me, you can not convince someone of this or you can not force someone to learn this" (V2)

It is through openness and awareness that the students let knowledge influence and thereby enrich their personal world. In good examples, a personal development begins in the learning reflection on the substance of caring science. The students argue that the ethics of caring science stimulates reflection and reconsideration, and is something that they cannot avoid. Caring science theory has, thus, the potential of supporting an increased level of maturity and a feeling of security on a personal as well as a professional level. Caring theoretical substance brings with it a content that gives the caring context a conscious meaning, which supports the development of new understanding. This process includes new issues that stimulate and which bring energy to the search for new knowledge.

A Potential of Caring Science in Learning

Despite the emphasis on "common sense" and the problems with the "unuseful" theoretical knowledge there is an intimation of a positive potential of the theoretical knowledge, if it can confirm the students' life experiences. If this is possible, it means that their lived experiences have validity, and at the same time the "common sense" is illustrated. As one student expressed:

Yes, you get it confirmed then, and I dare to get further with my experience and then I dare to use it. What I personally have felt, I get that confirmed in the class. Then I have confidence to use it in a certain situation. Because then it is not merely my experience, but a more general knowledge (3D)

In the interviews it was clear that the potential of caring science in learning always is connected with a *but*, "caring theories are good, but .....". This obstacle relates to theoretical knowledge being understood as rigid and lifeless, and that it must come alive in order to have an active influence in the learning. The students are longing for meaningful knowledge, because they are not really satisfied with merely learning the "doing" of caring. They express a need to live the theoretical knowledge in the caring context and to comprehend and understand it. The theoretical knowledge must relate more vividly to the students world of experiences in order to be accessible: "It requires more adjustment and feed-back in order to get more life in those structures. You must feel that it is fun to use them, when you enter the practice" (1B). The difficulties in using the theoretical knowledge in caring practice awaken feelings of distress and dissatisfaction in the learning.

Caring science knowledge has, however, the potential to support the students' learning. The graduate students describe how they, with help of caring science concepts, discover and make caring phenomena visible in practice. One example:

When I began my studies, all pieces were put together in a particular way. It was in the concrete situations that I could apply the theory and the whole caring science. It was the suffering of the human being, where I have to consider the wholeness and act as those "jack of all trades", who have a very broad knowledge in order to be able to perceive and help the whole person. I got a completely new understanding of the person in the industrial health service. I think that the theory of suffering has helped me to that understanding (V3).

In these examples, students perceive that they are able to develop patterns of knowledge and that their understanding of caring becomes greater due to caring science theory. The contribution of theoretical knowledge brings their experiences of caring to a deeper and broader context, which increases the possibilities of getting answers to the questions of "what and why", as one of the interviewed students pointed out.

Solitary Learning

The positive potential of caring science will not be realized if the students are left to utilize this potential by themselves. Unfortunately there was a lack of support from teachers, mentors or advisors in analyzing and working through theories in relation to their lived experiences. The interviewed students described how they are alone in their learning, which caused feelings of insecurity about their understanding of caring phenomenon, "I never know if I have learned something in a correct way, if it is right or wrong". And, "… several teachers are very anonymous. It is hard to get in contact with them to ask and discuss things that I would like to have clarified" (1B).

In the clinical field they could receive support from nurses who had teaching abilities. Such experiences provided the students with a sense of being confirmed that strengthened their self-confidence. It was also positive that at the same time they could identify their own actions in relation to the professional nurses, which gave them satisfaction: "Then I felt as I was a nurse. I felt good and successful about what I had achieved …there is no doubt about the importance of getting confirmation on what you have done" (2B)

Unfortunately this type of confirmation does not appear to be sufficient according to the students. They tell stories about events in the caring context that have concerned them and even made them upset, but that teachers or nurse supervisors have not paid attention to the students' needs. The events have never been discussed or reflected upon. In these types of situations the students have feelings and thoughts that might be hard for them to cope with:

The nurse told me that I had to hurry up and I was not allowed to stay with the patient. But I saw how sad the patient was and that she needed to talk. I couldn't understand why I had to learn to be stressful. I was very, very confused about that, but the nurse never mentioned this situation afterwards and we never discussed it. I had many questions about that and was disappointed, and had to discuss it with my friends (2A).

Without confirmation of either the lived caring experience or the theoretical knowledge, the solitary learning is strengthened. It appears to be particularly difficult for the nurse supervisors to support the linking of caring science to caring practice. Even among the graduate students, who otherwise are not expressing the same feeling of loneliness in their learning of caring science as the undergraduate students, there is this feeling of loneliness in the caring practice, in their workplaces. In that environment they do not have the possibility of discussing and reflecting on caring phenomenon in relation to caring science, because their colleagues are not familiar with that field of knowledge, but have a suspicious attitude towards theoretical knowledge. Thus it could be said that these nurses might have experiences of being outside the care communion at their working places.

Model Learning as the Educational Idea

Caring science knowledge is not implemented in caring practice, is not sufficiently alive in the learning relations between students and their clinical supervisors, and this has consequences for the students' learning. The shortcoming appears clearly in and is strengthened by traditional model learning, which inhibits the integration process of caring science in theory and practice and its fusion with the students' lifeworld. The model learning focuses on "doing" in a way that a reflected and more conscious development of knowledge will not occur.

Model learning is a significant educational model in caring practice according to the interviews. From the students' view, the clinical nurses are experts, and the learning is characterized by the "doing" in different caring situations. The model learning has three meanings, *unreflective imitation, more caring than learning, a triad.*

The students learn how to care through imitation. They start with observing how the nurses are acting and then they repeat the procedures, whilst being monitored by the nurses, until they have developed the ability to perform different assignments. The focus is on the issues of "how" and "doing". In this way the learning process is almost unreflective. The students describe nurses that perform nursing care in an excellent way, who are good models for the students. Those experienced nurses could also be good in teaching and supervising, if they had a clear structural framework for the care they give, which at the same time could be a clear structural framework for the students' learning. The clearness makes the meaning visible in the caring situation and the student can grasp the meaning of nursing care in a better way. In an ongoing dialogue the students get feed-back on their caring activities and sometimes there is also time for reflection. This learning provides joy and pleasure,

> ……..It was fun in another way. Because it is not fun if everything is confusing, like a chaos and everybody is running around without knowing how to do and how to cooperate with the others (1B)

The focus in the model learning is, however, mostly on the care and consequently the learning takes second place. The "doing" and how to do things correctly are of highest priority. One student expressed how she took care of and consoled a daughter to a patient who had died. The student's narrative showed a natural attitude without any reflection and critical thinking in relation to the specific situation. Relating to this, in model learning, the natural caring attitude is strengthened as a basis for learning, because the starting point for learning is unreflected experiencing and acting in the caring context. The idea to interweave caring science theory with caring experiences is not given attention and has no value in this kind of learning.

The learning process in the caring context is of a complex nature. The student has two relationships simultaneously in this context, and both are important for the learning. The nurse, the patient and the student constitute a triad. This triad means a certain interaction that might make the learning more difficult. The dependent relationship to the nurse becomes more problematic when the patient is involved in the learning situation. For example, the students feel a kind of insecurity in conversations with patients.

> ...It doesn't feel good for me as a student to console a patient when the nurse is behind me, observing and monitoring me, or in other types of conversation when I collect information from the patient. It feels ridiculous when the nurse is behind my shoulder (1C)

The students perceive that they do not have the opportunity to practice responsibility in the caring relationship. They have this problem throughout the training and they feel that they do not know what it means to take responsibility in the caring relationship. At the same time the interviews show that in open and trustful relationships with a patient the student dares to practice and develop caring skills. Thus the caring relationship can play a central role in the students' learning process and accordingly the students want to create good relationships with the patients, with the aim for the patients to be able to feel secure and to trust the students and their abilities. Such relationships require confidence in the students that they do not think they can obtain in contexts where there is a lack of supportive mentors as well as of the opportunity for interweaving theory in a practical context. It is thus very important that the supervision is formed in such a way as to create a secure atmosphere for both the patients and the students.

CONCLUSION AND DISCUSSION

From the present research we can conclude that reflection must be understood as an integrated and embodied process, in which all the senses of the body are involved (cf. Merleau-Ponty, 1995). Consequently, the urge to consider the reflection process as a separate cognitive act in the students' development of knowledge is an insufficient description. In reflection, memories, feelings and other experiences participate, and learning can, thus, never merely be a study of theories. Learning in the caring context must include an experiential dimension, i.e. the lived knowledge in its context, as has been shown in the present research. This means that the "subjective body", which plays a central role in the reflection, must be considered in the choice of teaching methods in order for the students' learning process to be supported. To experience with the whole body in a living context might be of crucial importance if the aim is to develop a deep personal knowledge of caring science.

Furthermore, the importance of the lifeworld perspective is seen as a foundational aspect of learning. The students' learning process starts in their lifeworld. A learning context is thus where teachers, supervisors or other mentors are able to meet the students in their world of experiences, and in dialogue create an understanding of how each student thinks about, reflects on and adopts the new knowledge in the caring context. The knowledge content is thus adjusted to the lifeworld of the students, which in practice means that the teacher must present the knowledge in relation to the student's pre-understanding in order to facilitate what Gadamer (1989) terms "a fusion of horizons", which entails a greater understanding. This is, however, a process of mutual adjustment between the student and the substance of caring, and in this the student needs support. If there is no adjustment, which can occur when the teacher enters the teaching context with a theory that cannot be applied to the students' lifeworld, the students are unable to grasp the new knowledge and it ends up with the students claiming that the knowledge is incomprehensible, and not usable. In teaching, we must realise that it is not sufficient just to possess the subject of knowledge, but that we must also be aware of how the knowledge encounters the students' lifeworld in a way that starts a favourable learning process. It is how the students think and cope with the knowledge that is crucial in this context. This perspective of teaching calls for strategies that enable the learning process of each student to become visible to the teacher, which of course has consequences for nursing education. Variation within the teaching context in order to meet the different learning profiles of different students is thus necessary. Further, teaching that allows for the "body as a subject" must also be developed. However, other research has shown how teaching methods easily take over and rule the teaching/learning enterprise (Ekebergh, et al, 2004). A conclusion is thus that all methods must always be related to the learning substance, the students' lifeworld and the learning context.

From the present study it is possible to draw an ideal picture of learning as reflection in caring practice. Reflection as a lived phenomenon is part of the students' experiences of different caring contexts, as reflection of on-going caring activities, as well as the opportunity to review the activities after they are performed (Andrews, 1996; Johns, 1998; Rolfe, 1998). Through simultaneous reflection on the caring performance the student and the teacher/supervisor have a reflective conversation about the actual caring situation, when it is actually happening, which can have a positive influence on the learning situation (Schön, 1995) and on a reflective approach in nursing care. Reflection on performed activities is characterised as an even more careful consideration of the situation. The students' intentionality is directed towards their world of feelings, dreams, hopes, and thoughts, which through reflection, not least if self-reflection is included, can become structured and articulated. If a reflective dialogue between caring theory and caring practice takes place, which includes a movement between nearness and distance to the present caring situation, it can be particularly beneficial for nursing education. On this point the present research findings are comparable to other reports from studies within nursing education, that emphasise a holistic approach of learning and the importance of experiences for learning to integrate theory with practice (Perry, 2000; Welch, et al, 2001).

To be a student could be something wonderful but it could also be difficult and complicated. Nursing students must live with expectations from different directions that sometimes can be in conflict with each other. The expectations from the caring practice field are not always congruent with the goals of the nursing study programme and the levels of competence required. Furthermore, the student meets a great number of persons during clinical training, for example, patients and their families, supervisors and other mentors, physicians, other nurses and caregivers, who all might have different expectations of the students. The latter try to adjust to the expectations that they perceive in different caring contexts. They want to fit into the caring culture, to be able to feel companionship and get confirmation of their worth, as persons as well as students.

This is, however, a laborious process of adjustment, where the students have to use great strength in order to be able to respond to all the criteria and demands of being a good nursing student. They can never completely share their experiences with someone else because they are in a position of dependence and the caring culture determines what is acceptable to talk about. This in turn determines what the students dare to discuss with their supervisors, other caregivers and patients. The students are vulnerable in this struggle to adapt to the caring culture and from this position they must encounter patients who are also in vulnerable positions. The students and the patients have thus in this sense some common characteristics, for example, dependence on expertise and competence, the student for his/her learning and the patient for his/her health. The present research shows how important it is that we are able to encounter the experiences of security/insecurity in being a student in caring contexts, because the results of the students' experience, in some way or another, influence how students in the future understand and approach their patients.

Central aspects of the present research have clear implications for the teaching and educational theory within caring science. If the caring science perspective is to provide a distinct framework for the students' learning and development within nursing education, the teaching strategies must be congruent with the substance of the subject, as has been seen in earlier research (Dillon & Wright Stines, 1996; Higgens, 1996; Hughes, 1998). The teaching must always be subordinated to the caring science substance to fulfil the goals of the education. Teaching or learning activities must thus be "substance oriented", instead of "activity" or "motive centred" as has been seen during some decades of the last century. Students' reflection should thus take place in relation to the substance.

In the present research most of the learning situations had their focus on *doing*, without a link to theory. The learning process in the clinical context is, according to a study of Pilhammar Andersson (1997), often totally separated from the theoretical substance of knowledge, and it is up to the students to link the experiences with the theoretical substance. This problem has also been highlighted by Jacono and Jacono (1994). They emphasise that it is the teachers who constitute the teaching method themselves and therefore must be ready to influence the students' learning in a positive way. Consequently, every teacher, supervisor or other mentor in nursing must have an integrated caring science perspective, which will be expressed in their attitude in the learning and caring situations. This entails an attentive listening approach to the students' needs and experiences in relation to caring and learning. If the teacher/supervisor is open and sensitive to the student's lifeworld and supports a secure atmosphere, the students might dare to take learning initiatives in a way that the learning process is promoted.

The predominant educational model in clinical nursing studies seems, however, still to be *model learning*. This is a well-known method, which is often seen as utilising a behavioural approach (Bandura, 1969). In the present research this model focuses on learning behaviours and skills. Diekelmann and Diekelmann (2000) maintain that when learning is reduced to a behavioural activity there is a risk that learning is perceived as being measurable in relation to skills. The nurses' professional work becomes a measure of what the student should learn, while reflection and discussion are perceived as tiresome and difficult in the learning situation and are thus avoided. It is, however, through observing the nurse as a model that the student gets a clear picture of what the profession means. Consequently the educational idea of model learning plays an important role in nursing education. It is necessary, however, to reflect on what kind of learning is desirable in this context. There is research that shows positive aspects of this type of learning. Nelms, Jones and Gray (1993) have studied how model learning plays a crucial role in learning a *caring perspective*. An important feature in the present research is that demands are made on the supervisor to have an integrated caring approach, which is to be expressed in the relation with the student. Model learning is not only a way of learning skills, but also a way of learning an approach, which presupposes an ideological foundation that is congruent with the content of the learning (ibid.). Consequently model learning might be an appropriate educational model if it is based on the caring science perspective and includes the lifeworld approach with a conscious reflective dimension.

REFERENCES

Andrews, M., 1996. Using reflection to develop clinical expertise. *British Journal of Nursing* 5, 508 – 513

Bandura, A., 1969. *Social learning and personality development*. Holt, Rinehart and Winston, London.

Brasell, B. & Vallance, E., 2002. Clinical practice/education exchange: Bridging the theory-practice gap. *Nursing Practice in New Zealand* 18(1), 17 – 26

Dahlberg, K., Drew, N. & Nyström, M., 2001. *Reflective lifeworld research*. Studentlitteratur, Lund.

Dahlberg H, Dahlberg K., 2003. To not make definite what is indefinite: A phenomenological analysis of perception and its epistemological consequences in human science research. *Paper presented at the 21:th International Human Science Research Conference*, Victoria, Canada

Dahlberg, K., 2006. The essence of essences. - the search for meaning structures in phenomenological analysis of lifeworld phenomena. *QHW –International Journal of Qualitative Studies of Health and Well-being*, 1(1), 11 – 19

Dahlberg, K., Ekebergh, M. & Ironside, P.M., 2003. Converging conversations from phenomenological pedagogies: Toward a science of health professions education. In: Diekelmann, N. & P. Ironside (Ed.), *Teaching Practitioners of Care: New Pedagogies for the Health Professions,* vol.2, 22 – 58. University of Wisconsin Press, Madison. WI.

Davhana – Maselesele, M., Tjallinks, J.E & Norval; M.S., 2001. Theory-practice integration in selected clinical situations. Curationis: *South African Journal of Nursing*, 24(4). 4 – 9.

Diekelmann, N.L., 1995. Reawakening thinking: Is traditional pedagogy nearing completion? *Journal of Nursing Education* 34, 195-196.

Diekelmann, N.L., 2001. Narrative pedagogy: Heideggerian hermeneutical analyses of lived experiences of students, teachers, and clinicians. *Advances in Nursing Science* 23(3), 53-71

Diekelmann, N. & Diekelmann, J., 2000. Learning ethics in nursing and genetics: Narrative pedagogy and the grounding of values. *Journal of Pediatric Nursing* 15(4), 226 – 231

Dillon, R.S. & Wright Stines, P., 1996. A phenomenological study of faculty-student caring interactions. *Journal of Nursing Education* 35(3), 113 – 118

Ekebergh M., 2001. *Tillägnandet av vårdvetenskaplig kunskap - Reflexionens betydelse för lärandet. (Acquiring of caring science knowledge - the importance of reflection for learning)* Department of Caring Science, Åbo Academys Press, Åbo.

Ekebergh M, Lepp M, Dahlberg K., 2004. Reflective learning with drama in nursing education – a Swedish attempt to overcome the theory praxis gap. *Nurse Education Today* 24: 622 – 628

Fealy G M., 1999. The theory-practice relationship in nursing: the practitioners' perspective. *Journal of Advanced Nursing* 30(1): 74 – 82

Gadamer, H - G., 1989. *Truth and method*. The Crossroad Publishing Corporation, New York.

Gallagher, P., 2003. Re-thinking the theory-practice relationship in nursing: an alternative perspective. *Contemporary Nurse* 14(2), 205 – 210.

Gassner, L-A., Wotton, K., Clare, J., Hofmeyer, A. & Buckman, J., 1999. Theory meets practice. Evaluation of a model of collaboration: academic and clinician partnership in the development and implementation of undergraduate teaching. *Collegian: Journal of the Royal College of Nursing Australia* 6(3), 14 – 22.

Giorgi, A., 1985. Sketch of a Psychological Phenomenological method. In: Giorgi, A. (ed.), *Phenomenology and psychological research*. Duquesne University Press, Pittsburg, PA.

Giorgi, A., 1997. The theory, practice, and evaluation of the phenomenological method as a qualitative research procedure. *Journal of Phenomenological Psychology* 28(2), 235 – 260

Higgins, B., 1996. Caring as therapeutic in nursing education. *Journal of Nursing Education* 35(3), 134 – 136.

Huges, L., 1998. Teaching caring to nursing students. *Nurse Educator* 20(3), 3 – 4.

Jacono, B.J. & Jacono, J.J., 1994. Holism: the teacher is the method. *Nurse Education Today* 14, 287 – 291.

Johns, C., 1998. Illuminating the transformative potential of guided refection. In: Jones, C. & Freshwater, D. (Ed.), *Transforming Nursing through Reflective Practice*. Blackwell Science Ltd, Oxford.

Merleau-Ponty, M., 1995. *Phenomenology of perception* (trans. C Smith. Orig. title: *Phénoménologie de la Perception*. 1st. ed. 1945). Routledge, London.

Nelms, T.P., Jones, J.M. & Gray, D.P., 1993. Role modeling: A method for teaching caring in nursing education. *Journal of Nursing Education* 32(1), 18 – 23

Perry, I., 2000. *Building Bridges To Clinical Practice*. Kaitiaki Nursing New Zealand February, 18 – 20.

Pilhammar Andersson, E., 1993. Det är vi som är dom. Sjuksköterskestuderandes föreställningar och perspektiv under utbildningstiden. (Nursing students' perspective of their education, a Doctoral thesis). *Studies in Educational Science* 83. Acta Universitatis Gothenburgiensis, Göteborg.

Pilhammar Andersson, E., 1997. *Handledning av sjuksköterskestuderanden i klinisk praktik. (Supervision of nursing students in clinical practice)*. Acta Universitatis Gothoburgensis, Göteborg.

Rolfe, G., 1996. *Closing the theory-practice gap. A new paradigm for nursing*. Butterworth-Heinemann Ltd, Oxford.

Rolfe, G., 1998. Beyond expertise: reflective and reflexive nursing practice. In: Jones, C & Freshwater, D. (Ed.). *Transforming nursing through reflective practice*. Blackwell Science, Oxford.

Schön, D., 1995. *The reflective practitioner - How professionals think in action*. (First edition. 1983). Arena, Aldershot, Hants, England.

Welch, L.J., Jeffries, R.P., Lyon, L.B., Boland, L.D. & Backer, H.J., 2001. Experiential Learning - Integrating Theory and Research Into Practice. *Nurse Educator* 26(5), 240 – 243.

In: Nursing Education Challenges in the 21st Century
Editor: Leana E. Callara, pp. 309-319

ISBN 1-60021-661-7
© 2008 Nova Science Publishers, Inc.

Chapter 13

FORMAL AND INFORMAL LEARNING OPPORTUNITIES OF FIRST-LINE NURSE MANAGERS

Karran Thorpe

School of Health Sciences, University of Lethbridge,
4401 University Drive, Lethbridge, AB, Canada T1K 3M4

INTRODUCTION

Dramatic changes in personnel, positions, roles, and responsibilities are rampant within the Canadian health care system. The first-line nurse manager's (F-LNM's) role has altered significantly, despite the dependence upon this role in realizing quality of patient care, quality of work life for staff nurses, as well as organizational effectiveness and efficiency. The literature suggests that little support is afforded F-LNMs in terms of both orientation to this changing, demanding role and educational opportunities. Further, there has been little research documenting the challenges and learning needs of this important health care professional.

The question guiding the research reported here is, "What is the impact of health care system restructuring upon the roles, leadership models, knowledge, skills, and competencies of first-line nurse managers?" The research program exploring the selection, training, development, and support systems of these F-LNMs entails Personal Interviews and a Delphi Study. In-depth, personal interviews, conducted with 26 F-LNMs, provide the basis for this paper, which focuses upon their experiences regarding formal and informal learning opportunities and needs.

RESEARCHING THE ROLE OF FRONT-LINE NURSE MANAGERS

McGillis Hall and Donner (1997), in a recent review of the literature, explain that the nurse manager's role has altered from "a narrow unit-based nurse model to that of a manager with 24-hour responsibility for one or more patient care units or programs" (p. 14). The changes they describe include: perception of role, relationship to job satisfaction of others, educational preparation, and dissonance between clinical and administrative duties. They conclude that "nurse managers will need support and education if they are to be successful in these new multidimensional roles and if they are to feel satisfied with their careers" (McGillis Hall and Donner, p. 28). Further, because the effect of the changing health care system is just beginning to be realized, research is needed to explore the role of F-LNMs for purposes of assisting health care organizations throughout this transition. Accordingly, McGillis Hall and Donner suggest that "leadership cannot be provided by nurse managers unless they feel competent and clear in their role" (p. 22) and, currently, several writers indicate that "nurse managers struggle with their role in decentralized structures" (p. 24).

Saunders, Bay, and Alibhai (1999) compare trends in hospital utilization of Alberta residents, provision of acute care services by the 17 Regional Health Authorities (RHAs), and patient transfers between RHAs between 1991/2 and 1996/7. They observe that the "province-wide ALOS [average length of stay] fell by 21% (from 6.8 to 5.4 days), . . . while the average case intensity rose by 8.7% (from 1.04 to 1.13 RDRG [Refined Diagnostic Related Group] weight units" (Saunders et al., pp. 41-42). The increase in patient intensity is not surprising given that less acutely ill patients tend to be treated in community centres and outpatient services. Nevertheless, the increase in patient acuity in hospital settings imposes a greater demand on F-LNMs and their staff nurses. This factor, alone, challenges F-LNMs in terms of numbers of staff on each shift and the ensuing incidences of stress associated with nursing shortages.

Some writers focus upon effective strategies (Aroian et al., 1997), educational needs (Ziegfeld, Matlin and Earsing, 1997), and specific managerial roles such as case manager (Conti, 1996). A few writers acknowledge the changing role of F-LNMs directly. For example, Manion, Sieg, and Watson (1998) explore the nature of managerial partnerships, adding some key steps and principles to achieve a successful outcome. Ingersoll, Cook, Fogel, Applegate, and Frank (1999) interviewed nine midlevel nurse managers to examine the effect of implementing a patient-focussed redesign on their roles and responsibilities. In one instance of major system integration, Formella and Bahner (1999), describing role transitions for vice-presidents of patient care, indicate that the nurse manager role was eliminated and replaced by a staff role of patient care coordinator, "combining some nurse manager functions and some charge nurse functions" (p. 13). These examples indicate that each situation is unique and, generally, that the F-LNM's role is increasing in complexity and demand.

F-LNMs face increased expectations and demands from their supervisors and staff nurses. Therefore, between these two groups, Persson and Thylefors (1999) explain that nurse managers confront role overload, role conflict, and role ambiguity. From the perspective of 33 Swedish ward managers, Persson and Thylefors identify "survival" of their units as the greatest challenge (19 of 33) as well as a "lack of time and resources [and] too much administrative work" (20 of 33 [p. 72]) as the major dissatisfying factors. Beairsto Goddard and Spence Laschinger (1997) compare the perceptions of access to job-related power and opportunity among 91 Canadian middle and first-line managers. Although "both groups reported having the least access to resources; followed by support, and information . . . . [and the] greatest access to opportunity" (p. 58), "first line managers in this study had lower scores than middle managers on all eleven characteristics of personal power" (Beairsto Goddard and Spence Laschinger, p. 59). They conclude that empowerment of managers and work effectiveness is dependent upon access to support, resources, information, and opportunity.

From the perspective of a practicing F-LNM, Carnevale (1997) contends that the "'nature' of nursing management is essentially misunderstood" (p. 9).

Learning, a concept central to this chapter, may be defined as an active process enhancing the "exploration, discovery, refinement and extension of the learner's meanings of the knowledge" (Billings and Halstead, 1998, p. 212). Effective learning may result in changed observable behaviour or unobservable mental processes. Importantly, learning can only be accomplished by the individual and "is influenced by a person's intellectual ability, background, knowledge and experience, and by the type of learning activities and the degrees of participation in the teaching-learning situation" (Billings and Halstead, p. 212). Further, learning is deemed to be a lifelong endeavour in the information age. Thus, lifelong learning is

A continuously supportive process which stimulates and empowers individuals . . . . to acquire all the knowledge, skills and understanding they will require throughout their lifetimes . . . and to apply them with confidence, creativity, and enjoyment in all roles, circumstances, and environments. (A National Learning, 1997, p. 8, cited in Duyff, 1999, p. 538)

Senge (1990) extends the notion of individual learning to encompass organizations. He espouses that only learning organizations will survive in a competitive market. Learning organizations constantly assess their situations and strive to create innovative approaches to attain their goals. Senge also discusses adaptive learning, which refers to maintaining the status quo or coping, and generative learning, which reflects creating innovative opportunities in anticipation of organizational growth and success.

EXPLORING FRONT-LINE NURSE MANAGERS' PERSPECTIVES ON THEIR LEARNING OPPORTUNITIES

Grounded theory provides an appropriate methodological design for this research because it supports a systematic and rigorous approach to a relatively unexplored phenomenon. Since the F-LNM role has received little attention, it is reasonable to explore and describe this social phenomenon with the intention of generating rather than testing theory. As Glaser (1999) states, "grounded theory refers to a specific methodology on how to get from systematically collecting data to producing a multivariate conceptual theory. It is a total methodological package" (p. 836). Furthermore, Strauss and Corbin (1994) suggest that researchers, in using grounded theory, are "interested in patterns of action and interaction between and among various types of social units (i.e., 'actors') . . . . [and] reciprocal changes in patterns of action/interaction and in relationships with changes of conditions either internal or external to the process itself" (p. 278). As Glaser explains, "Grounded theory tells us what is going on, tells us how to account for the participants' main concerns, and reveals access variables that allow for incremental change. Grounded theory *is what is*, not what should, could, or ought to be" (p. 840).

Hearing Front-line Managers' Voices

From a provincial directory of health care organizations, a list was created of acute and long-term care institutions with 100 or more beds (Canadian Healthcare Association, 1999-2000). A random sample of institutions was made from that listing. The sample included all F-LNMs working within those randomly selected institutions. From the list of names provided by senior health care administrators, another random selection determined the F-LNMs to be included in the Personal Interviews. It was anticipated that 30 to 50 F-LNMs would participate in the Delphi Study and 20 to 30 F-LNMs would participate in the Personal Interviews study.

Analyzing their Talk

Typically, Personal Interviews were conducted in the F-LNM's office or a quiet room chosen by, and at a time convenient to, the manager. The interviews were tape recorded and transcribed verbatim. Data collection and analyses occurred simultaneously, along with an ongoing review of the literature. However, a systematic approach to data analyses continued after data collection, using NUD*IST (1997). The unit of analysis was generally a sentence of text as codes and themes emerged. The Delphi Study, not reported here, sought consensus about their roles among F-LNMs and senior health care administrators.

The sample comprised 26 F-LNMs. All participants were in positions that could be labelled as F-LNMs, albeit with considerable diversity in titles. All but one of the participants was female; with a mean age of 47 years, ranging from 34 to 60 years (n = 21); 4 were single, 17 were married, and 5 were divorced (n = 26); and 10 managers had children at home. On average, the F-LNMs had been in their current positions 6.76 years (ranging from .5 to 20), worked in the organization for 12.13 years (ranging from 1 to 29), and anticipated 9.98 years to retirement (ranging from 1 to 20). The F-LNMs supervised nurses (i.e., registered nurses, licensed nurses, personal care aides), as well as other health care professionals (e.g., social workers, psychologists, recreational and occupational therapists, orthopedic technicians, educators, and physicians), porters, housekeeping personnel, unit clerks and assistants, and security guards.

The F-LNMs reported their previous experiences and educational qualifications in a straightforward manner. The majority of F-LNMs had worked in numerous positions and clinical areas prior to accepting their current position. Their learning opportunities were readily categorized as either formal or informal. Their comments also indicated the level of support received by senior administrators within their institutions and their future learning needs.

Formal Education

Educationally, 5 F-LNMs held diplomas, 16 had or were completing baccalaureate degrees (one had a prior degree), and 5 had or were completing master's degrees (i.e., two were nursing and two were management, with one manager holding two graduate degrees). For instance, one manager noted, "I obtained my diploma in [place]. . . . and have completed several management courses." Several managers proudly announced that they were within one semester of completing their baccalaureate nursing programs. Five F-LNMs spoke enthusiastically about their graduate programs. Two F-LNMs had completed their graduate-level management programs prior to commencing their managerial roles in their current institutions. All F-LNMs related benefits of their graduate studies to their work as managers; one commented:

> It's probably one of the hardest things I've ever done, is doing this job and going to school. But they really help each other. My work helps me contribute to my studies and my studies, in turn, help keep me current in my work and keep me thinking about how to make things better.

This comment was echoed by a F-LNM who observed that "Generally, I found educational programs are giving you the latest in research so you're able to understand the terms that people are using and stay current." Another F-LNM described how disappointed she was in having to take a term off from her program to meet the demands of her role. She vowed to return to her graduate studies as soon as possible, observing that the program provided a wonderful stimulus for personal and professional growth.

Most managers had completed courses or workshops in managerial, supervisory, and clinically-oriented topics. When seeking employment and considering a managerial position, one F-LNM reflected, "then I took that management program and I took a coronary care program." For the most part, the experienced managers explained that they had completed several management or supervisory courses when they were new to the role. Some of those programs are no longer available. However, most managers noted that they appreciated attending workshops or courses that were focussed on a specific topic, such as conflict management.

Informal Education

Other learning opportunities occurred for these F-LNMs as they interacted with colleagues, read current articles, and sought to meet individual needs. For instance, one F-LNM observed that, while willing to assist new managers, time and demanding workloads often prohibited collegial collaboration. Nevertheless, an experieced F-LNM remarked, "I had excellent people working around me; that's been such a bonus for me. I mean, you learn from others." A few managers discussed learning opportunities that resulted because of a change in their unit focus. In one example a unit was changed from a medical to a long-term care unit with tremendous learning curves created for not only the F-LNM but also staff members. To achieve this transition, the F-LNM stated, "I got the knowledge I felt I needed, brought that knowledge back to the unit to develop that team and to see the care change." She continued:

> I know that I'm internally motivated, so I need to find within me what it takes to get that goal, that vision that I see. . . . I think that there are a lot of people out there who have the same goals. So, if we communicate and identify needs and concerns, we can get there.

In these words, the F-LNM alluded to seeking information about current nursing practices through library searches and asking experts in the field, and ultimately, sharing the knowledge with staff nurses and other health care professionals.

Concomitantly, F-LNMs accepted responsibility for identifying and meeting the learning needs of their staff members. Reflecting upon this idea, one F-LNM noted that the lack of individuals in educational roles did not relieve her of the responsibility to "provide teaching and learning opportunities at the workplace . . . . It is just a foregone conclusion that you will get done what needs to be done. You will just kind of evolve into fulfilling those roles." Another F-LNM described how she provided learning experiences for staff members so that they may position themselves for future advancement in their nursing careers. She explained,

> There's a real culture here against continuing education . . . . So, I've actually given people the opportunity to come forward and get that experience over the past two years. So, if they've taken advantage of that they're going to have the preparation for these new postings.

F-LNMs not only contemplate their own learning needs but also consider the learning needs of their staff members. In all instances, they seek to creatively address those learning needs.

Support from Senior Administrators

Overall, the F-LNMs made a number of observations regarding support that they obtained, or did not obtain, from senior health care administrators regarding their learning needs. The level of support, on a continuum, ranged from no support to considerable support. In several instances, managers felt supported by senior administrators when pursuing change or when undertaking something new. "At times, I felt emotionally supported, like 'You're doing a good job.' But I haven't felt supported with, actually, the nuts and bolts that I need to do a good job."

Specifically, several F-LNMs suggested that they did not fully comprehend the budgeting process, because someone outside the unit established the base budget while F-LNMs supplemented and monitored their unit budgets. One F-LNM commented, "I most certainly appreciate her doing my budget. But because I'm not doing my own budget, I feel that there's a lack of knowledge there and a lack of experience." Several F-LNMs also stated that they learned how to use computers during their baccalaureate programs, not through any assistance provided within the work setting. In terms of support offered by employers to assist managers to become skillful and knowledgeable, one F-LNM commented: "Embarrassingly little [is offered.] There are expectations that you will produce spreadsheets for budget discussions without any help to understand Excel etc. [and with a short turn around time frame.]" It was expected that the manager would figure it out, being "a high achiever and a self-starter, you'll figure it out, at great cost, perhaps, but you will. . . . I would say that considering the complexities of the manager's job, that the training, or the education, doesn't support it at all, very, very far apart."

F-LNMs addressed their future learning needs thoughtfully and openly. Many of the managers identified assistance in learning about computers as critical to their work. As one manager stated, "PCs are a luxury; the only reason we got PCs is because one of our responsibilities is monitoring staffing." One manager said, "I think I am going to need greater skills in financial management and I'm going to need greater skills in negotiations…. [as well as] political knowledge and politics of the workplace." This same manager suggested that she would probably pursue a master's degree, to gain credibility and respect at the table. Human resource management knowledge and skills were significant to several managers because they were being asked to address issues of this nature with their unit employees. For instance, a F-LNM suggested that "managers should have had skills and training to fulfill that new HR function that's arrived on my doorstep. But that just doesn't happen."

To summarize, the F-LNMs took their learning opportunities seriously. They recognized the need for baccalaureate and graduate education and accepted responsibility for completing those formal programs of study. Furthermore, they acknowledged the necessity of ongoing, informal learning opportunities that assisted them with specific tasks in management, such as financial reporting. One F-LNM simply stated, "Learning is a lifelong thing with me." This perspective toward learning was shared by all participants in this research.

WHAT FRONT-LINE MANAGERS HAD TO SAY ABOUT THEIR LEARNING OPPORTUNITIES

Learning is an active, challenging, and ongoing process. Accordingly, Duyff (1999) explains the benefit to professional advancement when she suggests that the process of lifelong learning "stimulates and empowers people to acquire knowledge, values, skills and understanding that are needed in life . . . in enhancing their professional competence and career decisions" (p. 538). Professionals who establish career paths realize they can not achieve their goals without engaging in lifelong learning.

The F-LNMs participating in this research provide evidence that they are intelligent, keen, capable, insightful, knowledgeable, energetic, caring, expert clinicians, and visionary leaders. They get their work done by starting the day early and staying late. In addition to having a sound knowledge base in nursing, management, and technological theory, they identify critical thinking, sound analysis, time management, problem solving, decision making, and conflict resolution skills as essential to their roles. They accept responsibility for lifelong learning, concurring with Duyff (1999) who notes that learning is "self-initiated, self-directed, and self-evaluated" (p. 539).

Formal Education

Learning was important to these F-LNMs. With enthusiasm, they discussed both formal and informal learning opportunities as well as their future learning needs. A common definition of formal education is any learning opportunity that results in a diploma, certificate, or degree. The F-LNMs discussed their formal educational programs as critical to their success as managers. Further, they often referred to formal learning programs when providing examples of how they managed different tasks, functions, or activities. For instance, a few F-LNMs observed how their programs assisted them in how to communicate intended messages clearly and how to manage conflict. They readily identified topics important to nursing management such as financial matters, computer skills, and human resources management. Interestingly, managers' learning needs today closely match those listed by Pfoutz, Simms, and Price for nurse executives in 1987, such as, learning opportunities "in financial management, bargaining, reimbursement policies, data management and computer applications" (p. 141).

From their comments, one might infer that a baccalaureate degree is minimum educational requirement for the challenging roles of F-LNMs in today's health care environment. This level of formal education establishes a foundation on which to build, especially to accommodate management theory and practice within nursing and health care sciences. One might also infer that a baccalaureate education supports F-LNMs in managing adaptive learning opportunities, to use Senge's (1990) words. F-LMNs with graduate degrees or experienced managers seemed to convey a sense of balance in their roles. Perhaps their learning, both formal and informal, positioned these F-LNMs to achieve a level of proficiency. Senge suggests "personal mastery is the discipline of continually clarifying and deepening our personal vision, of focusing our energies, of developing patience, and of seeing reality objectively" (p. 7), a discipline essential to organizational success.

Informal Education

Informal learning was prevalent among all managers. In several instances, F-LNMs were required to take on an additional unit or area of responsibility. This finding is consistent with that of Persson and Thylefors (1999) who suggest that increased expectations and responsibilities can lead to role overload and role ambiguity. F-LNMs in this research described these additional role expectations as challenges and they prepared themselves to address their own learning needs as well as those of their staff members. They commented about reading constantly to learn more about issues confronting them daily. They often sought "self-help" books to meet specific needs. They welcomed opportunities to confer with colleagues within their own institutions and with colleagues who were working in other institutions, but in similar areas. F-LNMs recognized that their colleagues, albeit willing, were busy people and were not always free to assist them.

The F-LNMs in this research described both formal and informal learning opportunities that pertain to the individual. All learning situations contributed to their ability to understand their roles better; to complete numerous functions, tasks, activities with knowledge and skill; to conduct themselves appropriately in various interactions with staff members, colleagues, physicians, senior administrators, and the public; and to contribute to their organizations so that each enhances the achievement of organizational goals. The F-LNMs are to be commended for their efforts in pursuing both formal and informal learning. However, from an organizational perspective, their efforts are isolated and uncoordinated.

Support from Senior Administrators

Learning was related to personal and professional growth and development. F-LNMs mentioned that it was often difficult to pursue formal education while working full-time in such a demanding role. They appreciated informal learning opportunities that were offered to them by senior administrators. Through these learning opportunities, senior administrators encouraged F-LNMs to embrace change, take risks, and support institutional goals. Clearly, attending to these learning needs of the F-LNMs is key to successful organization development. In discussing organization development and learning, Korth (2000) relates, "More than 20 years later, organizations have not yet stabilized, and the interest in organizational learning and innovation has escalated" (p. 88).

Central to this notion of organizational learning is the concept of team development and learning. F-LNMs shared this perception; that is, they believed discussing issues with their colleagues would lead to sound resolutions. However, they were more likely to describe instances of working alone in solving problems and decision making. Nevertheless, senior administrators have a responsibility to foster the development of the teams, such as a team of F-LNMs, in their organizations. "The intelligence of the team exceeds the intelligence of the individuals in the team . . . . When teams are truly learning, not only are they producing extraordinary results but the individual members are growing more rapidly than could have occurred otherwise" (Senge, 1990, p. 10). Importantly, through organizational learning the capacity for generative learning is enhanced. It is through this approach to learning that the individuals and the institution obtain the greatest benefit. It is within this environment that F-LNMs are best able to champion quality of patient care, quality of work life for staff nurses, and organizational effectiveness and efficiency.

IMPORTANT LESSONS ABOUT FRONT-LINE NURSE MANAGERS' LEARNING NEEDS

A few recommendations are offered for educators and senior health care administrators.

Educators

1. Relate theory to practice so that learners can make connections between what they are reading in a text and what they observe in various practice settings.
2. Use as much flexibility as possible when offering courses, to attract all learners; that is, use creative scheduling and diversity in learning experiences.
3. Reduce residential requirements to encourage full-time workers to participate in courses and programs that will enhance their career planning objectives.

Senior Health Care Administrators

1. Offer practical learning workshops to assist employees with work-related learning needs.
2. Assist employees, through payment of tuition fees, to complete management certificate programs.
3. Support employees through establishment of mentorship or coaching relationships with colleagues or senior health care administrators.

CONCLUSION

In conclusion, the F-LNMs in this research indicated a desire and willingness to pursue career and related lifelong learning. They recognized that formal learning activities enhanced their career options while informal learning opportunities enhanced their abilities to address the challenges inherent in their roles. Given the constantly changing health care system, with particular emphasis upon the changing organizational structures, these F-LNMs identified a need for tangible support from their senior health care administrators. Put another way, they need to be brought into the 21st century of lifelong learners who work within learning organizations. It is no longer appropriate for individual employees to address their own learning needs in isolation of the learning needs of the organization.

Accordingly, Peter Senge (1990) remarks:

> Real learning gets to the heart of what it means to be human. Through learning we re-create ourselves. Through learning, we become able to do something we never were able to do. Through learning we extend our capacity to create, to be part of the generative process of life. There is within each of us a deep hunger for this type of learning. (p. 14)

To move beyond the individual learning perspective, Senge explains that a learning organization is "an organization that is continually expanding its capacity to create its future. For such an organization, it is not enough to merely survive" (p. 14).

REFERENCES

Aorian, J.F., Horvath, K.J., Secatore, J. A., Alpert, H., Costa, M.J., Powers, E., and Stengrevics, S.S. (1997). Vision for a treasured resource Part 1, Nurse manager role implementation. *Journal of Nursing Administration, 27*(3), 36-41.

Beairsto Goddard, M., and Spence Laschinger, H.K. (1997). Nurse managers' perceptions of power and opportunity. *Canadian Journal of Nursing Administration, 10*(2), 40-66.

Billings, D.M., and Halstead, J.A. (1998). *Teaching in nursing A guide for faculty.* Philadelphia, PA: W. B. Saunders.

Canadian Healthcare Association. (1999-2000). *Guide to Canadian healthcare facilities.* Ottawa, ON: Author.

Carnevale, F.A. (1997). The practice of management in nursing From novice to expert. *Canadian Journal of Nursing Administration, 10*(2), 67-80.

Conti, R.M. (1996). Nurse case manager roles: Implications for practice and education. *Nursing Administration Quarterly, 21*(1), 67-80.

Duyff, R.L. (1999). The value of lifelong learning: Key element in professional career development. *Journal of the American Dietetic Association, 99*(5), 538-543.

Formella, N.B., and Bahner, J. (1999). Role transition for patient care vice presidents From a single entity to a system focus. *Journal of Nursing Administration, 29*(4), 11-17.

Glaser, B.G. (1999). Keynote address from the Fourth Annual Qualitative Health Research Conference. The future of grounded theory. *Qualitative Health Research, 9*(6), 836-845.

Ingersoll, G.L., Cook J-A., Fogel, S., Applegate, M., and Frank, B. (1999). The effect of patient-focused redesign on midlevel nurse manager's role responsibilities and work environment. *Journal of Nursing Administration, 29*(5), 21-27.

Korth, S.J. (2000). Single and double-loop learning: Exploring potential influence of cognitive style. *Organizational Development Journal, 18*(3), 87-98.

Manion, J., Sieg, M.J., and Watson, P. (1998). Managerial partnerships The wave of the future. *Journal of Nursing Administration, 28*(4), 47-55.

McGillis Hall, L., and Donner, G.J. (1997). The changing role of hospital nurse managers: A literature review. *Canadian Journal of Nursing Administration, 10*(2), 14-39.

NUD*IST. (1997). *QSR NUD*IST 4 user guide* (2nd 3e.). Thousand Oaks, CA: Sage.

Pfoutz, S.K., Simms, L.M. and Price, S.A. (1987). Teaching and learning: Essential components of the nurse executive role. *IMAGE: Journal of Nursing Scholarship, 19*(3), 138-141.

Persson, O., and Thylefors, I. (1999). Career with no return: Roles, demands, and challenges as perceived by Swedish ward managers. *Nursing Administration Quarterly, 23*(3), 63-80.

Saunders, L.D., Bay, K.S., and Alibhai, A. A. (1999). Regionalization and hospital utilization: Alberta 1991/2-1996/7. *Healthcare Management Forum, 12*(1), 38-43.

Senge, P. (1990). *The fifth discipline The art and practice of the learning organization.* New York, NY: Doubleday/Currency.

Strauss, A., and Corbin, J. (1994). Grounded theory methodology. In N. K. Denzin and Y. S. Lincoln (Eds.), *Handbook of qualitative research.* Thousand Oaks, CA: Sage.

Ziegfeld, C., Matlin, C., and Earsing, L. (1997). Nurse manager orientation: Guidelines to meet the challenges of a rapidly changing role. *The Journal of Continuing Education in Nursing, 28*(6), 269-275.

INDEX

D

E

feet, 202
FES, 94
fidelity, 71, 262
financial support, 274
Finland, 297
first-line nurse managers (F-LNMs), xiii, 309, 310, 312
fitness, 255
flexibility, 317
fluid, 29, 45, 46, 292
focus groups, 63, 125, 199, 200, 201, 212, 218
focusing, 43, 154, 161, 250, 285, 316
food, 205, 254
Ford, 59, 60, 61, 92, 93, 102
formal education, 56, 124, 245, 315, 316
framing, 292
freedom, 65, 69, 98, 180, 245, 247, 261
frequency distribution, 67, 226
friendship, 234
frontal cortex, 30
frontal lobe, 30
frustration, 265
fulfillment, 253
funding, 12, 54, 57, 197, 277, 278, 279
fusion, 52, 300, 302, 304
futures, 162

G

gender, 251
general intelligence, 28, 29
general knowledge, 300
generation, 142, 218
genetics, 27, 244, 306
Geneva, 5, 13, 269
gifted, 227
girls, 203, 210
glass, 43
globalization, 255
glucose metabolism, 28
goals, 12, 33, 43, 155, 176, 234, 239, 248, 256, 260, 278, 304, 305, 311, 313, 315, 316, 317
God, 118, 139, 183, 189, 202, 207, 210, 211
gold, 8, 10, 170
governance, 71, 196, 273
government, ix, 21, 49, 53, 54, 56, 58, 61, 92, 93, 97, 98, 99
government policy, ix, 49, 56, 61, 98
GPS, 87
grades, 20, 144, 202, 204, 223, 232, 236, 237, 240
grading, 236, 278
graduate education, 315
graduate students, 300, 301, 302

grants, 276, 277, 279
Great Britain, 219
greek, 267
grounding, 306
group identity, xi, 196, 197, 198, 212, 214, 215, 216
group processes, 219, 235
group work, 234, 237
grouping, 67
groups, xi, 9, 16, 24, 30, 43, 63, 69, 72, 75, 76, 82, 100, 125, 136, 161, 174, 177, 190, 195, 197, 198, 199, 200, 201, 212, 213, 214, 215, 216, 217, 218, 229, 231, 234, 235, 236, 246, 249, 251, 261, 263, 265, 276, 297, 310
growth, xi, 4, 25, 26, 32, 34, 41, 138, 154, 156, 174, 190, 221, 222, 238, 258, 259, 273, 311, 313, 316
guidance, vii, 8, 35, 40, 53, 54, 59, 61, 124, 148, 244, 263, 276, 299
guidelines, 9, 10, 20, 161, 235, 245, 248, 275, 298
guiding principles, 246

H

habituation, 34
hallucinations, 167
hands, 123, 124, 125, 138, 141, 202, 210, 238
happiness, 291
harm, 71, 124, 130, 147, 197, 262, 263
Harvard, 44, 47, 242
hate, 185
head, 181, 204, 285
healing, 172, 190, 251, 256
Health and Human Services, 5
health care, vii, xiii, 1, 2, 12, 38, 55, 83, 138, 139, 156, 160, 165, 166, 168, 170, 175, 233, 242, 244, 250, 251, 253, 256, 257, 261, 262, 263, 264, 265, 266, 272, 276, 278, 309, 310, 312, 314, 316, 317, 318
health care professionals, 2, 139, 312, 314
health care system, xiii, 244, 309, 310, 318
health education, 170, 217, 254
health problems, vii, 2, 3, 7, 40, 42, 154, 164, 167, 169, 172, 174, 177, 187, 233, 256
health services, xii, 2, 156, 157, 160, 165, 169, 170, 263, 271, 272, 273, 274, 275, 276, 277, 278, 279, 281
health status, 141, 254, 255
height, 27
helplessness, x, 34, 171, 174, 184, 259
herbs, 249
heredity, 256
heritability, 46, 47
high school, 46

U